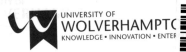
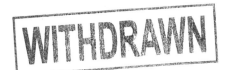

Virtual Gender

As yet there has been relatively little published on women's activities in relation to new digital technologies. *Virtual Gender* brings together theoretical perspectives from feminist theory, the sociology of technology and gender studies with well designed empirical studies to throw light on the impact of ICTs on contemporary social life.

A line-up of authors from around the world looks at the gender and technology issues related to leisure, pleasure and consumption, identity and self. Their research is set against a backcloth of renewed interest in citizenship and ethics and shows how these concepts are recreated in an online situation, particularly in local settings.

With chapters on subjects ranging from gender-switching online, computer games and cyberstalking to the use of the domestic telephone, this stimulating collection challenges the stereotype of woman as a passive victim of technology. It offers new ways of looking at the many dimensions in which ICTs can be said to be 'gendered' and will be a rich resource for students and teachers in this expanding field of study.

Eileen Green is Research Professor of Sociology and Director of the Centre for Social and Policy Research, University of Teesside. **Alison Adam** is a Senior Lecturer at the Information Systems Institute, University of Salford.

Virtual Gender

Technology, consumption and identity

Edited by Eileen Green
and Alison Adam

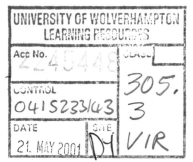

London and New York

First published 2001
by Routledge
11 New Fetter Lane, London EC4P 4EE

Simultaneously published in the USA and Canada
by Routledge
29 West 35th Street, New York, NY 10001

Routledge is an imprint of the Taylor & Francis Group

Typeset in Galliard by The Running Head Limited, Cambridge
Printed and bound in Great Britain by TJ International Ltd,
Padstow, Cornwall

British Library Cataloguing in Publication Data
A catalogue record for this book is available from the British
Library

Library of Congress Cataloging in Publication Data
Virtual gender: technology, consumption, and identity/edited by
Eileen Green and Alison Adam.
p.   cm.
Includes bibliographical references and index.
1. Women–Effect of technological innovations on. 2. Computers
and women. 3. Technology–Social aspects. 4. Technological
innovations–Social aspects. I. Green, Eileen, 1947– II. Adam,
Alison.
HQ1233.V57   2001
306.4′6–dc21   00–047056

ISBN 0–415–23314–3 (hbk)
ISBN 0–415–23315–1 (pbk)

Contents

Contributors

Alison Adam is a Senior Lecturer in the Information Systems Institute, at the University of Salford, UK. Her research interests include gender and information systems and computer ethics. Her book, *Artificial Knowing: Gender and the Thinking Machine*, was published by Routledge in 1998.

Jennifer Brayton is a doctoral candidate in the Department of Sociology at the University of New Brunswick, Canada. Her research focuses on the social aspects of ICTs. The focus of her PhD dissertation is on how people using virtual reality give meaning to their personal experiences and how these experiences shape their definitions of this technology. She is also the PAR-L technical support person for the Policy Action and Research List devoted to women-centred policy issues in Canada.

Elaine Graham is Samuel Ferguson Professor of Social and Pastoral Theology at the University of Manchester, UK. She is also Academic Director of the Centre for Religion, Culture and Gender, Department of Religions and Theology.

Eileen Green is Research Professor in Sociology and Director of the Centre for Social and Policy Research at the University of Teesside, UK, where she is grant holder (with Alison Adam) of the ESRC-funded research seminar series, Equal Opportunities On-Line. She has a long-standing research interest in interdisciplinary perspectives on gender and technology. She is co-author of *Women's Leisure, What Leisure?* (with Sandra Hebron and Diana Woodward, Macmillan, 1990) and *Gendered by Design? Information Technology and Office Systems* (with Jenny Owen and Den Pain, Taylor and Francis, 1993). Her current research interests include gendered use of ICTs in the household and the impact of innovative health technologies on older women's health and well being.

Nicola Green is working on a mobile telecommunications project with the Digital World Research Centre at the University of Surrey, UK. She is interested in the intersections between bodies, technologies and cultures of all kinds.

Maria Lohan is a Research Fellow at the Employment Research Centre (ERC) at the Department of Sociology, Trinity College, Dublin. Her main area of research expertise is in the sociology of science and technology with special reference to ICTs and transport technologies. She has a particular interest in gender (masculinities as well as femininities) and technology.

Krissi M. Jimroglou is a trainer and Virtual Training Institute programme co-ordinator for a non-profit agency in Washington DC called HandsNet. She trains non-profit professionals on how to integrate the Internet effectively into their programme and policy work. Jimroglou is a graduate of the inaugural class of Georgetown University's Communication, Culture and Technology programme.

Karen Littleton is a Lecturer in Psychology at The Open University, UK. She has also held research posts at the Universities of Nottingham and Southampton. She has completed an ESRC personal research fellowship. Her research interests include collaborative learning and gender and IT.

Greg Michaelson teaches Computer Science at Heriot-Watt University near Edinburgh, UK. His research interests include the design and implementation of functional languages, parallel functional programming, and gender in information technology.

Nelly Oudshoorn is Professor at the Centre for Studies of Science, Technology and Society at Twente University, The Netherlands, and a Lecturer at the Department of Science and Technology Dynamics at the University of Amsterdam. Her main research interests include the mutual shaping of gender and technology, particularly medical, and information and communication technologies. She is the author of *Beyond the Natural Body: An Archeology of Sex Hormones* (Routledge 1994) and co-author of *Localizing and Globalizing Reproductive Technologies* (Ohio University Press 1999).

Malcolm R. Parks is Associate Professor of Speech Communication and Assistant Vice Provost for Research at the University of Washington.

Margit Pohl studied Computer Science and Psychology in Vienna. Currently she works at the University of Technology, Vienna. Her main areas of interest are hypertext, educational software, human computer interaction and gender studies.

Leslie Regan Shade is an Assistant Professor in the Department of Communication at the University of Ottawa, Canada. Her research and teaching focuses upon the social and policy issues surrounding ICTs, with a particular focus on access, gender and public interest perspectives.

Lynne D. Roberts is a PhD student in the School of Psychology at Curtin University of Technology, Australia.

Els Rommes has a degree in public administration and public policy (MA). She is a PhD student in the field of gender and information technology at the Centre for Studies of Science, Technology and Society at Twente University, The Netherlands. Her research focuses on gender aspects of the design and use of digital cities in The Netherlands.

Anne Scott is a Lecturer in Women's Studies at the University of Canterbury, New Zealand. She has published a number of articles on women, health and alternative medicine. Now developing an interest in gender and technology, she is studying feminist activists' use of the informational and electronic media, and is also looking at theoretical and policy issues relating to reproductive technology.

Lesley Semmens is a Senior Lecturer in Computing at Leeds Metropolitan University, UK. She has worked at East Leeds Women's Workshops and her previous research area was the integration of formal notations into traditional software development methods.

Linda Stepulevage works in the Department of Innovation Studies at the University of East London, UK. She has an educational background in the social sciences and computer science and has worked as a computing professional. Her teaching is situated within interdisciplinary degree programmes and deals with women's relationship to ICTs and with the development of technical skills, such as database design. In her current research, she is especially interested in sexuality and gender–technology relations.

Ellen van Oost is an Assistant Professor in the field of gender and technology at Twente University, The Netherlands. She has a degree in mathematical engineering (MSc) and wrote a sociological-historical thesis on gender processes in the emerging occupational structure of computer science. She is currently active in a nationwide research project on the history of information technology. Her present research interests also concern contemporary and future influences of ICT on societal gender relations.

Marja Vehviläinen is an Academy of Finland researcher in the Computer Science department at the University of Turku, Finland. She has a background in research in information systems, social sciences and women's studies and has studied gender and information technology in the context of working life, citizenship and information technology and the history of computing.

Kate White is the Head of Black and White Communication, Inc., a communications research company based in Ottawa, Canada. Its focus is on risk and society, health and society, and gender issues in networking. She has also been the Canadian President of UNIFEM.

Michèle White is a visiting faculty member in the Art History department at the University of California Santa Cruz, USA. In 1997–8 she was a visiting professor in the Visual and Media Arts department at Emerson College. She teaches new media, contemporary visual culture, and gender theory. She completed her PhD in Art History at the Graduate Centre of the City University of New York in 1999. Her dissertation, entitled 'The virtual museum', considers nineteenth- and twentieth-century museums that do not have physical walls or material objects. Her article on MOO museums, entitled 'Cabinet of curiosities: finding the viewer in a virtual museum', appeared in the Autumn 1997 issue of *Convergence: The Journal of Research into New Media Technologies*. 'Where is the Louvre?', which describes web.museums, is forthcoming from *Space and Culture – The Journal*. She has spoken about technology in conferences at Barnard College, Cornell University, UC Berkeley, Duke University, and the University of Pennsylania.

Lynette Willoughby is a Senior Lecturer in Computing at Leeds Metropolitan University, UK. She has worked at East Leeds Women's Workshops and on the University WIT/Women Returners' project and was recently a partner in the EU Leonardo da Vinci Curriculum–Women–Technology project.

Simeon J. Yates is a Lecturer in Social Sciences at the Open University, UK. He is currently researching the impacts of new technologies and media on contemporary society. His research interests include gender and new technology, new media and television news production, language and CMC, and science in the media.

Gillian Youngs, an international political economist, is a Lecturer at The Centre for Mass Communication Research, University of Leicester, UK. Her publications include *International Relations in a Global Age: A Conceptual Challenge* (Cambridge: Polity Press, 1999) and the edited collection, *Political Economy, Power and the Body: Global Perspectives* (London: Macmillan, 2000). Her research interests include women and the theory and practice of the Internet and she has been a member of the UNESCO/Society for International Development of Women on the Net project since 1997.

Tables and figures

Tables

Figures

Preface

This edited collection arises from a special issue of the journal, *Information, Communication and Society*, and represents all the papers from that special issue plus a selection of specially commissioned chapters. These introduce debate and empirical research findings in the under-researched area of gender and information and communication technologies (ICTs). The rapid expansion of interest in ICTs in both industrial and academic circles has spawned a raft of research and writing on an exciting array of issues from virtual identities to cybercrime. Curiously, the gender dimension of these areas has received limited attention, historically often limited to discussions of women's absence from technical disciplines, their problems with office automation and their supposed 'technophobia'.

Having undertaken a variety of research and writing projects in the area for over ten years, we felt we knew the main authors in the discipline and the trajectories of current research. Having organized conferences and put together other edited collections, we knew the problems of adequately connecting empirical studies to solid theorizing and we also knew the problems of getting sufficient good material for publication in a research climate where authors often had to make their research interests in gender and ICTs secondary to what were often seen as more respectable mainstream research areas. This meant that we put out a call for papers for the special issue with some trepidation, knowing that we might well have had to trawl round our tried and trusted contacts should the response be thin.

In the event the response was overwhelming, demonstrating a wealth of theoretical and empirical work in progress across a broad range of academic disciplines where authors were able to demonstrate their confidence, not only in their empirical results but also in a range of different theoretical approaches, reflecting the high quality and innovation of ongoing international work in the field. It is heartening to see research on gender and ICTs coming out of the gender ghetto and also heartening to see so many talented researchers who are relatively new to the field. If the quantity and quality of papers for the special issue took us somewhat by surprise, so too did the subject matter of the papers we were offered. Although we realized that virtuality was becoming a hot topic throughout the whole spectrum of writing on information technologies – and this was reflected in the papers we received – we were surprised that we received few offers of papers on gender and work and education, areas which had traditionally been the mainstay of research on gender and ICTs. We rationalize this as relating to the segregation of the research area of gender and technology. As gender becomes a more mainstream topic in research on work and education, and as ICTs are becoming pervasive in the workplace and in educational settings, it may well be that gender in relation to work and education is less of a focus for gender and technology. Yet at the same time access remains a central issue in research on gender and ICTs, although now access is understood less in narrow physical or geographical terms and more as a less tangible though still restrictive concept. But there are also new themes to emerge. We are now beginning to understand consumption of information technologies along a gender dimension. At the same time this recognizes that analyses of ICTs as leisure technologies can be understood in gender terms. This also suggests that our use of ICTs may connect to our sense of identity and self that may be played out in new ways online. One aspect of identity that continues to receive much interest in the political sphere is that of citizenship and there is much speculation as to the possibilities of cyber-democracy and the concomitant ethical dimension of virtual life. All these new and relatively unexplored themes are reflected in the writing in this volume.

Themes and chapter descriptions

The book is structured around four main themes. Part I addresses the important issues of gendered access to ICTs and the Internet and the complex ways in which individuals' experience of such technologies are mediated by the social process of gender. Part II addresses the under-researched theme of technologies for leisure, pleasure and consumption, including five chapters which incorporate critical discussion of the use of ICTs which range from 'mundane' household items like the domestic telephone, to state of the art technologies such as virtual reality systems. Part III focuses upon citizens in the public sphere, at work and in the community, with three chapters which raise political and ethical concerns about technology as a product of social, political and cultural negotiations between designers, policy-makers and other groups. The final three chapters continue the focus upon ethical issues, by addressing the shifting boundaries between what we perceive as 'natural', 'human' and virtual realities or subjectivities.

Historical reflexivity and the biographical narrative are employed in Chapters 1 and 4, enabling the authors to insert themselves within the social relations of technology that they conceptualize as social process. The three authors of Chapter 1 analyse the early stages of a research project on women's relationship with the Internet. Placing them-selves within the process, Anne Scott, Lesley Semmens and Lynette Willoughby describe and deconstruct the political and academic story which they, as feminists from contrasting disciplines, brought to the project. Introducing three genres: 'the webbed Utopia', 'flamed into oblivion' and 'locked into locality', they argue that each genre has its own narrative logic but that all draw upon a common core of the male history and agree that while the ending is still open, it is rapidly clos-ing in.

A more intimate narrative has been selected by Linda Stepulevage in Chapter 4 which allows her to reflect upon her acquisition of tech-nological skills in childhood and use 'experience stories' to trace a girl's personal relationship with technology. In a most intimate and engag-ing manner she weaves conceptions of locally situated technological knowledge with familiar everyday practices in an effort to make visible the social relations of technology as process.

Two chapters in Part I draw upon quantitative data to explore the impact of gender upon the ways in which women and men approach and observe technology. Greg Michaelson and Margit Pohl argue con-troversially that email tends to disrupt and neutralize gender stereotypes found in face-to-face co-operative problem-solving among students. Their study found no statistically significant gender differences in email-mediated problem-solving in measures of message volume and of co-operation. In particular, they found that the gendered strategies that benefit men are disrupted by asynchronous communication. This emphasis upon gendered perceptions and use of ICTs is replicated in Chapter 3, where Kate White, Leslie Regan Shade and Jennifer Brayton draw upon the results of a trans-national study between New Brunswick, Canada, and Kenya in Africa. Testing the hypothesis that men and women approach and observe technology differently, they trace the social and economic barriers to access and use of ICTs, concluding that more research needs to be done on cultural differences.

In the final chapter of Part I, Gillian Youngs explores the nature of virtual communication and its link to reconceptualizing international politics through a discussion of the author's involvement in a 'Women on the Net' project. This project raises concerns as to the processes of 'relating internationally' especially with regard to the traditional invisibility of women in international politics and the question of boundaries which have been characteristic of state-centred approaches to international relations.

Part II opens with a chapter that also stresses the importance of social and cultural perspectives. In Chapter 6 Simeon Yates and Karen Littleton engage in an interdisciplinary debate about female attitudes and experiences in the area of computer games cultures. Drawing upon data from both psychological and sociological research, the chapter examines the role of the computer and computer games in the personal and interpersonal relations of the users. A cultural studies perspective enables the authors to explore the social relationships conducted around and via the computer in particular cultural settings. While acknowledging research which charts gender differences in the use of ICTs for leisure (Green and Adam 1998), the authors argue for the importance of listening to women and girls who actively use computer games if we are to understand fully the impact of gender in the field of computer gaming.

The next two chapters in Part II begin the theme of identity and subjectivity which is further developed in the final section of the book, themes which seem to dominate many of the contemporary theoretical debates around feminism and technology. Chapter 7 by Michèle White relates the textual processes of looking and gazing at multi-user object-oriented worlds (MOOs) to feminist theories of the gaze. Many users of MOOs want to believe that character descriptions offer a view that is like the 'real' body of the user. However, the author argues that the virtual look of certain characters, penetrating into any 'space' in order to examine other characters and determine their gender, renders an empowered gaze. This chapter suggests that MOO commands perpetuate a series of limiting identity constructs and establish some preliminary ways to interrogate these identity processes, while exploring at a more general level the ways that bodies, spaces and objects are constructed online.

The theme of virtual subjects is revisited in the next chapter, which explores the ways in which virtual reality systems become embedded in everyday life through leisure and consumption practices. Nicola Green discusses the practices of consumption which (re)produce and maintain bodily and subjective boundaries. Asking questions about the kind of new conventions of gender created in consumption relationships, she argues that immersive virtual reality technologies cannot be understood without considering the locales in which they are embedded and the social identities which they make.

The importance of understanding technologies within their 'everyday context' is a theme continued in the last two chapters, which emphasize the importance of concentrating on the meanings and perceptions of specific technologies within domestic settings. Focusing upon leisure as an everyday practice, in Chapter 9 Eileen Green explores the potential impact of ICTs upon leisure patterns within the household, suggesting the need for more research which asks questions about the extent to which differences, such as gender, affect the level and type of use of ICTs. Taking the view that technology is best understood as both a social and a technical process, the author argues that we need to know more about the ways in which 'ordinary people' appropriate 'ordinary technologies'. Technological artefacts may be marketed as 'leisure goods', but for an object or a technology to be accepted, it has to be found a space and a function within everyday arenas.

Men's perceptions of the 'mundane technologies' such as the telephone become the focus of the final chapter in this section, which analyses the diverse masculinities that become embedded in technological identities. In this chapter, Maria Lohan discusses the ways in which specific technologies become incorporated into our gender identities as men and women. Although a growing body of empirical research now exists on women's relationship to domestic technology, few investigators have explicitly focused upon men's perceptions and use of domestic technologies. Lohan argues that the apparently contradictory stance of looking at men in relation to a feminized and 'mundane' technology, such as the domestic telephone, is a useful research vehicle for examining the processes of variation and change both within genders and in gender–technology relations.

Part III explores aspects of citizenship and ethics in online gender relations. Alison Adam argues that the newly emerging discipline of computer ethics could benefit from insights into feminist theory, particularly feminist ethics, in regard to areas where there may be substantial differences in men's and women's experiences online. This is illustrated through a more extended analysis than is usually available in discussions of computer ethics by means of examples of 'cyberstalking', an extreme form of Internet-based harassment. This points to the inadequacy of current policy documents which advocate a liberal, free-market approach to the problem rather than seeing it as an issue with a strongly gendered dimension which therefore cries out for a gender analysis.

In Chapter 12, Marja Vehviläinen introduces us to the NiceNet group in North Karelia, Finland, an online women's community and a specifically located geographical group. In a national political environment which sets great store by its citizens having equality of access to ICTs, the women demonstrate their success and confidence in using web technology, becoming technically literate and reinforcing their own sense of community, largely through everyday leisure and work practices such as producing 'canning' labels. This is set against a backdrop that conceptualizes citizenship as carrying a wide range of rights, including those of access to technology.

The next chapter moves from Finland to The Netherlands and to the virtual city in an exciting attempt to analyse the social shaping of a digital city. Drawing upon a case study of Amsterdam, Els Rommes, Ellen van Oost and Nelly Oudshoorn use the concept of 'genderscript' to examine the gender relations embedded in the design. It is argued that in adopting an informal design process, the designers unconsciously projected their own masculine-biased interests on the future users who, despite the 'access for all' intent, emerge as overwhelmingly young, male professionals.

Part IV moves more explicitly from the concept of the citizen to the concept of the self and how this is manifest in different ways in online life. In Chapter 14 Lynne Roberts and Malcolm Parks explore this theme through the interrogation of the phenomenon of gender-switching on the Internet. Having suggested that the primary barrier to gender-switching is the belief that it is dishonest and manipulative, they argue that their data reveals it to be considerably more benign and practised by only a minority of MOO users for a small percentage of their time online. This chapter concludes that gender switching within MOOs of all kinds might best be understood as an experimental behaviour, rather than as an expression of sexuality, personality or gender politics.

The female bodily form is also the subject of the chapter by Krissi Jimroglou, introducing us to 'JenniCAM', a cyborg subject confined to her bedroom and created through the integration of the electronic image and the Internet. This creation, argues Jimroglou, exposes more than just flesh. JenniCAM reveals cultural tensions surrounding epistemological conceptions of vision, gender and identity and questions the role of technology in the representation and construction of gendered subjects. Using feminist film theory, she demonstrates how the construction and display of the female body via the digital camera transforms our readings of gendered bodies.

Elaine Graham's chapter explores the implications for feminist theory and praxis of a recovery of the goddess. Donna Haraway's 'cyborg writing' may have subverted many of the dualisms of western culture, but Graham warns of the dangers in rejecting the traditional gendered stereotypes associated with unreconstructed 'nature'. Drawing upon Luce Irigaray's work, she argues that some models of 'becoming divine' promise more radical configurations of the goddess, which offers an exciting addition to theories of cyberfeminism.

In beginning the exploration of these new themes which are crystallizing round the topic of gender and ICTs we are hopeful that this volume will spark more debate around the theme of gender and online life.

We would like to thank the regular members of the Equal Opportunities on Line: Gender and IT Economic and Social Research Council seminar series for their enthusiasm and excitement about the plans for the book. Many of them have become contributors during the process. Special thanks go to Flis Henwood, Gill Kirkup, Nina Wakeford and Barbara Cox (from CSPR at Teesside) for their support in organizing the seminar series that continues to be a 'creative ideas space' for exchange, networking and friendship. We are also grateful to Brian Loader, Editor of the Teesside-based journal, *Information, Communication and Society*, who was enthusiastic about us editing the special issue on which the book is based and encouraged us to enlarge it into an edited collection. Thanks also to Michelle Bacca and Edwina Welham at Routledge for their patience and support during the production process.

Last, but not least, we would like to acknowledge the support of our respective families. Ian and Craig put up with us 'disappearing for an hour' – which turned into three – mostly with patience and good humour. Thanks also to Sam, Zoë, Nicol and Sibyl who uncomplainingly put up with us on the numerous occasions when the writing overflowed into time reserved for them.

Eileen Green (e.e.green@tees.ac.uk) and Alison Adam (a.adam@salford.ac.uk)

Reference

Green, E. and Adam, A. (1998) 'On-line leisure: gender and ICTs in the home',
    Information, Communication and Society, 1 (3): 291–312.

Part I

Gendered access and experience of ICTs and the Internet

Chapter 1

Women and the Internet

The natural history of a research project

Anne Scott, Lesley Semmens and Lynette Willoughby

Abstract

This chapter represents a narrative, 'women and the Internet', as a women and technology origin story with a fixed beginning, a contested centre and an open ending. This chapter analyses our engagement with this narrative as a pilot study was conducted to look at women's perceptions of, and relationships to, the Internet. Although this story felt like a coherent and persuasive narrative, this was questioned as the outcomes of the pilot study were reflected upon. Women coming to the 'Net' led to a reconstruction of the questions that need to be addressed in researching gender and information technology. This chapter begins by describing and deconstructing the motivating story that was brought to this research project. Three genres are introduced – 'the webbed Utopia', 'flamed out' and 'locked into locality' – which are seen as forming the contested centre of this narrative. While each genre has its own narrative logic, all of them draw on a common tale of historical origins. From each of these perspectives 'women and the Internet' has an ending which is still open, but is rapidly closing.

Three questions are then identified which have been raised by analysis: what do we mean by 'access'?, what do we mean by 'the Internet'? and 'which women'? The seeming simplicity of these questions disguises serious difficulties which research in this area must address.

Introduction

We are three academics – a software engineer, a social scientist, and a microprocessor engineer – in the early stages of a research project on women's relationship to the Internet. We wish to explore means of increasing the access of ordinary women to some of the most powerful of the new communication and information technologies (ICTs). We also wish to discern why previous efforts to improve women's ICT access have been less than successful. We are feminists, and all three members of our group have a history of involvement in projects to improve women's access to technology, to education and to social power.

This chapter is a reflection on the pilot stage of our questionnaire-based study. It was expected that the pilot study would generate, primarily, methodological refinements and empirical data, but the results presented a rather unexpected set of outcomes. Rather than generating answers, it was found that the study was generating questions. In analysing the preliminary results, we began to reflect on the assumptions we had brought to this project, and on the way these assumptions are embedded in a story which is becoming established as the feminist account of women's relationship to the Internet and other new ICTs. This narrative then became the primary focus of our attention.

It is, perhaps, unsurprising that the 'facts' for which we were looking could not be disentangled from a narrative in which we were deeply, if rather unreflexively, embedded. Feminist epistemologists have established that all knowledge, including our own, must be contextualized (Lloyd 1984; Harding 1991; Alcoff and Potter 1993; Code 1995). As Haraway has noted:

> the life and social sciences . . . are story-laden; these sciences are composed through complex, historically specific storytelling practices. Facts are theory-laden; theories are value-laden; values are story-laden. Therefore, facts are meaningful within stories.
>
> (Haraway 1986: 79)

In this chapter, we would like to begin describing and deconstructing the political and academic story – a story we have entitled 'women and the Internet' – that we brought to this research project. We believe that this story has become familiar to feminists with an interest in gender and information technology; it is becoming – to borrow another of Haraway's terms – an 'origin story' (Haraway 1986). We will be representing 'women and the Internet' as a story with a fixed beginning, a contested centre and an open ending. It was an engagement with this origin story that catalysed our research interests and that informed our questionnaire design in the study's pilot phase. A lack of firm results then inaugurated a process of reflection that has highlighted the discursive construction of that story. It is these reflections, and the consequent rethinking of 'women and the Internet' as a narrative, that will be the subject of the rest of this chapter.

Women and the Internet – a women-and-technology origin story

A near-consensual beginning

'Women and the Internet' is a story that – notwithstanding a few feminist attempts to highlight the nineteenth century activities of Ada Lovelace (Toole 1996; Plant 1997a) – generally begins with the military–industrial complex. Numerous histories describe the development of the first computers during the Second World War to crack enemy codes and to calculate missile trajectories. Large mainframes later began to be used for scientific research and in business for payroll and databases. The linked network now known as the Internet is also described as having had its origins in the US military (Quarterman 1993; Panos 1995; Salus 1995). During the early days of the space race the US Department of Defense created the Advanced Research Projects Agency (ARPA). Part of ARPA's remit was to improve US military communications and, in 1969, four ARPANET computers were connected; these four nodes constituted the origin of the Internet.

Supported by the National Science Foundation (NSF) in the US (Loader 1997: 6), academics and industrialists began connecting to the network. By the time NSF support ended in 1995, the commercial potential of the Internet in the form of the World Wide Web was beginning to be realized, and the Internet had emerged as a globalized communication system (Harasim 1993a; Castells 1996). It was catalysing new means of engaging in politics (Schuler 1996; Wittig and Schmitz 1996; Castells 1997; Tsagarousianou et al. 1998), of constructing identity (Stone 1995; Turkle 1995), of managing business, and of organizing criminal networks (Castells 1996, 1998; Rathmell 1998). Within the feminist tale of its origins, this world-changing technology has been said to have had its origins in a male world with four roots: the military, the academy, engineering and industry (Harvey 1997). Differing versions of this historical account have been used to underpin analyses of the exclusion of women and other minority groups from the Internet via, for example, search engine operation, Internet culture and the netiquette which governs acceptable online behaviour (Spender 1995; Wylie 1995; Harvey 1997; Holderness 1998; Morahan-Martin 1998).

Table 1.1 Women as percentage of users (GVU 1994–8)

	Europe	USA	World-wide
Jan. 94			5
Oct. 94			10
Apr. 95	7	17	15
Oct. 95	10	33	29
Apr. 96	15	34	31
Oct. 96	20	32	31
Apr. 97	15	33	31
Oct. 97	22	40	38
Apr. 98	16	41	39

Empirical surveys have consistently suggested that women are under-represented as users of the Internet. The numbers worldwide using the Internet have been regularly surveyed by the Graphics, Visualization and Usability Centre, Georgia Tech University (GVU) (GVU 1994–8). Table 1.1 shows the percentages of women participants over the period from January 1994 to April 1998. The early figures show a very low participation rate that rose, stabilized at about 30 per cent, and is now rising again. The US has the highest numbers of women on the Internet; European women, by contrast, represent only between 15 per cent and 25 per cent of Internet users while, according to Morahan-Martin (1998: 3), only 5 per cent of Japanese and Middle Eastern Internet users are female. Other surveys have tried to get a picture of the 'average' user. *Which?*, in its 1998 annual Internet survey, claimed that UK users have a distinct profile: 'They tend to be male, under 35, living in the south, more affluent, employed, with no children living in the household' (*Which?* 1998). This data has played a pivotal role in grounding this tale of women's relative exclusion from the electronic networks.

While 'women and the Internet' has had a wide variety of retellings, the themes noted here tend to make repeated appearances. The resulting narrative has acted as a coherent and motivating origin story for feminists with an interest in the new information and communication technologies. In it, these technologies – with enormous potential to diffuse information more widely, to increase democracy, to overturn the modernist conception of the sovereign (male) individual, and to improve women's everyday lives – seem to have been misused, misappropriated and squandered. The point that the ICTs are reinforcing the very inequalities they should be combating is hammered home. As

Spender argues in her influential *Nattering on the Net* (1995), the ICTs represent the new literacy, therefore many women are being rendered as twenty-first century illiterates.

What should be done?

As noted in the introduction, we have been thoroughly immersed in this story. As feminists committed to democracy and to women's full inclusion in the contemporary socio-technological revolution, we have been involved in practical efforts to change this situation. Two of the authors have done a series of conference presentations on women's exclusion from the Internet, described as 'a white male playground' (Semmens and Willoughby 1996). We have written about the increasing privatization of the electronic networks (Scott 1998a), noting the fact that – as military funding has dried up – they have been increasingly orientated towards the interests of commerce and the private sector. We have all been involved in efforts to develop more women-friendly forms of ICT education.[1] We have put our energies into these projects in the belief that, without positive action by interested feminists, the electronic networks will soon be, as Wylie put it, 'no place for women' (1995).

Like others working in this area, we have used actor network theory and social constructionist analyses of technology to argue that technological development is, in itself, a social process; it is an endogenous part of the wider development of society. The shape of technological artefacts is, in both subtle and not-so-subtle ways, influenced by cultural expectations, legal frameworks, institutional imperatives, global finance markets, implicit models of potential users, and social beliefs (Cockburn and Ormrod 1993; Akrich 1995; Franklin 1997; Pool 1997). Historically, if new technologies are to gain acceptance they must, in some way, have acted to construct a social and cultural context in which they 'make sense', and in which they are needed (Callon 1991; Cockburn and Ormrod 1993; Latour 1993).[2] Thus, to be successful, new technologies must be produced in conjunction with new social practices, new social forms and new social networks which are able to receive and utilize them. We have been committed to the construction of new socio-technical practices which are as gender-sensitive as possible.

As interrelationships between the actors developing the 'information society' become denser and more complex, the shape of the new actor network developing around the ICTs (Callon 1991; Latour 1993) will become less malleable and less reversible; a new techno-social reality will have been created:

> A fact is born in a laboratory, becomes stripped of its contingency and the process of its production to appear in its facticity as Truth. Some Truths and technologies, joined in networks of translation, become enormously stable features of our landscape, shaping action and inhibiting certain kinds of change.
>
> (Star 1991: 40)

If women do not 'fit' well within the new technological standards now developing, they will find themselves being marginalized within developing social practices and social forms. As Haraway has noted, 'not fitting a standard is not the same thing as existing in a world without that standard' (1997: 37–8). The gender and ICT problem thus seems to be an urgent one; once this new socio-technical reality has become firmly established, people who fail to fit well within it must either adapt to it or accept marginalization.

'Women and the Internet', as a narrative, is thus a story suffused with anxiety. New technological standards, protocols, products and structures are being developed at an incredible speed. New legal frameworks, social practices, economic models, organizational structures, institutional forms, cultural traditions, educational practices and forms of discourse are emerging to provide a context for them (Castells 1996; Hills and Michalis 1997; Loader 1997; Agre 1998). The process of development currently underway will thus have direct and far-reaching material consequences. Like many other feminists working within this area, we have seen it as imperative that women are not excluded from full involvement in the design, use and adaptation of the ICTs during this formative phase of their development.

So this story forms a context in which we believe it important to learn why women seem to be relatively excluded from the electronic networks. It was decided that we needed to ask women themselves how they felt about the Internet, about their preconceptions and, after trying the net for themselves, their perceptions. This was the starting place for the pilot study 'Women coming to the Net', in which women attending short courses on the Internet or related subject areas were asked to complete a questionnaire. The shape of the pilot study drew heavily on a bid to the Economic and Social Research Council's (ESRC) virtual society programme, which had been submitted earlier by two of the authors.

Story? Which story?

While 'women and the Internet' opens in a reasonably cohesive fashion, this feminist tale then splits into at least three, semi-competing, versions.[3] At the risk of over-simplifying and caricaturing a very complex literature, we might designate these accounts as: 'the webbed Utopia'; 'flamed out'; and 'locked into locality'.

These three versions of the 'women and the Internet' narrative differ sharply in the way they perceive women's relationship with the Internet. They range from an optimistic celebration of women's subversive activity via the electronic networks to tales of exclusion, harassment and violence. Indeed, these competing stories might be said to belong to different genres entirely.

Account one: 'the webbed Utopia'

Drawing on examples such as the famous case of the PEN network in Santa Monica (Wittig and Schmitz 1996), Light argues that the electronic networks offer women new possibilities for networking and for participative democracy. She insists that this vision is not 'a feminist Utopia like the science fiction worlds of scholars such as Sally Miller Gearhart (1983). Rather, it is realistic and practical; at its core is the concept of seizing control of a new communications technology' (Light 1995: 133).

Whether or not Light's assessment of practicality can carry the tale 'Women and the Internet' all the way to its conclusion, she has correctly identified her genre. 'The webbed Utopia' is heavily influenced by the recent flood of feminist science fiction and fantasy. Sadie Plant, for example, recently stated that the 'doom' of patriarchy is inevitable, and that it 'manifests itself as an alien invasion, a program which is already running beyond the human' (1997b: 503).

The optimism of the webbed Utopians has been reinforced by a number of contemporary examples in which activists have successfully employed the Internet for political ends. Systers, cyber-grrls and other feminist networks, for example, have worked to open up women-friendly spaces on the electronic networks (Camp 1996; Wakeford 1997). Political networking – primarily via email – was successful in influencing the outcome of the Fourth World Conference on Women in Beijing; the campaign influenced both the conference's primary agenda and the scope of its associated non-governmental organization (NGO) forum (Gittler 1999; Huyer 1999). Mexican Zapatistas have used the

Internet to elevate a local dispute into a national and international political issue (Castells 1997). Political activists in China and Malaysia have used Internet-based communication to push the authorities into a corner, thus generating a political backlash (*The Independent* 1998a: 15, 1998b: 18, 1998c: 18). Computer-mediated communication has been used to revitalize urban democracy in a number of cities (Brants et al. 1996; Day and Harris 1997; Tsagarousianou et al. 1998). The ease and cost effectiveness of publishing on the World Wide Web has also made it possible to develop an international women's listing magazine (Burke 1999). The use of the electronic networks has clearly enhanced both local and global networking, thus opening up new social and political possibilities.

'The webbed Utopia' is an account that can, however, remain wilfully blind to dramatic differentials in access to, and control of, the electronic networks. Plant's claim (1995) that the networked organization of the World Wide Web inherently supports feminist and democratic styles of working seems, in this Utopian tale, to give her epistemological logic of networking a precedence over the more material logics of economic and industrial power. While Utopian feminists are busy eulogizing the wonders of women-only alternative public spaces, they are failing to challenge the contemporary use of cybertechnology – by industrial giants, global criminal networks, military strategists, wealthy financiers and international racists – to evade social regulation, entrench political control, and concentrate economic power (Panos 1995; Castells 1996, 1998; Loader 1997; Fischer-Hübner 1998; Lyon 1998; Capitanchik and Whine 1999).

Account two: 'flamed out'

If 'the webbed Utopia' belongs to the genre of science fantasy, 'flamed out' belongs to the horror genre, complete with invisible lurkers, menacing intimidation, pornographers, and even cyber-rapists (Spender 1995; Hilton 1996; Herman 1999). Even in feminist discussions of the ICTs which are primarily devoted to other concerns, references to unprovoked sexual aggression on the Internet form a recurring theme. In a passing reference to pornography on the Net, two authors recently suggested that:

> In these cases, new communication technologies not only help to immortalize the product of a distorted view of sexuality within patriarchal societies, but also help predators to find new victims,

creating a reverse civil society, a community of the predatory violent. Rapists or paedophiles can connect with their like-minded friends and together they can create a virtual world in which the 'abnormal' becomes normal . . .

(Inayatullah and Milojevic 1999: 81)

In one study of 35 days' worth of contributions to an email list, both men and women reported 'being intimidated by the bombastic and adversarial postings of a small minority of male contributors who effectively dominated the discussions' (Herring et al. 1992: 225). Moreover, a two-day discussion of a feminist topic – during a five-week period in which the other 33 days had been dominated by men – resulted in angry accusations from some of the men that they felt silenced. In fact, according to those narrating this version of 'Women and the Internet', it is women who are being silenced. Studies by Kramarae and Taylor (1993), Herring (1996) and Ferris (1996) suggest that men tend to monopolize online communication, even when the topic of discussion relates closely to women's interests and experience. Clem Herman (1999) argues that sexual harassment on the electronic networks has the effect of silencing women users. These studies of online communication suggest that, to paraphrase Kramarae and Taylor (1993), computer-mediated communication is more a male monologue than a mixed-sex conversation.

The tactic of flaming (aggressive online behaviour) – directed at those who infringe a masculinized 'netiquette' (Sutton 1996) – can be used to harass and victimize women in cyberspace. Spender (1995) discusses at some length the hostile environment created for women by flaming on the net and by the highly masculinized atmosphere existing in some computer labs; these issues have also been highlighted by Kramarae and Taylor (1993), Brail (1996), Wylie (1995) and Herring (1994). 'Flamed out' is by no means, however, a story told exclusively by women. Rheingold (1994), Miller (1996) and Seabrook (1997) have all pointed to the destructive influence of 'flaming' on women's – and men's – ability to participate in computer-mediated communication. These concerns have catalysed the creation of women-only spaces which can act as a 'sanctuary on a hostile net' (Camp 1996: 121).

'Flamed out' highlights the fact that the use of male violence to victimize women and children, to control women's behaviour, or to exclude women from public spaces entirely, can be extended into the new public spaces of the Internet. This powerful and engaging story, however, is also rather one-sided. Within the genre of horror, women are often presented as helpless victims of violence; in this respect, 'flamed out' is true to its literary roots. Such portrayals can be politically paralysing. Furthermore, they are highly misleading; most net-users do have some means to control or avoid intimidation and violence (Hamilton 1999; Newey 1999). Helpless victimization is not the experience of most women, in cyberspace or elsewhere. This version of 'women and the Internet' can be counter-productive for feminists; if cyberspace is so dangerous, women might well come to believe that their daughters would be safer spending their time somewhere else.

Account three: 'locked into locality'

The third version of 'Women and the Internet' might well find a home in the genre of domestic drama developed by nineteenth century feminist novelists. Like these novels of historical realism, 'locked into locality' is suffused by a melancholy awareness that, while the social, political and economic action is taking place in a distant public space, most women are still shut away at home.

The electronic networks have been repeatedly described as a 'new public space' or even as a new 'public sphere' (Harasim 1993b; Schuler 1996; Samarajiva and Shields 1997). Women, however, are said to be under-represented in these spaces, trapped in a shrinking 'private' sphere of print and of proximate, face-to-face contact:

> After five hundred years, women were just beginning to look as though they were drawing even with the men. They have reached the stage in countries like Australia where, for the first time, more women than men have been gaining higher education qualifications. But this success has been achieved in an education system still based on print . . . And just when it looks as though equity is about to be realized – the rules of the game are changed. The society (and soon the education system) switches to the electronic medium.
>
> (Spender 1995: 185)

The world of literature offered Victorian feminists in a few countries an escape from socio-political exclusion, domestic confinement and stifling mental decay; the electronic networks beckon to turn-of-the-millennium women around the world with a similarly inviting glow. As Arizpe recently noted, 'the Global Age has quietly been ushered in':

Women who have been forced to live in a confined space, in their houses or in their heads, get the shock we all received when suddenly facing images of other women freely organizing their lives with their partners, participating in political processes, and giving voice to their demands and dreams.

(Arizpe 1999: xv)

In the nineteenth century, the world of print allowed geographically isolated feminists to connect with each other, and thus build nationwide political networks (Lacey 1987; Alexander 1994). By turning inwards with a pen, Victorian feminists could upturn the constraints of the private sphere, and make an impact on the public world of ideas. They could subvert the geographies of public and private. ICT – by dramatically redefining contemporary notions of public and private (Rich 1997: 226; Gumpert and Drucker 1998) – may offer similar opportunities to twenty-first century feminists.

The heroines of 'Locked into locality' must do battle with the prejudices of their contemporaries regarding women's place, women's capabilities, and women's desires. They must struggle to acquire necessary material resources: not a 'room of their own' (Woolf 1929), but a computer of their own and the software, education, training, time and space needed to use it. Women are often identified with local identities and the particularity of place (Enloe 1989; Castells 1997). As these geographies of place and locality are subverted by new geographies of information flow, women face a double challenge: they must defend their local spaces against the threat posed by a disembodied globalization, and they must also create spaces within the new electronic media for their own voices (Escobar 1999).

'Locked into locality', as an account, is thus highly sensitive to the material constraints of time, space, money, educational background, cultural expectations, and employment opportunities, which act to limit women's opportunities and aspirations in relation to the ICTs. Research conducted by those constructing this tale suggests that the obstacles women must overcome to gain full access to these networks are still substantial. Grundy (1996) points out that men are more likely than women to be in jobs providing access to the Internet; Adam and Green (1997) further note that constructions of women's work as 'less skilled' can be used to justify the granting of lower levels of autonomy in women's use of ICTs at work. The use of ICTs at work can reinforce expectations of accessibility and flexibility, which are often imposed on women (Markussen 1995; Wagner 1995). Boys tend to dominate computer clubs and gaming networks (Haddon 1992; Spender 1995). During the Internet's recent growth spurt, there has actually been a decline in the numbers of women studying computing in universities (Wright 1997). In a study of the use of domestically owned PCs, Wheelock (1992) found that wives/mothers made less use of the machines than other family members. In an international survey of women's groups and individuals (APC 1997; Farwell et al. 1999), the most frequently cited barriers to women's ICT access were lack of training and the cost of equipment. Respondents also mentioned problems relating to equipment accessibility, lack of time, information overload, language constraints, lack of privacy and security, fear of backlash or harassment, skill deficiencies, and alienation.

Victorian feminists pushed for an extension of opportunities, so that a few women might be able to overcome the many obstacles in their path and forge public careers. Similarly, 'locked into locality' is, as a narrative, closely associated with the equal opportunities discourse of the WIT, the WISE, and the GIST programmes.[4] By working to create social support networks, to institute cultural changes, and to induce higher expectations of, and by, girls and women, these programmes have been notably successful in enabling some women to pursue scientific and technological careers (Whyte 1986; Swarbrick 1987). They have also, however, been criticized for their individualism. In assisting individual women who wish to 'make it' in the male worlds of science and technology without first problematizing economic and social structures, the public/private division, and the gendered cultures of contemporary technology, they run the risk of reducing structural issues to problems of individual deficiency (Kelly 1985; Cockburn 1986; Whyte 1986; Swarbrick 1997).

In spite of the problems associated with it, it is in the tale of 'locked into locality' that we have felt most at home. In its steady focus on material factors both the dangers and the opportunities posed by the Internet are placed in perspective. Its historically and socio-economically sensitive individualism is highly usable within an educational context. As a narrative it is both practical and flexible. Our own research project was embedded in this version of 'women and the Internet'.

Women and the Internet: questioning the tale

'Women coming to the net': a pilot study

Some time was spent putting together a questionnaire for the pilot stage of this project. We attempted to frame the questions in a way which was sensitive to the problems of time, space and material constraint which we believed would most affect women's experiences of the ICTs. In addition to addressing a number of demographic variables with relevance to the structure of many women's lives, our questionnaire asked respondents to discuss their perceptions of enabling and disabling technologies. We differentiated individual access and household, community-based, and work-based access; questions were also asked about the control and ownership of ICT equipment and software, in practice. Respondents were asked to identify their preferred environments for using the Internet, their preferred contexts for training, and their preferences regarding types and quantities of external support. We also asked our respondents to tell us for what purposes they used their computers and for what purposes they would like to use their computers.

As we started distributing our questionnaires, we felt that we had developed a pilot research instrument of some sophistication. The questionnaires were distributed on three short courses aimed at women with differing levels of ICT ability and confidence. When analysis began, however, we found to our chagrin that we had almost no data we could directly use. The answers on completed questionnaires reflected widely divergent readings of the questions, as well as a wide divergence in women's basic conceptualizations of ICT. There did not seem to be any patterns emerging at all. Two of us independently analysed the questionnaires and came to the same depressing conclusion: what had gone wrong?

Researching gender and IT

At this stage, some basic rethinking was required, and one member of the group took advantage of an upcoming departmental seminar to begin doing this (Scott 1998b). Problems seemed to stem from the fact that the question, as we had originally framed it, was unanswerable. The pilot study had been designed to address the question: what are the factors that limit and constrain women's access to the new ICTs? This is a question that emerges naturally from 'locked into locality', the version of the 'women and the Internet' story we favoured.

It assumes that women are a relatively homogeneous group, who have been prevented by material and cultural factors from gaining full access to an unproblematized, electronic, 'public sphere'. However there are at least three complicating problems hiding in this question: what do we mean by 'access'?, what do we mean by 'the Internet'?, and which women? We would like to address each of these in turn.

What do we mean by 'access'?

We began our study with a conceptualization of 'access' that challenged the notion that ICT users are – first and foremost – consumers. This conceptualization of ICT users is, of course, evident in the discourse of many private corporations; it may also be found in ICT policy papers emerging from the UK's former Tory government (CITU 1996) and the European Union (Federal Trust 1995; Campbell and Machet 1999). As long as 'access' means, as Wylie put it, access to 'the right to clerk and consume' (1995: 3), it is hard to counter the argument that greater equality of ICT opportunity can best be generated after a working network has been established by the more dynamic private sector.

By contrast, we have tended to configure ICT users as citizens – as social, political and cultural agents.[5] Our conceptualization of 'access' thus owes a great deal to the actor network analysis of technology, discussed previously in this chapter. The question we have been asking might thus be rephrased as follows: are women to be admitted to the electronic public sphere as consumers, as workers and producers, or as full citizens and social agents?

Our conceptualization of 'access', however, has also been blind to concerns that don't fit naturally into this narrative. Dutton (1998) argues that we cannot think about ICT access in a manner that simply adds it to peoples' existing capacities and resources. Instead, we must think about geographies of access: to what are people gaining access, and for what are these new connections substituting? People might surf the web instead of going to their local public library, for example; instead of putting their money in the NatWest on the high street, they might do their banking with First Direct; instead of spending their time chatting with a neighbour, they might make close friends with an email user in Tokyo. In short, social, economic and political networks that were once heavily based on geographic proximity are being replaced by a new 'space of flows' – networks based on affinity or the provision of specialized services (Castells 1996). However, since not everybody can afford 'tele-access',[6] this will result in holes being punched in communities of physical locality, while more socially and economically exclusive 'virtual' communities are created. These segmented communities will be less able to maintain a shared culture (Escobar 1999: 35). The meaning of 'community' is thus changing with those people fortunate enough to have access to the Internet now being able to create (in effect) privatized, fragmented and geographically dispersed communities.

The question of access, therefore, cannot be addressed on an individualized basis. Rather, it must be transformed into a question about the social relations of technology. As May puts it, 'technologies do not necessarily bring with them specific social relations antagonistic or co-operative. It is the use to which technologies are put that develops their social relations' (1998: 253). How will the new ICTs be integrated into everyday life? What new social networks will be created? Who will those networks include, and who will be excluded? How will everyday activities be transformed? How will people with varying levels of ICT equipment, software, training and interest find, or create, a way to manage the micro-power relations which have been thrown into some level of flux by the need to integrate these new techno-social forms? These questions cannot easily be addressed within the 'locked in locality' narrative, with its 'equal opportunities' focus on socially created material constraints that act on an individual level.

Moreover, our analysis of the data in our questionnaires suggests that the question of 'access' – even if we could develop an appropriate narrative frame for it – is simply too complicated to be usefully addressed via a short survey. The question of 'ICT access' must be embedded in a larger set of questions about ICT use which are, in turn, embedded in a set of questions about social institutions, social practices and social networks. Asking the respondents about the features on their computers told us little, for example, because we did not have contextualizing information relating to their reasons for having those features, the use they made of them, their conceptualizations of that use, and the way these practices were embedded in the larger structures of their lives.

What do we mean by 'the Internet'?

Our questionnaire included a number of questions about the features respondents had on their computers, the features they wished to have, and the use they made of their computers. These questions were designed to differentiate between active and passive use of the Internet. In keeping with the emphasis of 'Women and the Internet' on enrolling women into an active construction of new socio-technical relations, they were designed to differentiate cyberconsumers from cybercitizens. The data collected, however, came aground on a simple but thorny problem. Most artefacts begin to carry a multitude of meanings as they are appropriated by users and incorporated into their daily lives (Silverstone et al. 1992). This multiplicity, however, is greatly magnified in the case of both the personal computer and the Internet, whose very *raison d'être* is the manipulation and communication of symbolic meaning. We had fallen foul of the 'black box' fallacy (Grint and Woolgar 1997): proceeding as if the Internet, and the equipment used to access it, could be conceptualized as 'things' with a single, coherent and accessible meaning.

As we began to analyse our data, we realized that we really couldn't make sense of the personal computer, or of the Internet, as a single thing. The respondents were clearly conceptualizing both the PC and the Internet in dramatically varying fashions; perhaps the PC isn't a single thing. Our reflection and analysis leaves us with the uncomfortable conclusion that the computer/ Internet remains, at least, five different things. Politicians and employers tend to think of the computer/ Internet as a tool to keep track of money and stock, assist in marketing and publicity, transfer software and data, and improve management and administration. 'Locked into locality' draws heavily on this conceptualization of the computer/Internet. Artists, musicians and writers, by contrast, think of the computer/Internet as a publisher. All three versions of 'women and the Internet' have analysed the implications of the fact that people can publish on the web at little cost, and without going through publishers. This makes public platforms available to more people and catalyses the development of more democratic epistemologies; however, it also allows pornography and hate literature to be produced and disseminated via the Internet. In most homes, the computer/Internet is, first and foremost, a toy; it is primarily used for playing games (Haddon 1992; Wheelock 1992). As the computer/ Internet-as-toy tends to be male dominated, with violent and misogynistic games, this conceptualization plays a key role in the 'flamed out' discourse. To teachers, academics and parents, the computer/Internet is often conceptualized as a library, with uses in information storage and dissemination, technologies of learning, and academic publishing. The implications for educational practice make this conceptualization of key interest to the progenitors of 'locked into locality'. The computer-as-tool conception – which reigned almost undisturbed during the 1970s and 1980s – has come under pressure from a newly hegemonic understanding of the computer/Internet-as-social-centre. The astonishing development of lateral communicability – via fax, email, conferencing, electronic bulletin boards, discussion groups, multi-user-domains, chat groups, and the electronic transfer of large files – has, to a large degree, generated the optimism of 'the webbed Utopian' discourse.

Working within the 'women and the Internet' narrative, we wanted to understand how we might improve women's access to this 'thing' called the Internet. The answers respondents gave, however, were embedded in these very different understandings of what the computer and the Internet are. Without teasing out precisely with which conceptualization the respondents were operating – something which would have been difficult to accomplish in any short questionnaire – it was impossible to make sense of the answers to many of the questions asked. The research had come aground on a problem with no easy or obvious solutions. It may not be possible to create a coherent narrative about women and the Internet without first creating some kind of coherent cultural narrative about the computer/Internet itself.

'Which women?'

The story of 'women and the Internet' is, at its core, a narrative about the restricting of Internet access to men (and some women) of certain social groups. It highlights the problems created by the fact that Internet users tend to be male, white, younger than average, and to have high average incomes. Even within these restricted social groups, however, there are major demographic issues – bearing particularly on the way women organize their lives – which have been inadequately investigated. Are women, for example, with school-age children more or less likely to use the World Wide Web independently than other women? Do women living in same-sex households/relationships have more confidence with the new technologies than do those living with men? Are women more likely to engage with the new information technologies if they are also involved in community activities and/or in paid work? Are women Internet users more or less likely to be disabled than non-users, and are their impairments clustered within certain categories? In mixed gender households, who loads software, organizes the desktop and engages in other cyber-based nest-building tasks?

The 'locked into locality' narrative, with its deep sensitivity to the problematic construction of public and private in women's lives, is an ideal starting place from which to address these semi-demographic questions. We began our research in the belief that a large survey might usefully address such issues and, indeed, we found that these questions worked quite well on the questionnaire. A more widely distributed questionnaire which has come to terms with the other difficult issues raised above could be invaluable in this respect.

A more fundamental issue relates to our very choice of the Internet for study. Why has the 'women and the Internet' discourse focused on the Internet?

As Dutton (1998) noted in his recent study of pager use, there are some ICT technologies with a much more even demographic spread of users, in relation to gender, social class and ethnicity. His research showed that these cheaper and less glamorous technologies are being creatively used by women to reshape local social structures, reorganize social geographies and recreate social institutions. This informal activity, however, has been little studied; it has been tucked away into the more peripheral corners of the information revolution. If we are serious about exploring women's ability to remain socially and politically effective in an information age, we cannot narrow our attention too severely. We need to think more carefully about the geographies of the information revolution itself.

Conclusion – a retelling of the tale

The story of 'women and the Internet' has served as something of an origin story for feminists working in this field. Although it has been deeply contested – in genre as well as detail – this story has acted as a coherent and persuasive motivating myth. We began our research project from a standpoint firmly embedded within it. In the course of our analysis, however, we have come to question the way this story has been framed. A number of questions have occurred to us:

- How much have the Internet's military–industrial origins actually influenced women's current and future relationships with this technology?
- What does it mean to say that women have been excluded from this new medium?
- Is there any point in talking globally about women's relationship to the Internet?
- Why has this tale focused so closely on the Internet (as well as virtual reality and other 'sexy' new technologies) while tending

to ignore cheaper, more pervasive, and perhaps more democratic technologies such as the pager and the mobile phone?
- Can we conceptualize the 'Internet' as a single thing?
- How can we integrate the complex and seemingly incompatible threads of discourse from which this story has been woven?

It may be necessary to begin formulating a more reflexive and variegated origin story in relation to women and ICT. This new tale should address two key questions:

- How are the new social geographies of ICT access being gendered?
- How can we intervene to direct the shaping of new techno-social relations in more democratic, inclusive, and neutrally gendered ways?

Although this new story should be extremely gender-sensitive, it might not begin with women – as a homogeneous category – at all. The 'locked into locality' narrative is fundamentally concerned with the way citizenship is materially structured in relation to time, space and economic resources. A women and technology story which is adequate to its task should analyse the changing shape of these material geographies in the information age.

The story of 'women and the Internet' has catalysed wide-ranging research and valuable developmental work. Thus, rather than abandoning this narrative, we would suggest embroidering it with new texturing and a new reflexivity.

We need to problematize the recurring themes that have shaped this narrative. The narrative logic drawn on in our research matters greatly; it acts to shape the conclusions to be reached, for as noted at the beginning of this chapter, facts have meaning only within stories.

Notes

1 East Leeds Women's Workshop, Women into Technology (Open University, UK), Curriculum–Women–Technology project (EU), 'Community Development and the Internet' short course and module (Bradford University, UK).

2 For an example of the way this necessary process can be deliberately utilized to achieve social ends, see Randi Markussen's discussion (1996) of the Scandinavian participatory design tradition.

3 In fact, there are surely more than three competing versions of this tale. However, some of its strands – such as those arising from studies of the impact of IT on women's work, of international development and IT, or of the participatory design tradition – have tended to be rather peripheral to the early formulation of our research project, and are thus not discussed in this chapter.

4 Women into Technology, Women in Science and Engineering, Girls into Science and Technology.
5 This conceptualization has found some expression in national ICT policy where it has come into conflict with the dominant, more conservative, conceptualizations (LIC 1997; DCMS 1998). The Libraries and Information Commission's new document (LIC 1997) emphasizes that access must be free at the point of use if the ICTs are to be used to increase social inclusiveness and to strengthen representative democracy.
6 Or desires it: see, for example, Umble's discussion (1992) of the Pennsylvania Amish community's response to the telephone.

References

Adam, A. and Green, E. (1997) 'Gender, agency, location and the new information society' in B. Loader (ed.) *The Governance of Cyberspace: Politics, Technology and Global Restructuring*, London: Routledge.

Agre, P. (1998) 'The Internet and public discourse'. Available online: http://www.firstmonday.dk/issues/issues3_3/agre/ (17 January 1999).

Akrich, M. (1995) 'User representations: practices, methods and sociology' in A. Rip, T. Misa and J. Schot (eds) *Managing Technology in Society*, London: Pinter.

Alcoff, L. and Potter, E. (1993) *Feminist Epistemologies*, London: Routledge.

Alexander, S. (1994) *Becoming a Woman, and Other Essays in 19th and 20th Century Feminist History*, London: Virago Press.

APC (1997) 'APC women's programme: survey findings (May 1997)'. Available online: http://community.web.net/apcwomen/apctoc.htm (17 January 1999).

Arizpe, L. (1999) 'Women's freedom to create: women's agenda for cyberspace' in W. Harcourt (ed.) *Women@Internet: Creating New Cultures in Cyberspace*, London: Zed Books: xii–xvi.

Brail, S. (1996) 'The price of admission: harassment and free speech in the wild, wild, west' in L. Cherny and E. R. Weise (eds) *Wired_Women: Gender and New Realities in Cyberspace*, Seattle, WA: Seal Press: 141–57.

Brants, K., Huizenga, M. and Van Meerten, R. (1996) 'The new canals of Amsterdam: an exercise in local electronic democracy', *Media, Culture and Society*, 18: 233–47.

Burke, K. (1999) 'AVIVA: the women's World Wide Web' in Liberty (ed.) *Liberating Cyberspace: Civil Liberties, Human Rights and the Internet*, London: Pluto Press: 187–97.

Callon, M. (1991) 'Techno-economic networks and irreversibility' in J. Law (ed.) *A Sociology of Monsters: Essays on Power, Technology and Domination*, London: Routledge.

Camp, L. J. (1996) 'We are geeks, and we are not guys: the systers' mailing list' in L. Cherny and E. R. Weise (eds) *Wired Women: Gender and New Realities in Cyberspace*, Seattle, WA: Seal Press: 114–25.

Campbell, P. and Machet, E. (1999) 'European policy on regulation of content on the Internet' in Liberty (ed.) *Liberating Cyberspace: Civil Liberties, Human Rights and the Internet*, London: Pluto Press: 140–58.

Capitanchik, D. and Whine, M. (1999) 'The governance of cyberspace: racism on the Internet' in Liberty (ed.) *Liberating Cyberspace: Civil Liberties, Human Rights and the Internet*, London: Pluto Press: 237–57.

Castells, M. (1996) *The Rise of the Network Society*, Oxford: Blackwell.

Castells, M. (1997) *The Power of Identity*, Oxford: Blackwell.

Castells, M. (1998) *End of the Millennium*, Oxford: Blackwell.

CITU (Central IT Unit) (1996) 'Government direct', HMSO: Green Paper.

Cockburn, C. (1986) 'Women and technology: opportunity is not enough' in K. Purcell et al. (eds) *The Changing Experience of Employment: Restructuring and Recession*, London: Macmillan.

Cockburn, C. and Ormrod, S. (1993) *Gender and Technology in the Making*, London: Sage.

Code, L. (1995) *Rhetorical Spaces: Essays on Gendered Locations*, London: Routledge.

Day, P. and Harris, K. (1997) *Down-to-Earth Vision: Community Based IT Initiatives and Social Inclusion*, London: IBM Corp.

DCMS (Department for Culture, Media and Sport) (1998) 'New library: the people's network', the government's response, London: HMSO.

Dutton, W. (1998) *Society on the Line: Information Politics in the Digital Age*, Oxford: Oxford University Press.

Enloe, C. (1989) *Bananas, Beaches and Bases: Making Feminist Sense of International Politics*, London: Pandora.

Escobar, A. (1999) 'Gender, place and networks: a political ecology of cyberculture' in W. Harcourt (ed.) *Women@Internet: Creating New Cultures in Cyberspace*, London: Zed Books: 31–54.

Farwell, E., Wood, P., James, M. and Banks, K. (1999) 'Global networking for change: experiences from the APC Women's Programme' in W. Harcourt (ed.) *Women@Internet: Creating New Cultures in Cyberspace*, London: Zed Books: 102–13.

Federal Trust (1995) *Network Europe and the Information Society*, London: Federal Trust for Education and Research.

Ferris, S. (1996) 'Women online: cultural and relational aspects of women's communication in online discussion groups', *Interpersonal Computing and Technology*, 4: 29–40. Available online: http://www.helsinki.fi/science/optek/1996/n3/ferris.txt (17 January 1999).

Fischer-Hübner, S. (1998) 'Privacy and security at risk in the global information society', *Information, Communication and Society*, 1 (4): 420–41.

Franklin, S. (1997) *Embodied Progress: A Cultural Account of Assisted Conception*, London: Routledge.

Gearhart, S. (1983) *The Wanderground, Stories of Hill Women*, London: Women's Press.

Gittler, A. (1999) 'Mapping women's global communications and networking' in W. Harcourt (ed.) *Women@Internet: Creating New Cultures in Cyberspace*, London: Zed Books: 91–101.

Grint, K. and Woolgar, S. (1997) *The Machine at Work: Technology, Work and Organization*, Cambridge: Polity Press.

Grundy, F. (1996) *Women and Computers*, Exeter: Intellect Books.

Gumpert, G. and Drucker, S. (1998) 'The mediated home in the global village', *Communication Research*, 25 (4): 422–38.

GVU (Graphics, Visualization and Usability Centre, Georgia Tech University) (1994–8). Available online: http://www.gvu.gatech.edu/user_surveys/survey-1998-04/#exec (17 January 1999).

Haddon, L. (1992) 'Explaining ICT consumption: the case of the home computer' in R. Silverstone and E. Hirsch (eds) *Consuming Technologies: Media and Information in Domestic Spaces*, London: Routledge: 82–96.

Hamilton, A. (1999) 'The net out of control – a new moral panic: censorship and sexuality' in Liberty (ed.) *Liberating Cyberspace: Civil Liberties, Human Rights and the Internet*, London: Pluto Press: 169–86.

Harasim, L. (ed.) (1993a) *Global Networks: Computers and International Communication*, London: MIT Press.

Harasim, L. (1993b) 'Networlds: networks as social space' in L. Harasim (ed.) *Global Networks: Computers and International Communication*, London: MIT Press: 15–34.

Haraway, D. (1986) 'Primatology is politics by other means' in R. Bleier (ed.) *Feminist Approaches to Science*, Oxford: Pergamon Press: 76–118.

Haraway, D. (1997) *Modest_Witness@Second_Millennium. FemaleMan©_Meets_OncoMouse™: Feminism and Technoscience*, London: Routledge.

Harding, S. (1991) *Whose Science? Whose Knowledge?: Thinking from Women's Lives*, Buckingham: Open University Press.

Harvey, L. (1997) 'A genealogical exploration of gendered genres in IT cultures', *Information Systems Journal*, 7: 153–72.

Herman, C. (1999) 'Women and the Internet' in Liberty (ed.) *Liberating Cyberspace: Civil Liberties, Human Rights and the Internet*, London: Pluto Press: 198–205.

Herring, S. (1994) 'Politeness in computer culture: why women thank and men flame' in Bucholtz, et al. (eds) *Cultural Performances: Proceedings of the Third Berkeley Women and Language Conference*, Berkeley: University of California: 278–94.

Herring, S. (1996) 'Posting in a different voice: gender and ethics in computer-mediated communication' in C. Ess (ed.) *Philosophical Approaches to Computer-mediated Communication*, Albany: Suny Press: 115–45.

Herring, S., Johnson, D. and De Benedetto, T. (1992) 'Participation in electronic discourse in a feminist field' in K. Hall, M. Bucholz and B. Moonwoman (eds) *Proceedings of the Second Berkeley Women and Language Conference*, Berkeley: University of California.

Hills, J. and Michalis, M. (1997) 'Technological convergence: regulatory competition: The British case of digital television', *Policy Studies*, 18 (3/4): 219–37.

Hilton, I. (1996) 'When everything has its price', The *Guardian*, 27 August.

Holderness, M. (1998) 'Who are the world's information poor?' in B. Loader (ed.) *Cyberspace Divide: Equality, Agency and Policy in the Information Society*, London: Routledge: 35–56.

Huyer, S. (1999) 'Shifting agendas at GK97: women and international policy on information and communication technologies' in W. Harcourt (ed.) *Women@Internet: Creating New Cultures in Cyberspace*, London: Zed Books: 114–30.

Inayatullah, S. and Milojevic, I. (1999) 'Exclusion and communication in the information era: from silences to global conversation' in W. Harcourt (ed.) *Women@Internet: Creating New Cultures in Cyberspace*, London: Zed Books: 76–88.

The Independent (1998a) 'China fires first shot in Internet war', 4 December.

The Independent (1998b) 'China uses jail threat to keep control of Internet', 13 December.

The Independent (1998c) 'Malaysia losing fight against cyber protest', 13 December.

Kelly, A. (1985) 'The construction of masculine science', *British Journal of the Sociology of Education*, 6 (2): 133–54.

Kramarae, C. and Taylor, H. J. (1993) 'Women and men on electronic networks: a conversation or a monologue' in H. J. Taylor, C. Kramarae and M. Ebben (eds) *Women, Information Technology and Scholarship*, Urbana: Center for Advanced Study: 52–61.

Lacey, C. (ed.) (1987) *Barbara Leigh Smith Bodichon and the Langham Place Group*, London: Routledge and Kegan Paul.

Latour, B. (1993) *We Have Never Been Modern*, Hemel Hempstead: Harvester/Wheatsheaf.

LIC (Libraries and Information Commission) (1997) *New Library: The People's Network*, London: Department of Culture, Media and Sport.

Light, J. (1995) 'The digital landscape: new space for women?', *Gender, Place and Culture*, 2 (2): 133–46.

Lloyd, G. (1984) *The Man of Reason: 'Male' and 'Female' in Western Philosophy*, London: Methuen.

Loader, B. (1997) *The Governance of Cyberspace: Politics, Technology and Global Restructuring*, London: Routledge.

Lyon, D. (1998) 'The world wide web of surveillance: the Internet and off-world power flows', *Information, Communication and Society*, 1 (1): 91–105.

Markussen, R. (1995) 'Constructing easiness – historical perspectives on work, computerization and women' in S. L. Star (ed.) *The Cultures of Computing*, Oxford: Blackwell: 158–80.

Markussen, R. (1996) 'Politics of intervention in design: feminist reflections on the Scandinavian tradition', *Artificial Intelligence and Society*, 10: 127–41.

May, C. (1998) 'Capital, knowledge and ownership: the "information society" and intellectual property', *Information, Communication and Society*, 1 (3): 246–69.

Miller, S. (1996) *Civilizing Cyberspace: Policy, Power, and the Information Superhighway*, New York: ACM Press.

Morahan-Martin, J. (1998) 'Women and girls last: females and the Internet', Bristol: IRISS 1998 Conference.

Newey, A. (1999) 'Freedom of expression: censorship in private hands' in Liberty (ed.) *Liberating Cyberspace: Civil Liberties, Human Rights and the Internet*, London: Pluto Press: 13–43.

Panos briefing (1995) *The Internet and the South: Superhighway or Dirt Track?*, London: Panos.

Plant, S. (1995) 'The future looms: weaving women and cybernetics', *Body and Society*, 1 (3–4): 45–64.

Plant, S. (1997a) *Zeros + Ones: Digital Women + The New Technoculture*, London: Fourth Estate.

Plant, S. (1997b) Extract from 'Beyond the screens: film, cyberpunk and cyber-feminism' in S. Kemp and J. Squires (eds) *Feminisms*, Oxford: Oxford University Press: 503–8.

Pool, R. (1997) *Beyond Engineering: How Society Shapes Technology*, Oxford: Oxford University Press.

Quarterman, J. (1993) 'The global matrix of minds' in L. Harasim (ed.) *Global Networks: Computers and International Communication*, London: MIT Press: 35–56.

Rathmell, A. (1998) 'Information warfare and sub-state actors: an organizational approach', *Information, Communication and Society*, 1 (4): 488–503.

Rheingold, H. (1994) *The Virtual Community: Finding Connection in a Computerized World*, London: Secker and Warburg.

Rich, B. R. (1997) 'The party line: gender and technology in the home' in J. Terry and M. Calvert (eds) *Processed Lives: Gender and Technology in Everyday Life*, London: Routledge: 221–31.

Salus, P. (1995) *Casting the Net: From ARPANET to Internet and Beyond*, Wokingham: Addison-Wesley.

Samarajiva, R. and Shields, P. (1997) 'Telecommunication networks as social space: implications for research and policy and an exemplar', *Media, Culture and Society*, 19: 535–55.

Schuler, D. (1996) *New Community Networks: Wired for Change*, New York: ACM Press.

Seabrook, J. (1997) *Deeper: A Two-year Odyssey in Cyberspace*, London: Faber and Faber.

Scott, A. (1998a) 'Reconceptualizing "equal access" in the informational society: two British policy models for the public provision of information technology', unpublished.

Scott, A. (1998b) 'Researching gender and IT', unpublished.

Semmens, L. and Willoughby, L. (1996) 'Will women be excluded from the "white male playground"?', unpublished, paper given at MediaActive Conference, Liverpool.

Silverstone, R., Hirsch, E. and Morley, D. (1992) 'Information and communication technologies and the moral economy of the household' in R. Silverstone and E. Hirsch (eds) *Consuming Technologies: Media and Information in Domestic Spaces*, London: Routledge: 15–31.

Spender, D. (1995) *Nattering on the Net: Women, Power and Cyberspace*, Melbourne: Spinifex.

Star, S. L. (1991) 'Power, technology and the phenomenology of conventions: on being allergic to onions' in J. Law (ed.) *A Sociology of Monsters: Essays on Power, Technology and Domination*, London: Routledge.

Stone, A. L. (1995) *The War of Desire and Technology at the Close of the Mechanical Age*, London: MIT Press.

Sutton, L. (1996) 'Cocktails and thumbtacks in the old west: what would Emily Post say?' in L. Cherny and E. R. Weise (eds) *Wired_Women: Gender and New Realities in Cyberspace*, Seattle, WA: Seal Press: 169–87.

Swarbrick, A. (1987) 'Information technology and new training initiatives for women' in M. J. Davidson and C. L. Cooper (eds) *Women and Information Technology*, Chichester: John Wiley and Sons: 255–80.

Swarbrick, A. (1997) 'Against the odds: women developing a commitment to technology' in M. Maynard (ed.) *Science and the Construction of Women*, London: UCL Press: 55–75.

Toole, B. (1996) 'Ada Byron, Lady Lovelace, an analyst and metaphysician', *IEEE Annals of the History of Computing*, 18 (3): 4–11.

Tsagarousianou, R., Tambini, D. and Bryan, C. (eds) (1998) *Cyberdemocracy: Technology, Cities and Civic Networks*, London: Routledge.

Turkle, S. (1995) *Life on the Screen: Identity in the Age of the Internet*, London: Phoenix.

Umble, D. (1992) 'The Amish and the telephone: resistance and reconstruction' in R. Silverstone and E. Hirsch (eds) *Consuming Technologies: Media and Information in Domestic Spaces*, London: Routledge: 183–94.

Wagner, I. (1995) 'Hard times: the politics of women's work in computerized environments', *The European Journal of Women's Studies*, 2 (3): 295–314.

Wakeford, N. (1997) 'Networking women and girrls with information/communication technology: surfing tales of the world wide web' in J. Terry and M. Calvert (eds) *Processed Lives: Gender and Technology in Everyday Life*, London: Routledge: 50–66.

Wheelock, J. (1992) 'Personal computers, gender and an institutional model of the household' in R. Silverstone and E. Hirsch (eds) *Consuming Technologies: Media and Information in Domestic Spaces*, London: Routledge: 97–112.

Which? (1998) Available online: http://www.which.net/nonsub/special/isp-survey/executive.html (17 January 1999).

Whyte, J. (1986) *Girls into Science and Technology*, London: Routledge.

Wittig, M. and Schmitz, J. (1996) 'Electronic grassroots organizing', *Journal of Social Issues*, 52 (1): 53–69.

Wright, R. (1997) 'Women in computing: a cross-national analysis' in R. Lander and A. Adam (eds) *Women in Computing*, Exeter: Intellect Books.

Woolf, V. (1929) *A Room of One's Own*, Harmondsworth: Penguin.

Wylie, M. (1995) 'No place for women', *Digital Media*, 4 (8): 3–6.

Chapter 2

Gender in email-based co-operative problem-solving

Greg Michaelson and Margit Pohl

Introduction

In the 1970s and 1980s, the question whether there are gender differences in face-to-face communication played an important role in feminist discussions. A considerable number of studies (for an overview see, for example, Trömel-Plötz 1984; Gräßel 1991; Tannen 1991) showed conclusively that such gender differences exist. In particular: men talk more than women, men tend to interrupt women more often and women encourage and support each other's topics more often than men. It is an open question whether similar phenomena can be observed in email communication. The study described here tries to clarify this issue.

In feminist literature the effects of email on gender differences in communication is still controversial. On the one hand, many women apparently have had fairly negative experiences on the Internet. Sexual harassment on the net produces a climate that does not encourage women to use the Internet (Spender 1995; Brail 1996). Furthermore, the rules of politeness governing face-to-face communication seem to be less binding when there is no physical presence; therefore a phenomenon like flaming is fairly common in electronic communication (Herring 1994; Spender 1995). It is argued that such aggressive behaviour favours men, who then dominate conversations, whereas women give up participating because of the lack of positive feedback. A major problem in this context is still the question of access. As long as there is no cheap and simple way to get online, people who are not male, white and middle class will have difficulties (to a larger or smaller extent) in accessing the Internet. However, recent technological developments that greatly cheapen and ease the use of communication technologies show that solutions to this problem are possible.

Susan Herring's research (Herring 1996) supports this negative view to some extent. Based on her empirical findings, she assumes that there are gender specific styles of email communication, with an aligned style predominantly used by women and an opposed style used predominantly by men. People who adopt the aligned 'variant' either support or at least appreciate other people's views and try to keep the conversation going. People who use the opposed variant criticize the views of their addressee. As Herring found, many messages that fall into the latter category close with a remark that the discussion should be ended as the topic is not relevant. This is very similar to findings from research into face-to-face communication which showed that women tend to keep the conversation going by encouraging people to speak whereas men tend to ignore or criticize utterances by other people. Herring, however, does not see these styles or variants as a strict dichotomy. Some women in her sample incorporated features of the opposed variant when participating in a discussion on a male-dominated mailing list, whereas men behaved in a more 'aligned' manner on female dominated mailing lists. She calls this phenomenon 'style mixing'. Based on her results one might conclude that gender associated styles of communication are not rigid and unchangeable but fluid and elusive.

Herring concludes that conventional stereotypes of gender roles which portray women as emotional and men as rational are misleading and cannot be substantiated by empirical evidence. Stereotyping women as 'emotional' suggests that they are unsuited to use 'rational' information technology, which by implication becomes identified as a male domain. Herring argues that such stereotypes 'exclude women by definition from the Information Age' (Herring 1996: 105) and that it is not surprising that in such circumstances women are reluctant to go online.

There are, on the other hand, researchers who focus on the opportunities offered by the Internet rather than on its negative effects. It seems that this strand of research has become more popular in the past few years. For example, Dale Spender (1995) had been very uncomfortable with computers but felt intrigued by email. Sherry Turkle (1995) argues that the Internet supports styles of interaction which are more 'feminine' than traditional programming. Kaplan and Farrell (1994) investigated the attitudes of young women who spend much of their time surfing the Internet. They found that there are apparently no intrinsic barriers to women in the Internet and that women can enjoy it as much as men do. Bergman and van Zoonen (1998) conducted a similar investigation. They analysed case studies of women who used the Internet for private and professional purposes. They conclude that all these women found the opportunity for activities which are relevant for them personally and which cannot be seen as part of a broader masculine culture. Sadie Plant (1996) sees opportunities for the dissolution of all forms of identity on the Internet. The Internet is a medium where an individual may construct actively their own persona, free from social stereotypes that are reinforced by physical appearance. In a subsequent publication, Plant presents Ada Lovelace, who might be called the first computer programmer, as a kind of a role model for present-day women using computers (Plant 1997). Despite her generally positive attitude towards computer technology she emphasizes the 'double-edged' character of the Internet: 'No matter how spontaneous their emergence, self-organizing systems are back in organizational mode as soon as they have organized themselves' (Plant 1997: 49).

Both approaches described above are probably legitimate, and both are supported by empirical evidence. It can be concluded that the Internet is a flexible technology that can be shaped to a certain extent by the people who use it. However, it is difficult to formulate consistent hypotheses based on the ambiguous results of the scientific literature. On the one hand, one might expect computer-mediated interaction to be similar to face-to-face communication; on the other hand one might conclude that the lack of physical, bodily presence of individuals leads to a weakening of gender roles.

In our 1995 investigation of email-based co-operative problem-solving (Pohl and Michaelson 1997) we found no important gender differences in co-operation within the overall group. On the other hand, within individual pairs some stereotypical behaviour could be observed. However, our 1995 study was based on only eight pairs which we felt was too small to permit more than tentative conclusions. Thus we decided to replicate our 1995 study with a further eight pairs, to enable more detailed analysis of possible gender effects in email-based interaction. Following Susan Herring (1996), in analysing the 1995 data, we focused on the degree to which the participants in paired email discussions co-operate. Our original hypothesis had been that gender differences would be observed along this dimension. In the light of our first experiment, we modified this hypothesis to propose that gender stereotypes tended to disappear in email conversation. Thus, in repeating the experiment in 1998 we expected to find a similar pattern to 1995.

The 1995 experiment and its analysis

The 1995 experiment is described in detail in Pohl and Michaelson (1997). Here we reprise its main features. Pairs of Heriot-Watt

University and Vienna University of Technology students were asked to co-operate in solving each other's tasks, using email in a single continuous afternoon session. The HWU subjects were asked to describe an afternoon in Vienna, visiting four interesting sites. Similarly, the VUT subjects were asked to describe an afternoon in Edinburgh, also visiting four interesting sites. Eight pairs took part, in two four-pair sessions, with all gender/location combinations represented twice. Subsequently, all email messages were analysed quantitatively, to identify gross patterns of email use by word count, and qualitatively to tease out interaction patterns in individual dialogues.

It might appear that cultural differences between Austria and the UK would have an impact on our study. While we acknowledge broad differences, rooted in different histories and languages, we think that these are largely irrelevant. Both societies are grounded in advanced industrial capitalism where young people share a common northern/western hemisphere mass culture that largely rejects comparable conservative national traditions. We also think that concrete contemporary differences, that might influence the gendering of information technology, tend to be self-cancelling. Thus, mass computer use is more widespread in the UK than in Austria, but Austria has more progressive equal opportunities legislation than the UK and may have less rigid social stereotypes associated with technology use. Finally, the higher education class and gender participation profiles are similar in both countries. As discussed below, the domicile of our experimental subjects does not appear to be significant in our study. Nonetheless, this is an interesting dimension for future investigation.

In our 1995 experiment (Pohl and Michaelson 1997) we introduced the idea of an 'own/other' ratio as a measure of co-operation. This is the ratio of words expended on a subject's own task to words expended on their partner's task. Note that this ratio measures relative overall effort, correcting differences in message frequency and length. We termed a ratio of less than 1 as 'altruistic', a ratio of 1 as 'balanced' and a ratio of more than 1 as 'selfish'. Using this measure, we found no gender or location differences between overall gendered/located groups and all displayed some degree of altruism. However, we did identify wide variations in individual co-operation within pairs. The latter finding complemented the qualitative analysis which identified a variety of gendered behaviour patterns across gender boundaries. Nonetheless, our conclusions (Pohl and Michaelson 1997) were necessarily tentative owing to the small sample size.

The 1998 experiment

In 1998, we repeated the experiment with another eight pairs of subjects under the same conditions as in 1995. Analysis of the 1998 pre- and post-experiment questionnaires showed that the 1998 subjects had greater email experience than those in 1995, and that the 1998 Edinburgh subjects were older than the 1995 Edinburgh subjects.

However, t-tests for independent samples show no significant differences at the 5 per cent level between the 1995 and 1998 sub-cohorts of Edinburgh women, Edinburgh men, Vienna women, Vienna men, all Edinburgh subjects, all Vienna subjects, and all women and all men, on all but one of our key indicators. There is a significant difference in total number of words between all 1995 and all 1998 women, with 1998 women sending significantly more words (t-test = –2.52; t = 2.145 at 5 per cent significance level with 14 degrees of freedom). On average, 1995 women sent 634.12 (standard deviation 398.93) words in 8.88 messages with an average message length of 71.45. On average, 1998 women sent 1,018.25 (standard deviation 164.69) words in 8.88 messages with an average message length of 114.73. Thus the 1998 women used consistently more words than the 1995 women.

Nonetheless, given that all measures other than this showed no differences, we feel confident in combining the results from the 1995 and 1998 sub-cohorts to make an overall analysis by gender and location.

Quantitative analysis

Text analysis

Email is unlike other forms of written language in that there is a tendency to use speech- and note-like constructs as well as more formal phrases and sentences. Here, all the words in a construct that is principally about one category are assigned to that category but in a complex construct, like a multi-phrase sentence, sub-constructs may be allocated to different categories. Personal details inserted from 'signature' files at the end of messages have been ignored as they represent no effort on the part of the sender. 'Subject' headers have also been ignored: it might be interesting to examine how they are used in more detail. Email also contains non-natural language constructs like smileys and uniform resource locators (URLs). In the present analysis, smileys have been ignored and URLs have been counted as one word. It would be interesting to investigate smiley and URL use by gender: for example, folklore has it that smiley use is predominantly male.

Each individual message is analysed to identify the number of words concerned with meta-communication, which involve the mechanics of interaction, personal communication, about themself and their partner, and task communication, which deals with their own and their partner's problem. In almost all cases, word categorization is straightforward. However, in a small number of exchanges, some ambiguities may arise between the 'meta' and 'personal' categories, and between the 'personal' and 'task' categories. For example, in an early message, Jim (Edinburgh) asks Ernst (Vienna), whose identity he doesn't yet know, 'What is your real name?'. Ernst tells him and Jim then starts all subsequent messages with 'Ernst'. We do not know Jim's intention in asking the question. It could be simply to establish how to write an appropriate 'meta' salutation or it could be an attempt to determine Ernst's 'other's personal' gender: its effect appears to be the former. Given our focus on task behaviour, such 'meta'/'personal' misclassifications are not so significant.

However, 'task'/'personal' ambiguities are more problematic as a misclassification may affect our co-operation measure which is based on a ratio of effort on one's own task to effort on both one's own and one's partner's task. For example, Alfred (Vienna) writes: 'I think it's a great idea to walk, because then one can see more than when you sit in a bus or even in the subway. By the way: do you have a subway in Edinburgh?'

The first sentence looks like an 'own personal' statement. Wendy (Edinburgh) replies: 'We don't have a subway, the only real public transport option is the bus. But the Royal Mile is actually almost exactly a mile, not too far to walk, although you might want to catch a bus (Number 1) back up the hill again after you have been to Holyrood – if you want to go there!' providing an 'other's task' response. The first sentence then functions as an 'own task' sentence. The second sentence is unambiguously an 'own task' question about transport in Edinburgh which might reinforce a response to the first as an 'other task' elicitation.

There are many inherent dangers in trying to attribute intentions retrospectively or reverse engineer a conversation, where 'common sense' categorization fails. One solution might be to carry out a number of independent categorizations of the text and then explicitly resolve differences. Other possibilities include video recording each subject during an experimental session using a talk-aloud protocol or interviewing subjects during text analysis to clarify classifications from their perspective.

Choice of indicators

The combined 1995 and 1998 results have been analysed for three principal indicators for each experimental subject: the number of messages they send, the overall number of words in their messages and a co-operation measure. The first two are self-explanatory, and can also be interpreted along the co-operative/unco-operative dimension, as people who 'talk' very much usually have little time to listen to others. However, for the co-operation measure we decided to replace the 'own/other' ratio used in our 1995 experiment (Pohl and Michaelson 1997).

To recap, all messages have their header and footers discarded and are then inspected to find the number of words about meta-communication, about the sender, about the recipient, about the sender's task, and about the recipient's task. The 1995 'own/own' measure was the ratio of the total number of words about the sender's task to those about the recipient's task. The intention in using a ratio was to compensate for individual differences in message length in making comparisons of allocation of task effort, for example enabling the comparison of verbose and taciturn people. In retrospect, this was an unsatisfactory characterization as information about proportional effort is lost. Instead, here we use the 'own/(own + other)' ratio; that is, the total words concerned with the sender's task as a proportion of the total words concerned with both the sender's and the recipient's tasks. As mentioned earlier, a ratio less than 1 indicates 'altruism', a ratio of 1 indicates 'balance', and a ratio of more than 1 indicates 'selfishness'.

Analysis by sub-cohorts

Comparisons between Edinburgh women and men, Vienna women and men, Edinburgh and Vienna women, Edinburgh and Vienna men, all Edinburgh and Vienna subjects, and all women and men are now presented.

It can be seen from Table 2.1, on average, that Edinburgh women sent fewer, longer messages than Edinburgh men. On average, Vienna women sent slightly fewer, shorter messages than Vienna men. All show a similar degree of 'altruism'. However, t-tests for independent samples show no significant differences at the 5 per cent significance level were found, on number of messages, number of words or the

Table 2.1 Indicators for Edinburgh and Vienna women and men

	Edinburgh women	Edinburgh men	Vienna women	Vienna men
No. of subjects	8	8	8	8
Total no. of messages	62	81	80	90
Average no. of messages	7.75	10.12	10.00	11.25
Total no. of words	6,850	4,807	6,369	7,451
Average no. of words	856.25	600.88	796.12	931.38
Average own/(own + other)	0.33	0.38	0.38	0.36

Table 2.2 Indicators for all Edinburgh, Vienna, women and men

	Edinburgh	Vienna	Women	Men
No. of subjects	16	16	16	16
No. of messages	143	170	142	171
Average no. of messages	8.94	10.62	8.88	10.69
No. of words	11,657	13,820	13,219	12,258
Average no. of words	728.56	863.75	826.19	766.12
Average own/(own + other)	0.36	0.37	0.36	0.37

own/(own + other) measure between Edinburgh women and men, between Vienna women and men, between Edinburgh and Vienna women, or between Edinburgh and Vienna men.

Moving now to whole location and gender sub-cohorts, it can be seen from Table 2.2 that on average Edinburgh subjects sent slightly fewer, slightly shorter messages than Vienna subjects. Similarly, on average women sent slightly fewer, slightly shorter messages than men. All show similar 'altruism'. Once again, t-tests for differences produced no significant results at the 5 per cent level for any indicators by location or by gender.

Analysis of co-operation by pair

With only four pairs for each gender/location combination, it is very hard to draw significant conclusions about co-operation patterns within pair groups. However, an overview is provided in Table 2.3.

In each sub-table, the first two columns show individual's own/(own + other) measures for each of four pairs of subjects. Plotting the own/(own + other) measures for each pair on a scatter graph – Figure

Table 2.3 Own/(own + other) by gender/location pair groups

(a) Edinburgh women and Vienna men				(b) Vienna women and Edinburgh men		
	EW	VM	Difference		VW	EM	Difference
Pair 1	0.69	0.67	0.02	Pair 1	0.28	0.32	–0.04
Pair 2	0.16	0.31	–0.15	Pair 2	0.36	0.60	–0.24
Pair 3	0.38	0.32	0.06	Pair 3	0.31	0.55	–0.24
Pair 4	0.16	0.35	–0.19	Pair 4	0.27	0.42	–0.15

(c) Edinburgh and Vienna men				(d) Edinburgh and Vienna women		
	EM	VM	Difference		EW	VW	Difference
Pair 1	0.43	0.21	0.22	Pair 1	0.63	0.88	–0.15
Pair 2	0.47	0.47	0.00	Pair 2	0.27	0.34	–0.07
Pair 3	0.05	0.42	–0.37	Pair 3	0.04	0.21	–0.17
Pair 4	0.20	0.13	0.07	Pair 4	0.30	0.42	–0.12

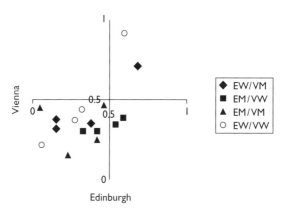

Figure 2.1 Own/(own + other) plot for gendered/located pairs

2.1 – shows no discernible pattern apart from the already noted overall tendency to 'altruism'.

In contrast, crude gender stereotyping of men as generally 'selfish'
and women as generally 'altruistic' would place woman/woman pairs
in the bottom left quadrant (EW and VW 'altruistic'), man/man pairs in
the top right quadrant (EM and VM 'selfish') and woman/man pairs in
either the top left (EW 'altruistic' and VM 'selfish') or bottom right
quadrant (EM 'selfish' and VW 'altruistic').

The third column in the tables shows the difference between the
Edinburgh subject's and the Vienna subject's measure. A negative dif-

ference suggests that the Edinburgh subject is more 'altruistic' than the Vienna subject: a positive difference suggests that the Vienna subject is more 'altruistic' than the Edinburgh subject. From Table 2.3 (a and b), it appears that in mixed pairs, women are more 'altruistic' than men, corresponding to the stereotype. Vienna women appear consistently more 'altruistic' towards Edinburgh men (Table 2.3 (b)) than Edinburgh women towards Vienna men (Table 2.3 (a)). In same sex pairs, Vienna women appear consistently more 'altruistic' than Edinburgh women (Table 2.3 (d)). Nonetheless, results from such small samples should be treated with considerable caution.

Conversation analysis

Conversation analysis, email and gender

Conversation analysis is a methodology for studying the organization of everyday conversation. One of its basic assumptions is that order is produced by the participants of a conversation according to rules that are very often applied instinctively and without conscious effort. One of the areas which has been studied extensively by conversation analysis is the so-called turn-taking process which ensures that only one speaker will talk at a given time and that speakers will take turns in conversation (Sacks et al. 1974). The turn-taking process may seem trivial and simple at first but careful analysis shows complex patterns of behaviour. One of these patterns is adjacency pairs (Nofsinger 1991), pairs of utterances which often occur adjacent to each other and which 'belong together'. Typical adjacency pairs are questions/ answers, invitations/acceptances, offers/acceptances, congratulations/ thanks, etc. In conversations, the second part of an adjacency pair usually follows the first. If the second part is missing, it is seen as something unusual and any interaction may break down as a consequence.

Conversation analysis in its original form does not consider the contents of any interaction but only its organization and its structure. It is not concerned with questions about how often particular phenomena occur, and there is no interest in the specific ethnographic features of the participants or the settings of a conversation (Psathas 1995). This assumption has been criticized frequently (Forrester 1996). Conversation analysis posits that the rules of any conversation are negotiated by the participants while the interaction is going on. For this negotiation process to be fair it is necessary that all the participants have the same social status and power. This is not always the case. Numerous studies in the past 20 years have shown that women are discriminated against in face-to-face discussions (see the Introduction).

Nevertheless, conversation analysis has been used occasionally in feminist studies of discrimination against women in verbal interaction (Fishman 1984). Several authors suggest the use of conversation analysis for email exchanges because of its attention to the social context of naturally occurring interaction (for example, Luff et al. 1990). Furthermore, conversation analysis can make several specific problems of email conversation visible that might not be detected by other methods of analysis. The following example is part of a conversation recorded during our second experiment in 1998, between a man in Vienna and a woman in Edinburgh (less important parts of the messages are omitted):

Heather's first message	'Looking forward to hearing from you about Vienna.'
Andreas' second message	'I guess you didn't read my first email yet.'
Heather's second message	'I see you managed to email me first. (Just ignore the other message)'
Andreas' third message	'hm. I already answered the other message, can't ignore it anymore'

As is obvious from the above example, email messages overlap. Therefore, a fairly rigorous structure of adjacency pairs is not possible. Nevertheless, in most cases people manage to keep an email conversation clear and understandable. Email is basically a mixture between spoken and written language (Yates 1996). Our empirical results show a tendency for the adjacency pair structure of spoken language to be preserved, especially if the people interacting use very short messages. On the other hand, some characteristics of written language also influence email, for example, when several questions are answered summarily in a long, rather complex piece of text. Both strategies lead to greater coherence. Still, the lack of non-verbal cues, the time-lags and the lack of mutual commitment (Hesse et al. 1995) can lead to considerable confusion.

Our basic hypothesis, tested by conversation analysis was, therefore, that strategies adopted by women and men to cope with this novel situation differ. Women refer to other people's messages more extensively, and they do this, for example, by answering questions more exhaustively. This form of behaviour might be called aligned. Nofsinger (1991) uses the term alignment to define activities that ensure mutual understanding and real interaction. In contrast, Herring (1996) uses the term only when the participants support each other and share each other's opinion to a great extent. In our analysis, we used the term more in the sense of Nofsinger. Nevertheless, it would be interesting to conduct our analysis in greater detail to test whether our empirical data conforms to Herring's main assumptions.

Our main focus in the analysis was question/answer sequences. Because of the particular nature of the conversations (students had to co-operate to develop tours through Edinburgh/Vienna with the help of their partners), questions and answers made up more than 50 per cent of all conversations. As described above, strict adherence to the question/answer structure of face-to-face conversations was not to be expected. We were especially interested therefore to see under which circumstances such a deviation from face-to-face communication happened and if any gender differences could be observed.

Results

In general, students tended to stick to the question/answer structure of normal communication, although with modifications. It was very seldom that only one question was asked or one answer was given in one email message. The sequential nature of adjacency pairs is lost in email conversations. Furthermore, a considerable number of questions were not answered at all, a phenomenon which would be rather strange in face-to-face conversation. There are several reasons why this happened.

Time-out (running out of time) is one of the most common causes of question/answer breakdown. At the end of the interaction, when it was clear that very little time was left, students did not bother to answer their partner's questions although the most conscientious ones answered questions until the last minute. There were technical problems with email reliability, especially in the 1995 experiment. In the middle of most conversations, tremendous time lags can be observed. People reacted very differently to these time lags. Some of them felt overwhelmed by the large amount of questions that kept pouring in after the time lag and either did not answer them at all or answered them quite summarily. The time lag also produced a considerable amount of chaos in some conversations, so that people could not keep track of which questions they had already answered: sometimes they answered questions twice.

Another category of questions are rhetorical questions (for example, 'Well, what do you think about it?', 'Any more questions?' etc.).

Students apparently did not think it was worth the effort to answer such questions. A very important category are personal or provocative questions. When Sarah (Vienna woman) and Digby (Edinburgh man) discuss pubs in Edinburgh, Sarah asks 'Are you there to have a drink too?' and, a little bit later, 'Why do you think arthurs seat sounds too boring for me?' (spelling as in the original). She gets answers to almost all of her other questions but not to these two. Still, this does not impede their discussion in any way. Apparently, it is easier to evade unwelcome questions in email than in face-to-face communication.

It is very difficult to make any quantitative statements about whether or not gender differences in question/answer sequences exist because our sample still seems too small for that. The way in which pairs interacted determined to a large extent how many questions were asked. If pairs got on well with each other then more questions were asked than when pairs had little in common. A larger sample is necessary to filter out this influence. Still, there is one interesting phenomenon: five women answered all of their partner's questions but only one man answered all those of his partner.

It is also interesting to look at single conversations and analyse whether they conform to gender stereotypes or not. In our study, there were two typically woman to woman conversations, one from 1995 and one from 1998. In both conversations, extremely few messages were sent and few questions were asked. Apart from that, the discussions are rather different. Victoria (Edinburgh) and Edith (Vienna) sent only short messages and did not really co-operate to achieve their goal. From her last message, it can be inferred that at least Edith was not happy with that situation. However, Nicole (Vienna) and Morag (Edinburgh) sent extremely long messages. They sent letters rather than email messages and told each other a great deal about their opinions and beliefs.

In contrast to that, Graeme (Edinburgh) and Paul (Vienna) show typical macho behaviour in their interaction: pornographic allusions, remarks about girls, long and frequent messages, remarks which show a strong competitive orientation and ironic and abusive remarks. This behaviour is probably produced as a joint effort, thus two men may be necessary for such an interaction and they reinforce each other.

Conversation analysis shows that email interaction is fundamentally different to face-to-face conversations in that women and men behave in similar ways in many respects. Nevertheless, if we analyse single cases, stereotypical behaviour can be observed. These cases show that gender stereotypes are very flexible and do not consist of a fixed set of traits.

The questionnaire

Before and after the experiment students had to answer a short questionnaire. The first part consisted of questions about the students (age, sex, computer and email experience, etc.) and the second part consisted of questions about the experiment (for example, whether most time was spent on their own task or on another's task, whether interacting in English was easy or not, etc.). In the following sections, we summarize salient results.

There was great variability in prior computer experience. One of the participants had only used the computer for two years. The maximum use, on the other hand, was 20 years. Fifty per cent had used computers for six to 12 years. All the participants were computer science students; therefore it can be assumed that their acquaintance with the computer is greater than that of 'normal' computer users. There is a significant difference between women and men as far as computer experience is concerned. Women on the average had used computers for 7.63 years. The same value for men was 11.31 years. This difference is significant on the 1 per cent level ($t = 2.46$).

There was more uniformity in email experience. Most people had less email experience than computer experience. Three participants, all from the 1995 experiment, had no email experience at all. One participant had seven years of email experience. Fifty per cent of the students had between one and five years of email experience. Overall, there was no gender difference in email experience. On average, women had 3.17 years of email experience and men 3.5 years. This difference is not significant ($t = 0.43$). On the other hand, there is a significant difference in email experience between participants of the 1995 and the 1998 experiments. The participants of the 1995 experiment had, on average, 2.06 years of email experience and the participants of the 1998 experiment had 4.6 years ($t = 4.43$). This is significant at the 1 per cent level. It is interesting that there is a significant gender difference in computer experience but not in email experience. This would support the hypothesis that women feel more comfortable with an interactive and co-operative technology like email than with computers as such (Spender 1995) although our sample is, of course, too small to generalize this result too much.

In the questionnaire which was filled in after the email session we asked how the students experienced interacting with their partner. There were no significant differences in perceptions of sessions by gender, apart from in perceived sizes of messages, where women answered significantly more often that their own messages were longer than their partner's messages (t = 2.55). One might argue that women talked more than men and that their impression was realistic but this is not supported by the facts. Men consistently underestimated their share in the conversation.

Conclusions

The results from the combined 1995 and 1998 cohorts provide sound confirmation of our 1995 findings. First of all, there are no significant gender differences in email-mediated problem-solving at a statistical level in measures of message volume and of co-operation. In particular, it seems that the gendered strategies that benefit men are disrupted by asynchronous communication. One tentative explanation might be that bodily presence is important in reinforcing gender-stereotyped behaviour. However, our results contrast with those from Herring's study, which showed that mail list behaviour tends to reflect the gender stereotypes in face-to-face interactions. We speculate that this may be due to a distinction between private and public discussions (Pohl 1996). In public discussion forums such as mail lists, peer and group effects may still act to reinforce stereotyped styles, even in the absence of bodily presence.

In contrast to a lack of group differences, we have found a range of gender differences in the strategies adopted by individuals in single pairs. Thus, while gross gender stereotypes are weakened in email exchanges, they are not displaced. Interactions necessarily involve strategies and familiar gendered strategies from face-to-face interactions, which overwhelmingly predominate in everyday life, are a fundamental source.

The participants in the experiment were surprisingly enthusiastic: indeed, many insisted on continuing interactions for much longer than originally had been planned for. In post-experiment debriefings, many participants expressed considerable interest both in the overall experimental findings and in staying in touch subsequently with their experimental partners.

Our study suggests a range of further research. As well as larger-scale replications to provide for robust analysis of patterns of pair behaviours, a variety of additional analyses of gender effects in email interactions might be useful, for example in 'meta' and 'personal' constructs. A more detailed analysis of question/answer patterns would enable further characterization of gender effects taken together. Finally, it may be fruitful to investigate how participants interpret the interaction, either through interviews or more detailed questionnaires, for example to what degree they felt confused/frustrated/motivated, etc. by the use of email for co-operative problem-solving.

This research has been conducted almost entirely by email – the authors have met face-to-face on only three occasions since the study began in August 1994.

Acknowledgements

We would like to thank all the participants in our 1995 and 1998 studies. We would also like to thank Nancy Falchikov for her helpful comments on this chapter.

References

Bergman, S. and van Zoonen, L. (1998) 'Fishing with false teeth: women, gender and the Internet', *Razón y Palabra*, 9 (2), Noviembre–Enero 1997–98. Available online: http://www.cem.itesm.mx/dacs/publicaciones/logos/anteriores/mes9/cities2.htm (18 January 1999).

Brail, S. (1996) 'The price of admission: harassment and free speech in the wild, wild west' in L. Cherny and E. R. Weise (eds) *Wired_Women: Gender and New Realities in Cyberspace*, Seattle, WA: Seal Press: 141–68.

Fishman, P. (1984) 'Macht und Ohnmacht in Paargesprächen' in S. Trömel-Plötz (ed.) *Gewalt durch Sprache: Die Vergewaltigung von Frauen in Gesprächen*, Frankfurt am Main: Fischer: 127–40.

Forrester, M. (1996) *Psychology of Language: A Critical Introduction*, London: Sage.

Gräßel, U. (1991) *Sprachverhalten und Geschlecht*, Pfaffenweiler: Centaurus-Verlagsgesellschaft.

Herring, S. (1994) 'Gender differences in computer-mediated communication: bringing familiar baggage to the new frontier', keynote talk at panel entitled 'Making the Net "Work": is there a Z39.50 in gender communication?', American Library Association annual convention, Miami, 27 June 1994 (unpublished manuscript).

Herring, S. (1996) 'Two variants of an electronic message schema' in S. Herring (ed.) *Computer-Mediated Communication. Linguistic, Social and Cross-Cultural Perspectives*, Amsterdam/Philadelphia: John Benjamin Publishing Company: 81–106.

Hesse, F. W., Garsoffky, B. and Hron, A. (1995) 'Interface-design für computerunterstütztes kooperatives Lernen' in L. J. Issing and P. Klimsa (eds) *Information und Lernen mit Multimedia*, Weinheim: Psychologie Verlags Union: 253–67.

Kaplan, N. and Farrell, E. (1994) 'Weavers of the web: a portrait of young women on the net', *The Arachnet Electronic Journal on Virtual Culture*, 26 July, 2 (3). Available online: http://www.lib.ncsu.edu/stacks/e/ejvc/aejvc-v2n03-kaplan-weavers.txt

Luff, P., Gilbert, N. and Frohlich, D. (1990) *Computers and Conversation*, London: Academic Press.

Nofsinger, R. E. (1991) *Everyday Conversation*, Newbury Park, London, New Delhi: Sage Publications.

Plant, S. (1996) 'On the matrix: cyberfeminist simulations' in R. Shields (ed.) *Cultures of Internet*, London: Sage: 170–83.

Plant, S. (1997) *Zeros + Ones: Digital Women + the New Technoculture*, London: Fourth Estate.

Pohl, M. (1996) *Geschlechtsspezifische Unterschiede im Sprachverhalten*, Frankfurt am Main: Peter Lang.

Pohl, M. and Michaelson, G. (1997) 'I don't think that's an interesting dialogue: computer-mediated communication and gender' in A. F. Grundy, D. Koehler, V. Oechtering and U. Petersen (eds) *Women, Work and Computerization: Spinning a Web from Past to Future*, Proceedings of the 6th International IFIP Conference, Bonn, Germany, 24–27 May, Springer: 87–97.

Psathas, G. (1995) *Conversation Analysis: The Study of Talk-in-Interaction*, Thousand Oaks, London, New Delhi: Sage Publications.

Sacks, H., Schegloff, E. and Jefferson, G. (1974) 'A simplest systematics for the organisation of turn-taking for conversation', *Language*, 50: 696–753.

Spender, D. (1995) *Nattering on the Net: Women, Power and Cyberspace*, North Melbourne: Spinifex.

Tannen, D. (1991) *You Just Don't Understand*, London: Virago.

Trömel-Plötz, S. (ed.) (1984) *Gewalt durch Sprache: Die Vergewaltigung von Frauen in Gesprächen*, Frankfurt am Main: Fischer.

Turkle, S. (1995) *Life on the Screen: Identity in the Age of the Internet*, New York, London, Toronto: Simon and Schuster.

Yates, S. J. (1996) 'Oral and written linguistic aspects of computer conferencing' in S. Herring (ed.) *Computer-Mediated Communication: Linguistic, Social and Cross-Cultural Perspectives*, Amsterdam/Philadelphia: John Benjamin Publishing Company: 29–46.

Chapter 3

Lives and livelihoods in the technological age

Kate White, Leslie Regan Shade and Jennifer Brayton

Introduction

This chapter summarizes results of the first phase of 'Lives and livelihoods in the technological age', developed by Black and White Communications Inc. 'Lives and livelihoods' is a pilot project whose goals are to provide research and policy perspectives on the impact of information and communication technologies (ICTs) on women's lives. It aims to derive strategic benefits through finding ways that women can feel connected to ICTs (and thereby helping their children, families, and communities). This includes economic growth, human development and aiding in social cohesion which are especially important given current trends towards a knowledge-based economy/society (KBE/S).

Although the emphasis of the project, to date, has been on women's lives, the project has also investigated how men conceive of and use ICTs. This follows from several recent policy recommendations, including the International Development Research Centre (IDRC) Gender and Information Working Group, and 'The canon on gender, partnerships and ICT development' presented by the Independent Committee on Women and Global Knowledge at the Global Knowledge 1997 Conference in Toronto. The IDRC Gender and Information Working Group stated that policy recommendations should account for several factors, including the information needs of both men and women to 'foster an understanding of the mutual benefits to be gained by society' (IDRC 1995: 279). It also recommended that approaches should be participatory, encouraging community-wide participation in the design and management of initiatives and that the first phase of this project (the retreat) should be characterized by this methodology. The canon (Independent Committee on Women and Global Knowledge 1997), in emphasizing that 'gender equity must be embraced in all facets of engineering, design, development and delivery if the new information technologies are to be fully effective' also encouraged respecting 'equal partnerships of men and women in development'.

This chapter will first outline the theoretical background to the project, followed by the project objectives and methodology of the retreats. The summary findings of the two retreats will be detailed, with separate analysis of the results of the Canadian and African retreats with respect to issues regarding barriers to access. The chapter then concludes with a comparison of the two international groups and with recommendations and suggestions for further action.

Theoretical foundations

> Despite the belief of some individuals, the computer is not a toy; it is a site of wealth, power and influence, now and in the future. Women . . . and indigenous people, and those with few resources . . . can not afford to be marginalised or excluded from this new medium.
>
> (Spender 1996)

A significant body of academic research has looked at the gender issues surrounding technology. Henwood (1993), Balka (1996), Gilbert and Kile (1996), Plant (1997), Hawthorne and Klein (1999) and Wakeford (1999) among others, have published books and articles addressing the gendered dimensions to the societal understanding and acceptance of new computer technologies. With respect to information and communications technology, studies range from the different programming skills of men and women, what has been dubbed 'epistemological pluralism', to interpersonal skills in computer-mediated communication in the work of linguist Susan Herring (1996). Some work has also looked at the gendered discourse surrounding media presentations of computerization (Millar 1998) and women's stake in the prevailing socio-economic realities of computerization in developed and developing countries (Eisenstein 1998; Harcourt 1999).

Many theorists and authors are on the forefront of acknowledging the real life physical and social barriers that can prevent certain social groups from being able to access and participate comfortably in our new technological age (Loader 1998). While computers may be viewed as a technological tool open for use by any member of society, gender and other aspects of social location, such as race, class, age and physical ability, can influence and shape one's expectations of these new information technologies (Ebo 1998). Technology is typically conceptualized in society as a neutral tool whose use determines whether it is positive or negative. But public understanding of technology is also shaped by the meanings and metaphors that are already in the social landscape. Buzzwords such as the 'World Wide Web', 'cyberspace' and the 'information highway' may be intimidating and anxiety-producing to those who define themselves as being non-users or new computer and Internet users. These socially held values and beliefs about technology may act as barriers to using computers and the Internet in the way that finances can act as a physical barrier for many members of society (McChesney 1999; Schiller 1999).

Objectives and methodology

The project involved organizing two day-long retreats to look at how men and women conceive of ICTs. The first retreat was held in Fredericton, New Brunswick, Canada, and the second retreat was held in Nairobi, Kenya, Africa; both were held in March 1998. The agenda was developed and planned from focus groups and expert knowledge in each of the countries, and with local partners. The African Women in Crisis (AFWIC) group, an initiative of The United Nations Development Fund for Women (UNIFEM), was the facilitating partner for the Kenyan retreat. The participants of the retreats were chosen with the help of a selection committee. Interviews were conducted to determine each participant's basic comfort and knowledge levels with technology, as well as personal and professional interests. At each retreat, participants introduced themselves to the group and provided background information regarding their technological experiences. Based on this information, rapporteurs recorded each participant's interaction, comfort level and enthusiasm for the technology. Women and men were separated from one another for the day and were given separate conference rooms for the discussion and web introduction sessions.

The retreats were designed to provide a forum where women and men could address their fears – and dreams – surrounding technology, how technology could be comfortably introduced into their lives, what innovations/changes they would bring to existing ICTs, and how technology could be used to mediate elements of their lives. The retreats provided participants with introductory technological information and Internet experience, as well as the opportunity to discuss their own experiences with computers and technology with members of the same sex.

Based on the theoretical materials pertaining to the gendered dimensions of technology, our initial hypothesis was that men and women would approach and observe technology differently. The purpose of the retreats was to address the cultural differences between men and women and their different approaches to technology. In determining the comfort level, expectations and perceptions of the value of technology, the project had as its main goal the determination of targeted measures to improve, enrich and strengthen ICT training programmes and to contribute to public policy via qualitative data.

For the Fredericton retreat, a survey was constructed by the research team asking the respondent to provide personal information, such as age group, education attained, structure of the family household and language. Additional questions on technological ability were also provided, detailing one's comfort levels using computers as well as the Internet, and the applications most commonly used by the participants. The full day retreat on technology was hosted by Black and White Communications at the Smythe Street Community College in Fredericton, New Brunswick.

The two groups were segregated by sex and each had its own facilitator of the same sex. There were 12 participants in each segregated group, chosen by the co-ordinators on the basis of cross-representation of class, age, ability, education, household structure and technological experience. Each group was given the opportunity to discuss their feelings about computers in their lives and perceived barriers to their access online. Each group was also asked to design an ideal computer system and to develop an advertising slogan for the system. Two research assistants, one female and one male, were hired for participant observation and workshop recording of each of the segregated groups. Two male videographers were also present to video the activities of the separate groups and digitally photograph the participants at each session. This provided the research team with both qualitative and quantitative data for cross analysis and comparison.

UNIFEM's regional office for eastern Africa collaborated with Black and White Communications for the Nairobi retreat. Prior to implementing the retreat, UNIFEM sought partnership with the World Bank (WB), United Nations Information Centre (UNIC), Intermediate Technology Development Group (ITDG) and Africa Online. Representatives of these groups constituted a steering committee that co-ordinated the implementation of the project. The retreat brought together various nationalities living in Nairobi, including Kenyans and people from neighbouring communities. Twenty-four different grassroots organizations, government institutions and church groups were contacted to nominate a participant. Before the retreat, interviews were conducted with all participants to obtain basic knowledge about their computer experience, cultural background and area of work. Overall 20 participants (11 men and nine women) participated in the interviews and retreat. As a further component of the Kenyan retreat, a videographer was present in order to document the process and support the reporting and follow-up initiatives. The retreat was held at the UN compound at Girgiri where access to conference rooms and a computer facility was facilitated by UNIC. The agenda for the retreat was designed to facilitate qualitative discussions as well as to give some learning inputs.

The Fredericton retreat

Barriers to access

Overall the research findings indicate several common barriers to access and participation for women and men. Psychological comfort was indicated as problematic for both women and men. Anxiety and fear were described as the feelings towards an increased use of computers in the respondent's everyday lives. One of the access barriers also cited was the economic cost of computers – as one respondent stated: 'people just can't afford them'. Another impediment was the constant need to upgrade computers: 'a level of difference separates those who can keep up and those who can't. If a person can't keep up, they become obsolete'. Respondents were concerned that this barrier could create a profound class difference in users. Within both groups, the use of computers and participating online was primarily the activity of men and children in the home. Computers were viewed by women and men as having both positive and negative roles relating to social relationships. Three areas of concern pertaining to computers were security and privacy, the appropriateness of technology in everyday life, and age. Women and men overlapped in some areas of concerns and had different concerns in other areas.

Psychological comfort

Similar topics and concerns were raised within the groups. Computers, and technology at a more general level, seem to exist in an uneasy and ambiguous space for most participants as they can simultaneously ease as well as erode human social relations. Computers are perceived as quick and efficient yet also capable of invoking anxiety and fear. While the range of participants in the workshop were broad in scope, ranging from non-users to heavily involved users of the technology, consensus was attained regarding the need for computers to be improved and made more accessible to all members of society. Where the groups diverged was in the meaning, emphasis and attention given to these shared concerns. The same issues were raised and put on the table but women and men allocated different value to these issues.

For women and men alike, computers exist in an uneasy societal space. Computers are socially constructed as being more efficient and quick at providing information, a benefit to our society and a fundamental feature of the new technological landscape. Many of the participants initially used such terms as 'convenient', 'interesting', 'stimulating' and 'amazing', suggesting they too are part of the social world that has been socialized into accepting computers as something new and thus also positive and beneficial. Both groups suggested common elements to the positive uses of computers in society such as for communication, better education, as a resource and a tool for gathering information, for increasing productivity and for entertainment value.

However, computers are also anxiety-inducing. Computers are scary because they are new and still unknown. For women, one might make a mistake and break the machine. This first dimension to fear pertained to self-blame – that, as a result of being unknowledgeable, the women might hurt or destroy the technology. Men seemed less concerned with fear over damage and more concerned about learning to adapt to be marketable. This was the second perceived dimension to fear as a category. Computers were felt to be taking away jobs from people and the reliance on technological computer skills in the workplace created anxiety for those who identified as being new to computers. Having these skills was seen positively as increasing employability, but the constant upgrades and new programs were seen as impossible to keep up with. A third dimension to fear surrounding computers had to do with fear for others. Women showed a higher degree of concern for the content of the Internet and the exposure of children to sensitive or explicit material and were afraid of what computers would bring into the home for their family. This might be explained by the sample selection of women and men – all the men were childless and half the women lived with children, thus making them more sensitive to issues of safety in the home. In all three dimensions, the common theme was that fear and anxiety were connected to a lack of personal control over the impact computers have on our lives. While other technologies, such as television, can be regulated by the user, computers have been introduced and accepted into our social climate without any sense of control over the process.

Economic access

Women and men both realized that the potential consumer is fundamentally limited by financial access, and that the cost of computers can be a barrier. Having access to computers requires money to buy or rent the technology. While the men tried to design a computer to appeal to those with access to money, the women were more focused on designing features that would make the technology less expensive to maintain and upgrade. The women were concerned with the overall cost of buying a computer and were frustrated by the pressure to have top quality computer systems that were unaffordable. In addition, the societal pressure to have top quality means that the consumer constantly needs to upgrade hardware or purchase new software products. This was seen by the women as a never-ending drain on family finances.

By contrast, the men also felt finance was a barrier to computers, but were more concerned that this made it more difficult to become skilled and limited their marketability for work. Continuous upgrades and planned obsolescence of computers affect work opportunities, as the example of one respondent's father who lost his job to a more computer-knowledgeable worker illustrates. One must have the money to learn about computers initially as well as keep up with the constant cycle of improvements and additions to programs, software and design.

Although women identified finances as contributing to a further division between those with information and those without, men connected finances with limited access in different ways. For women, the tension involved the way that money was needed to always upgrade computers when computers are already available and functional. Having to upgrade continuously was a source of frustration for women. The cycle of constant upgrades and advances was also a source of frustration for men, but more attention was focused on how publicly available computers, like those in libraries or community access centres, were not accessible since they were typically not up to current market standards. Having no access to top computer systems was seen as a barrier to participation and advancement of marketable computer skills. In both cases, the cycle of upgrades was seen as inevitable and continuous, and while frustration was felt at this cycle, it was also framed as being related to growth, change and advancement.

Social relationships

Social relationships with others can be profoundly affected by computers, although again, there is ambiguity over whether computers ease or erode relationships. In the women and men's groups, arguments and feelings for both points of view were put forward. Computers do not facilitate or damage relations but rather contain both features depending on the user and the context. Again it was the emphasis on which issues were of greater importance that seemed to differ between the groups, and not the issues themselves. Men first defined computers as being positive for communication where they could speed up the exchange of information. It was also felt that computers mediated communication and that it was less threatening and scary when one was not face to face with someone. Women also saw the potential for computers to ease social relations, but constructed this in a different manner. They felt computers could support communication where they could use them to reach distant family and friends. Women were quick to note that computers could act as a bond of similar interest between people.

However, the greatest fear for women was that the computer would hinder social relationships, especially with the family. More time using a computer was seen as less time committed to the family. Heavy users of technology were discussed by the groups in negatively coded language, such as 'too focused' or 'addicted'. This indicated a degree of discomfort with computers in terms of taking time away from other aspects of life. Men also defined addiction, where people could spend too much time online, as a possible negative consequence. For men, the more negative consequence of computer-based communication was the lack of physical body language cues that also communicated meaning.

Issues of concern

There are three major identifiable areas of concern regarding computers in everyday social life. The first dimension pertains to privacy and security of personal information, where certain aspects of computers were seen to facilitate an invasion of privacy and personal space. One of the female respondents indicated that the ease of communication by computer also allowed strangers to communicate easily with you. For instance, one of the respondents had received a graphic photograph of slain people via email from a stranger in a chat room. This experience terrified her and ruined her appreciation of communicating in chat rooms.

While men were also concerned with security and privacy issues, this was manifested in a different manner. The men expressed concern over who was the overall organizing body on the Internet. But while the women wanted to have this information to satisfy their need for accountability regarding privacy violations, the men framed their concern in terms of control and ownership. The men seemed more concerned over who had power on the Internet, and had negatively assumed they had to conform to established rules to which they could not contribute. Both women and men seemed surprised to discover that there was no unifying and governing body that regulated the structure and content of the Internet.

The second major issue related to the appropriateness of computer technology in the social realm. The men and the women in the separate sessions showed similar values and beliefs surrounding the appropriateness of computers in certain aspects of their social lives. Both groups felt that computers were not appropriate in many social circumstances. Each group tried to find ways to change the way computers are built as well as how to make computers more mobile and marketable. The women perceived that there were certain social situations, where computers were seen as currently acceptable, that posed problems for them as mothers, i.e., issues of public versus private space. In particular, women were more wary of having computers in the home relegated to private areas, such as the bedroom, and felt more comfortable with the idea of having computers in public shared spaces, such as the living or family room. This meant families would have more control over what their children were accessing over the Internet. Unlike television which has restricted times for viewing, potential sensitive and/or offensive material is available online 24 hours a day. Women were more concerned than men with the availability of inappropriate material on the Internet. Content issues of offensive and/or pornographic material were simply not raised by the men's group. The men seemed more focused on ways that computers could be introduced to all aspects of society with no concern as to the repercussions, feasibility or necessity of having technology available.

While women raised security and the ease of accessing inappropriate materials online (pornography and drug literature) as issues of concern, men discussed age as a real barrier to their participation. This third area of concern was only raised by the men. As one respondent commented, the 'younger pull the older', and as services and systems become increasingly computerized, the need to redefine and augment skill sets becomes more imperative for older men in the workplace in order to compete. Knowing and understanding computers was viewed as the domain of younger men, and older men felt threatened at possibly losing out in the job market owing to their age and lack of technological knowledge.

These common threads of concern illustrate how computers at present are still not as personally accessible as would be suggested by contemporary social discourse. Economic barriers, such as finances, can affect one's ability to be able to use and to be comfortable with computers. But as the findings from both groups indicate, in order to participate in the new technological climate, one must also have a certain degree of comfort and technological knowledge. As the differences between the groups indicate, women and men have the same concepts and issues regarding computers but the emphasis varies in the differences in concern. For instance, one main question raised is whether women have less time to use ICTs because of their traditional gender roles and duties in the household.

The Nairobi retreat

Barriers to access

As in the Fredericton retreat, women and men in the Nairobi retreat indicated several similar barriers pertaining to ease of access and participation with computers. Issues relating to psychological comfort in experiencing computers, economic factors and social relationships were shared concerns with the Canadian group. However, barriers to computer access relating to language, basic availability of telecommunications in Africa, relationships between the north and south, and educational possibilities were unique to the Nairobi retreat. Both women and men in Nairobi questioned the wisdom and feasibility of investing in Internet technology when, in many cases, communities in Africa do not even have access to basic telephone services. Both men and women articulated concerns centred on who are the primary beneficiaries of technology transfer, and whether or not technology transfer benefits the foreign manufacturers, bankers and foreign communication media rather than rural and urban communities in Africa.

Psychological comfort

Most respondents felt positive towards the Internet. Their perception was that access to the Internet (and especially email) would facilitate their work. Computers in the workplace were only being utilized for basic tasks, which could be expanded: 'The computers are not used for anything other than typing, storing information and retrieving it. [They are used for] Internal communication . . . but not used for outside communication.' One respondent representing an NGO stated that the Internet should be introduced as a marketing tool in Kenya: 'Women in Kenya have so many resources they could market their soap stones, etc.' The Internet was also seen as being positive in terms of access to new information: 'If we had Internet access it would make a difference both internally and externally. We would become better informed.' The Internet was felt to bring the world to Africa, giving Africans the opportunity 'to see what is happening in other parts of the world'.

While some felt comfortable towards the technology, others felt alienated. One respondent suggested that her resistance and discomfiture towards computers stemmed from her Swahili background. The newness of computers and the Internet meant, to many respondents, that it was too early to tell the impact of computers on their lives: 'It is not possible to know whether the Internet will turn out for the good or for the bad because so little is known about it yet.'

Economic access

Given that the economic situation in Kenya is getting worse, priorities for getting online are simply not as important as maintaining a basic livelihood. Accessing the Internet is far too expensive. Because of the high cost of telecommunications equipment, few Africans can afford such ICT devices as mobile phones or the Internet. All the respondents expressed a need for cost reduction on ICTs. Concern was raised over the cost of computer technology leading to an increase in the gap between the rich and the poor. Many male respondents questioned the value and relevance of ICTs for all people and especially for poor people who struggle to meet their basic needs: 'I have little use for Internet resources. Look at people in the slums – they have very little use for it!'

There was some disagreement as to whether or not the government should provide support for allowing women to get online: 'The problem with the government funding facilities is not because of lack of abilities but because of corruption. Women with access get very selfish and lock up other women.' Most of the women respondents mentioned that access depends on economic and social status, and that advantaged women should help the not-so-advantaged: 'Some women are underprivileged. Our challenge is to make sure that she benefits. She is affected by global politics.'

Social relationships

Female respondents positively stressed that the Internet could be used as a useful tool for creating awareness about women's issues and gender equality. 'Right now it is the men's story . . . we are reading it. It is a challenge for the African woman to have her story told. We should use the Internet to tell our stories.' These respondents also mentioned that the Internet can create a forum for debate and communication: 'The Internet brings an opener where our girls can discuss the issues globally.' One of the statements made by a female respondent was illustrative of the computer's utility as a lifelong companion: 'It feels like the lap-top is a co-wife!'

By contrast, the male respondents expressed fears and worry about the content of material on the Internet: 'You can get anything. So if anybody is thinking of committing a crime he can get anything. The bottom line is the influence. Another thing is that there are photographs of all actions.' Other male respondents were more positive but still worried about inappropriate information and use by children: 'In the case of children, computers shouldn't be thought of as [a] toy for games. This is unfortunately how it is. Children should have access, but shouldn't use it for games or pornography.'

With respect to perceptions of gender differences in the use and participation of ICTs, many respondents pointed out that many more women then men are exposed to ICTs through their employment as clerical workers. However, it was also noted that the actual managers and owners of the technology often are, or are perceived to be, male. It is also significant that these men don't carry the technology home to their wife and kids. It was seen as a problem that most computers are placed in offices. One of the men made a link to women's household duties: 'A woman is disadvantaged by the role she plays in the home. She can only access computers in her workplace. She is too busy outside her work. This is even more significant in rural areas.'

Although the male respondents recognized that existing economic and social structures are discriminatory to women, they also recognized that they must assist women to have access and use of the Internet: 'We must include women in regard to access to the Internet. The Internet is a powerful weapon. You can work on it yourself . . . it is a powerful tool for development.' Gender insensitivity was also an issue raised by the female respondents. While acknowledging that gender insensitivity can be imposed upon women by women, it was recognized that it is men who most need sensitization.

Language

Lack of education and thus little or no knowledge of the English language is a major deterrent for getting Kenyan women online. Many illiterate women only speak their own tribal language.

Basic telecommunications access

One of the main barriers to access to the Internet is access to basic telecommunications facilities. All the male respondents expressed frustration with the basic telecommunications system: 'We need to improve the reliability, availability and costing of national infrastructure, particularly with respect to the telephones.' Respondents indicated that support mechanisms should be facilitated by political support. In addition, the costs of the basic telephone service should be decreased. Male respondents felt that because Kenya's telephone company has a monopoly on telecommunication networks, liberalization could help decrease the charges, but the concern is that 'privatization of national ICT utilities may lead to foreign ownership'.

Rural and urban access to ICTs varies but the predominant concentration of ICTs is within urban environs. All the female respondents agreed that there was a difference between rural and urban access, given that many rural communities do not even have a basic phone connection. Many of the male respondents agreed that ICTs could be very useful for the rural population: 'Information is poor. Look at the average man in a village . . . what kind of information can he get? . . . only what is available. If people from far provinces would be connected they would be able to get their newspaper like everybody else and not have to wait one week for the daily newspaper.'

The north/south divide

Another barrier to use and participation is the perception that the technology is developed and designed in the north for export to the south. Some female respondents emphasized the need for more African influence on technology: 'It is necessary to Swahilitize computer programs.

Swahili increases the feelings of Nationalism.' The male respondents were equally concerned that the design, development and diffusion of ICTs was led by the north without adequate involvement of African countries. Many respondents felt that Africa's lack of influence was a serious problem that could lead to increased inequalities between the north and the south: 'Loss of local or tailored content will lead to alienation and disempowerment.' Respondents were concerned that access to and participation with ICTs is important for attaining national advantage. Many respondents recognized that information is important for development: 'Whoever has the technology has the power. Technology/ information is the same.' Other respondents expressed sadness at the technological imperative. As one male respondent said: 'It is inevitable . . . then it is very hard to put up conditions. We have decided we need it, so what do we do? We cannot block it out. You know the phones are there. I feel very sad.'

Education

Both groups were in agreement that education is the way to make computer technology accessible. Education and awareness campaigns of the advantages of the Internet were felt by the female respondents to be a good way to get more women (particularly entrepreneurial women) and young girls online. 'Advocacy on Internet is important to change the attitude of girls. Girls are not dropouts. It is lack of facilities that favour boys. We need to change the way of thinking and people's attitudes. If girls are educated then ours will be the last generation of disadvantaged women.' Male respondents also mentioned that in order for communication technologies to become relevant for people, more education is needed before introducing ICTs. Development of a user's guide was suggested by the men as a way to control abuse of new technologies.

Comparisons between the Fredericton and Nairobi retreats

Respondents from both international groups expressed frustration at their lack of knowledge concerning both technical, social and policy developments surrounding ICTs. Given both the swiftly changing nature of technological development and the increased move towards a knowledge-based economy/society, it is surprising that not much consultation has been done by either industry or governments on the needs, desires and aspirations of ordinary men and women in both developed and developing countries. One of the benefits of the Fredericton and Nairobi retreats has been a fostering of communication concerning the relationships between men, women and ICTs. The concerns surrounding economic growth, human development, and aiding in social cohesion are crucial elements that need to be looked at at the start of this millennium.

There were some striking contrasts with respect to perceived use, benefits and the value structure of ICTs between the Fredericton and the Nairobi groups. Given that developed countries such as Canada are now more oriented towards developing various 'information highways' through targeted government and private-sector funding, and that the rhetoric of the 'knowledge-based economy/society' is well entrenched in most OECD countries, it is not surprising that the men and women in the Fredericton retreat had a certain presumption towards ICTs. For both men and women, the computerization of their workplaces, educational institutions and domestic spaces for both work and leisure activities will be an inevitability. The Nairobi respondents, however, were more circumspect about the computerization of their society, particularly given their socio-economic status and their questioning of the inherent value of ICTs in their everyday lives. As well, the continued dominance of the Internet by the English language (Fishman 1998–9) was felt to be an obstacle to overcome in order to encourage community-wide participation. The Nairobi women also perceived that access to ICTs was an opportunity to enhance their socio-economic position within society and to promote both their entrepreneurial activities and their indigenous knowledge. Indeed, women activists and NGOs have found that utilizing ICTs enhances their communication power (Mansell and Wehn 1998: 249–52). However, ongoing concerns persist surrounding access barriers, including the transformation of work and the need to enhance, rather than detract from indigenous knowledge (Shade 1997).

Unlike the Fredericton groups, the Nairobi groups seem to have reached more consensus on issues that impact on their country. In particular, both female and male groups were very concerned about the increasing division between the north and the south in terms of access to telecommunications infrastructure.

Conclusion

The final project report of 'lives and livelihoods' recommended that further retreats be established nationally across Canada to determine access to and participation of ICTs. The research model will include men and women from a variety of demographics, cultures and ability levels. Its primary objectives would be the creation of strategic partnerships to support and disseminate project outcomes, the identification of the cultural differences between men and women and their approaches to and acceptance of technology, the determination of the comfort level, expectations and perceptions of the value of technology to men and women and the development of targeted measures to improve, enrich and strengthen training programmes.

Several proposed methodologies to accomplish these goals have been enumerated, including the creation of a guidebook to implement technology training programs for the marginalized, taken directly from the participants' recommendations, and the provision of a continuing forum for public consultation. Other suggested methodologies include developing future scenarios and social impact statements.

Future scenarios, or scenario planning, is a methodology that was utilized by Pamela McCorduck and Nancy Ramsay (1997). They used future scenarios to explore four different alternatives for the future of women. Within each scenario, current events, demographics and social trends were coupled with future technological promises. According to McCorduck and Ramsay, scenarios begin with examining the work of census takers and demographics and then examining the trends (short- to long-term) with the scenarist, considering which trends might persist and which might be anomalies. Future scenarios was also used by IDRC and the United Nations Commission on Science and Technology for Development in their recent publication (Howkins and Valantin 1997).

Social impact statements (SIS) can be used to describe ICT systems and their benefits, disadvantages and barriers for use and also to acknowledge concerns and address fundamental principles. SIS are a form of public participation, specifically related to design issues. In particular, SISs describe the system and its benefits through an identification of goals, stakeholders and benefits. They address concerns and potential barriers such as changes in employment, security and privacy issues, accountability and misuse, biases, individual versus societal benefits, access and democratic principles and outline a development process for specific projects regarding design, evaluation and implementation (Shneiderman and Rose, 1997).

Based on the information garnered from the Fredericton and Nairobi retreats, it is clear that several recommendations for future research should be considered in the realm of access to the technological and social infrastructures (economic barriers and domestic versus workplace issues), employment and workplace issues, content issues (creation, cultural sovereignty and indigenous knowledge) and design issues (user-centred designs and participatory design).

References

Balka, E. (1996) 'Women and computer networking in six countries', *Journal of International Communication*, 3 (1): 66–84.

Ebo, B. (ed.) (1998) *Cyberghetto or Cybertopia: Race, Class, and Gender on the Internet*, Westport, CT: Praeger.

Eisenstein, Z. (1998) *Global Obscenities: Patriarchy, Capitalism, and the Lure of Cyberfantasy*, New York: New York University Press.

Fishman, J. A. (1998–9) 'The new linguistic order', *Foreign Policy*, 113: 26–40.

Gilbert, L. and C. Kile (1996) *Surfer Grrrls: Look Ethel! An Internet Guide for Us!*, Seattle, WA: Seal Press.

Harcourt, W. (ed.) (1999) *Women@Internet: Creating New Cultures in Cyberspace*, London and New York: Zed Books.

Hawthorne, S. and Klein, R. (1999) *Cyberfeminism: Connectivity, Critique and Creativity*, Melbourne: Spinifex Press.

Henwood, F. (1993) 'Establishing gender perspectives on information technology: problems, issues, and opportunities' in E. Green, J. Owen and D. Pain (eds) *Gendered by Design: Information Technology and Office Systems*, London: Taylor and Francis.

Herring, S. C. (1996) 'Gender and democracy in computer-mediated communication', *Electronic Journal of Communication*, 3 (2).

Howkins, J. and Valantin, R. (1997) *Development and the Information Age: Four Global Scenarios for the Future of Information and Communication Technology*, Ottawa: International Development Research Centre. Available online: http://www.idrc.ca/books/835/index.html

IDRC Gender and Information Working Group (1995) 'Information as a transformative tool' in *Missing Links: Gender Equity in Science and Technology for Development*, Gender Working Group, United Nations Commission on Science and Technology for Development, Ottawa: International Development Research Centre.

Independent Committee on Women and Global Knowledge (1997) 'The canon on gender partnerships and ICT development', presented at the Global Knowledge 1997 Conference, June 22–25, Toronto, ON. Available online: http://www.postindustrial.com/morewomen

Loader, B. D. (ed.) (1998) *Cyberspace Divide: Equality, Agency and Policy in the Information Society*, London and New York: Routledge.

Mansell, R. and Wehn, U. (1998) *Knowledge Societies: Information Technology for Sustainable Development*, Oxford: Oxford University Press.

McChesney, R. (1999) *Rich Media, Poor Democracy: Communication Politics in Dubious Times*, Urbana: University of Illinois Press.

McCorduck, P. and Ramsay, N. (1997) *The Futures of Women: Scenarios for the 21st Century*, New York: Warner Books.

Millar, M. S. (1998) *Cracking the Gender Code: Who Rules the Wired World?*, Toronto: Second Story Press.

Plant, S. (1997) *Zeros + Ones: Digital Women + the New Technoculture*, New York: Doubleday.

Schiller, D. (1999) *Digital Capitalism: Networking the Global Market System*, Cambridge, MA: MIT Press.

Shade, L. R. (1997) 'Post-Beijing and beyond: gendered perspectives on access' in R. Lander and A. Adam (eds) *Women in Computing*, Exeter: Intellect Books.

Shneiderman, B. and Rose, A. (1997) 'Social impact statements: engaging public participation in information technology design' in B. Friedman (ed.) *Human Values and the Design of Computer Technology*, Stanford, CA: CSLI Publications/Cambridge University Press.

Spender, D. (1996) *Nattering on the Net: Women, Power and Cyberspace*, Toronto, ON: Garamond Press.

Wakeford, N. (1999) 'Gender and the landscapes of computing in an Internet café' in M. Crang, P. Crang and J. May (eds) *Virtual Geographies: Bodies, Space and Relations*, New York and London: Routledge.

Chapter 4

Becoming a technologist

Days in a girl's life

Linda Stepulevage

Abstract

Studies of the gender relations of information and communications technologies (ICTs) seldom deal with these relations as experienced in early childhood, except as located in schooling. The construction of identity in relation to technology is negotiated from an early age. In this chapter a technological strand is identified in childhood using 'experience stories', writing about specific situations or events on a specific theme, with the focus of analysis being on the theme, rather than on the individual. In reflecting on this technological strand of childhood the chapter tries to make sense of how everyday experiences serve as sites for constituting our relations with ICTs, and more personally, how they constitute social relations for a young, white, working-class girl. This chapter also hopes to make visible technological acts that are essentialized and/or made invisible in later years.

This chapter draws on a multi-layer definition of technology and uses conceptions of locally situated knowledge and practices to explore how a young girl might develop a familiarity with technology as part of everyday living. Class and race relations as well as gender relations are significant in early conceptions of 'knowing and doing' and in later awareness of constructions of technology and technological identities and subjectivities. This chapter therefore attempts to identify these relations within the experience stories.

By applying a concept of technology that encompasses the knowledge, skills and practices in the everyday life of a young girl, I hope to contribute to a richer understanding of the gender, class and race relations implicit in what is recognized as technological knowledge and to contribute to a more inclusive understanding of the social relations of ICTs.

Remembrance of things past: the cleaning of paint brushes

In the late summer of 1996, I hired a painter to paper and paint my high front room ceiling. As he was washing out his rollers, he said, 'This is the job I hate most.' I continued the conversation with him, saying that my uncle was a house painter and when I was a child I had spent many summer days observing and listening to him as he worked. I told him that I had learned about how important the quality and care of brushes was and wondered whether it was the same with rollers. Later, when I thought about why I felt the need to expand on this process, I realized that I consider the cleaning of painting tools as a significant part of the act of painting. I saw painting as a technology; I possessed knowledge about paints, techniques, types of brushes and their care and I took a perspective grounded in technological skills and knowledge. I realized the commonality between me and the painter and how my reaction was rooted in my subjectivity as a technologist.

Introduction

In reflecting on the association made between early childhood experiences and painting, I identified the connection between technology as a concept and the daily-lived experience of technology in a working-class childhood. Childhood experiences were linked with an immersion in technology, especially how technological artefacts and skills in using them were a part of my daily life outside school. This chapter explores my experiences of technology as lived in childhood and therefore is a reconstruction by the adult me, working in academia and concerned with gender–technology relations. I am trying to make sense of how I, as a young, white, working-class girl, began becoming a technologist. In reflecting on this construction of my own past experiences, I hope to contribute to an understanding of how gender, class and race relations might constitute current and possible future social relations of ICTs in our daily lives.

Class is especially significant in this analysis of my experience stories. There is a tendency to demonstrate simply the negative effects of technological development for the majority working-class population, rather than the diverse aspects of human engagement with technology in our daily lives (Yoon 1996: 176). Hakken and Andrews (1993), in their study of technology and working people in Sheffield, UK, raised an important question regarding class–technology relations. How do people think about themselves in relation to technology – as agents, acting on or with technology, or as acted upon? They found in their study that ICTs are 'important new terrain over which various social groups are struggling to accomplish their basic goals' (p. 231), a negotiation rather than a simple binary of actor and acted upon. With regard to gender and class relations, Walkerdine (1996) notes constructions of an acted upon working-class in some feminist approaches to class and gender. She argues that we need to move away from notions of working-class femininity that construct it as more conservative, stereotyped and passive, and resistant to feminist change, and begin exploring a diverse set of questions regarding working-class subjectivity in relation to assumptions about education, career, consumption, etc. (p. 357). As Walkerdine argues, we need to look at specificities of class such as the relation between historical context and power, knowledge, desire and survival (p. 358). By situating technology within specific accounts of a working-class girl's childhood I hope to present some of these diverse aspects.

This exploration of the construction of a technologist takes the form of an autobiographical narrative. The construction of identity in relation to technology is negotiated from an early age, yet these experiences have seldom been explored outside formal school settings. I would like to explore the positioning of women as technologists using what Widerberg (1998: 196) calls 'experience stories', i.e., writing about specific situations or events on a specific theme, with the focus of analysis being on the theme, rather than on the individual. In this case the theme is the interrelationship of technology and daily life in childhood. These experience stories are used within the tradition of the large body of feminist work in this form which explores the intersection of social structure and personal agency rather than focusing on individual experience (Stanley 1992; Swindells 1995). The 'small, concrete details' of a person's life can enable the spinning out of lines of inquiry into larger-scale social structures and processes (Glenn 1997). Glenn names some of these structures and processes as 'the labour market, technological change, and the geographic and social movements of populations' (p. 82). Using experience stories that reconstruct the small concrete details from my early life, the structures and processes I explore are those of the labour market, education, i.e., both formal and informal learning, and the discursive practices of everyday life. Smith (1998) cites a method used by Matsuda that I have found useful in understanding the interactions of the relations of gender, class and race in these structures and processes. Matsuda calls it 'ask the other question . . . When

I see something that looks racist, I ask, "Where is the patriarchy in this?" When I see something that looks homophobic, I ask, "Where are the class interests in this?" ' (Smith 1998: 139).

The use of artefacts like paintbrushes is one aspect of technology touched upon here, but engagement with technology as situated knowledges and practices is the focus of this exploration. These aspects of technology are especially important in identifying and understanding our relations with ICTs in their various forms. In the following sections a brief description of the concept of technology that informs these experience stories is provided, then a discussion of how approaches and concepts drawn from feminist work on systems development provides a framework within which to consider the stories. Next in sequence are the experience stories themselves; they are followed by an analysis of gender, race and class intersections that can be seen in the experiences and practices that constituted my developing technological identity. The identity 'black' is used to represent African-American people in the stories, an identity that came into use during the time period.

Technology as a concept

The concept of technology underlying my experience stories encompasses various layers of meaning: technology as a form of knowledge, as human activities and practices, and as physical objects or artefacts (Wajcman 1991: 15). In Lerman's study of the reciprocal shaping of technological knowledge and social structure in mid-nineteenth century Philadelphia, the city in which my experience stories are grounded, she asserts that the study of technological knowledge should place 'people making and doing things – from cooking to carpentry' at the centre of our focus' (1997: 31). Lerman situates her study within a particular landscape, another important layer of meaning for technology. It is technology as people making and doing things within local settings that is the focus of my experience stories.

Fourez's definition of technological literacy (1997) also helps make sense of the social relations of technology found in my stories. His definition is concerned with the empowerment of the individual within the political, economic and cultural context of the present world. He defines a person as scientifically and technologically literate when their knowledge enables them to have autonomy, rooted in the humanistic goal of each individual realizing their potential, to have a capacity to communicate about technology, for example, to be able to explain the problem you're having with an office software application, and to have a capacity to cope with specific situations and negotiate over outcomes (pp. 904–6).

An early childhood learning experience clearly demonstrates the relationship between autonomy and technological knowledge and skills. A combination of spatial awareness, hand and finger dexterity, understanding of directions and sheer determination to learn so that I could dress myself completely on my own are the technical and social aspects of the first technological skill I remember achieving: tying my shoelaces. This seemingly straightforward process was constituted as a complex social relation. I remember my mother teaching me first. Her method was to shape one lace in a loop and encircle it with the other; I found it very difficult and was having problems with it. My father taught me a method he presented as being easier; it was to form two loops and tie them together. I eventually learned both and decided to use my mother's method; I remember being very pleased with myself at mastering the complexity of it. I also remember learning why my father considered his method easier. He was partially ambidexterous, having been forced to become right-handed at school.

Valuing the invisible: insights from systems development research

In focusing on technology from a perspective which brings skills and knowledge to the fore and in which technology is an intrinsic part of any learning process, I made use of the concept of articulation work, 'work that gets things back "on track" in the face of the unexpected . . .' (Star 1991: 84). This concept is relevant to my exploration of technology in that it highlights the skills and knowledge developed and practised in situations where they are usually unrecognized and unacknowledged. Suchman (1994) presents a powerful account of design work with information workers which demonstrates the concept of articulation with relation to gender. In a law firm, a senior attorney characterized the type of coding of legal documents that information workers were responsible for as 'ideally, you hire chimpanzees to type in From, To, Date. And then, ideally, you then have lawyers go through it again and read each document, with their brain turned on' (p. 14). She explored the complexity of the workers' practices and the situated and shared knowledge and decision-making that was required and, by implication, the construction of knowledge about legal practices that these workers developed. As Webster (1996) points out, since the position of women office workers in jobs classified as low status, low paid and low skilled differed from researchers and/or feminist systems developers who wished to work with them, it cannot be assumed that professionals' understanding of skills and knowledge and situated work practices coincide with those of the office workers. In the legal office example, however, researchers' collaboration with the workers was effective in determining appropriate technological artefacts to support situated work practices.

The concept of articulation work acts as a frame within which we can redefine the 'keeping things going' of daily life as facets of technological practice. Suchman and other researchers (for example, Clement 1991; Green et al. 1993; Holtgrewe 1994; Balka 1997; Ramsay et al. 1997) argue that much of the work women do is invisible to others. In reframing this 'invisible' work as articulation work, there is an acknowledgement of the judgement, practical reasoning, knowledge and skillfulness that such work requires (Suchman 1994). Use of the concept articulation work highlights the idea that nothing is as simple as it seems. A 'simple view' is mediated through gender, class and race relations that constitute what is considered to be technology. With its commitment to acknowledging the invisible in workers' situated activities, articulation work is directly relevant to my experiences of learning as a working-class child.

The learning experiences of my everyday life were usually invisible in formal school settings yet these experiences, on reflection, were more significant in constituting my technological identity. By applying a perspective that recognizes shared knowledge, situated activity and local agency, I began to see how rich my childhood was in relation to learning about technologies and becoming a technologist. The knowledge I acquired grew out of shared activities: the performing of tasks, playing, listening, talking, watching and being situated in a neighbourhood where the sights, smells and sounds of large-scale industrial production were physical backdrops to my life among people who seemed to be constantly 'doing'.

Learning by doing

Education is an important aspect of everyday life as a child. Research by Jarvis and Rennie (1996) concludes that technology as taught in English schools within the National Curriculum is mainly 'design and make' or model-making (p. 48). They note it has a tendency to parallel industrial processes and to offer no wider context nor address technological knowledge and application of concepts (p. 50). This contemporary conception of 'learning by doing' might be seen to reconstitute vocational training for what are considered to be working-class jobs.

As the experience stories I use are about learning to become a technologist through experiences of everyday life, this requires conceptualizations of both learning and technology outside the formal structures of education. Saljo (1999) makes the point that technology tends to be disregarded in dominant perspectives of learning that see knowledge as purely mental or as material and independent of human activities. He presents a socio-cultural understanding of human learning that takes both thinking and acting into account (p. 149). In taking this perspective, we can reclaim the doing and thinking implicit in everyday activities, such as writing a note with pen and paper, as technologies.

There is a strand of systems development that has applied a related concept, that of design by doing. Design by doing aims to enrich understanding and gain knowledge of the situated practices of workers' jobs (Ehn 1993). It is seen to enable an articulation of 'tacit' knowledge, the 'knowing how' knowledge required to get a job done (Adam 1998). In that sense, it is related to the concept of articulation work. Design by doing has been identified as a site of learning as well. It has been shown to deepen the understanding of systems designers not familiar with certain work practices. It also provides a framework in which working-class people's knowledge and skills can be recognized and acknowledged. From a working-class perspective, 'doing' needs to be reclaimed as a significant and enriching learning aspect of a working-class education that takes place outside formal schooling.

Some of the practices and experiences we learn from and continue doing are constituted as technological skills and knowledge; others are not. In this chapter I attempt to identify the roots of skills and knowledge that as an adult I can recognize as technological but that have been constituted through relations of gender, class and race that twist and turn them into different forms, in different situations, at different times. It is an extension of other feminist work which explores the reciprocal relations of gender and technology but, in this instance, I wish to look at how, in childhood, we might develop a firm grounding in technological competence in spite of the asymmetrical gendered relations identified by so many researchers (examples include Cockburn and Ormrod 1993; Aune 1996; Ramsay et al. 1997). A firm grounding, of course, does not imply that technological skills and knowledge will remain firmly grounded in all situations at all times but what I hope to uncover is conceptions of technological skills and knowledge that are usually unnamed in discussions of technology. Just as in systems design, the practices and knowledge of the dominant actors name the technologies and skills, so too in childhood, research demonstrates that while girls may be successful in gaining technological skills and knowledge, technology is perceived as in the boys' domain (Elkjaer 1992; Rasmussen 1997; Volman 1997; Dixon 1998). Articulation work and design by doing demonstrate that work situations are rich sources of learning, experimenting, adjusting, interpreting, abstracting and making technology. These experience stories demonstrate that technological practices are also part of the social relations of everyday living in many other locations.

The roots of my experience stories

My parents were born in a coal mining region in north-eastern Pennsylvania in 1917–18; my mother the daughter of Italian immigrants, my father the son of Lithuanian immigrants. They both left school at 14 or 15 years of age to earn money; my mother in a factory, my father, in a coal mine. My mother became a 'housewife' once she started to have children (first my sister, myself four years later, my brother nine years later) but she sometimes worked in a factory when my father was out of work. My father worked briefly at Ford in Detroit, then in various skilled factory jobs in Philadelphia. When I was about five years old he was out of work and began training as a welder. When he finished the training, that included making various metal artefacts, the process of which would be part of supper time conversation, he couldn't find a permanent job in welding. He did get a job training to become an engine lathe operator and he carried on doing this work in the same factory until his retirement. This very brief history of my parents conceals within it a high level of technological skills and knowledge which I attempt to articulate in a set of experiences stories that demonstrate how the contingencies of daily living and the need for food, shelter and clothing constitute a grounding for their development and for alternate readings of gender–technology relations, for example, men's vulnerability in relation to technology within an employment context (Brewer 1996). As approaches to the development of technological systems have shown, however, the background is not complete without providing some details of its location.

These stories are situated in the USA in the 1950s to 1960s, in times I remember as being dominated by military machinery, that of the Korean conflict, 'the cold war', and the Cuban missile crisis. They were also times, in the southern United States, of voter registration drives and challenges to segregation in buses, schools and universities. Philadelphia, a northern city with a large percentage of black people, had its own forms of segregation; my earliest experiences related to housing. The housing pattern was similar to that in Chicago in the 1950s: one of 'block busting, distinct racial and ethnic neighbourhoods, and white flight' (Weber et al. 1997: 236). White European first and second generation working-class people, mainly Roman Catholic, lived in our section of the city. Ethnic identity for Catholic people was partially assumed in early childhood via schooling. There were Irish, Italian, Polish and Ukranian parishes in our neighbourhood; we went to the Italian parish and school. My sense of being Italian deepened through living with my Italian grandmother. While the part of the city in which we lived was a white section, our immediate area was an exception. Black people lived on two streets parallel to ours and had done so even before the houses on our street were built. While I cannot remember anything ever said directly about associating with black people when I was a child, it was clear to me that we children would not play on those streets nor be friends with black girls and boys. It wasn't until I attended high school that I had social conversations with black people.

The high school I attended, a Catholic girls' school, was centrally located and enrolled students from working-class parishes throughout the city. My high school yearbook with its photographs of the 1965 graduating class of 633 students shows that 80 per cent of the students were white and 20 per cent were black. While I was in high school, a few attempts were made by black families to purchase houses and live on some of the streets in our section of the city. These were immediately and violently challenged by some white residents, constituting a subject position in which white working-class people could assume power. The situation was debated in the city newspapers but there was no enforcement of black peoples' rights to live safely in their homes. In the 1980s, black people finally began to settle in the area. My father died before our own block was integrated and my mother remained in the house on her own, on a street where she now has white, black and Hispanic people as neighbours but where 'white flight' is still practised by some.

Technology and paid work

My earliest associations with technology at work are the steel and iron slivers in my father's skin, the heavy steel-tipped work boots that needed to be resoled every month because of cuts and tears from scraps of iron and the greasy and oily clothes that he took to the laundry because my mother thought they might ruin her washing machine. When my father spoke about the technologies he worked with, he situated his experiences locally: relations with the foreman and co-workers, the influence of the weather and the relationship between materials and piece rates. A millimetre off in a cut was especially significant to particular pieces of steel because of their value; the temperature outside affected the process and materials inside. It was difficult and dirty work and we, his daughters, were supposed to, and did, want something 'better'. We were expected to marry men who had less oppressive jobs and to have children; until then we should work in a job that was less oppressive than factory work. This technology of engine lathe work was constructed by my father as masculine and as undesirable but also as highly complex and skilled work, as work involving many variables, much problem-solving and varied social relations.

During the intervals when my father was on strike or was laid off owing to a slow period at work, my mother would work at the factory around the corner from our house. The company was a manufacturer of very expensive ladies shoes that used hand-sewn lasts. She didn't have special work clothes or get splinters in her skin. She talked about the work as not being very demanding: the gluing of an inner sole into the shoe. Permanent workers did the more skilled work that involved handling of the leather and my mother, being a part-time temporary worker, performed a task reserved for the expendable female workforce.

Her status as a paid worker was reactive for reasons other than the state of the expensive shoes market, however. She only did paid work when my father was out of work as he disapproved of her being in employment. He saw it as his responsibility to earn enough money to support us all. My mother did not dispute this and when we as children asked her about it, she would say she had enough to do at home. My father supported this rationale by sometimes naming all the 'jobs' she did, including being 'the banker'. My father handed my mother his pay every week and she gave him money for his expenses which usually consisted of petrol for the car and cans of drink from the machine at the factory. She made sandwiches for his work-time meal.

The complexity of the gendering of technology is evident in these relations. While my mother saw her job as unskilled, she told us about the skilled work that other women did and she situated the skill demands of her position locally in relation to a reserve labour force. The articulation work of the home, on the other hand, was highly valued by my father and in the presence of us children, my mother was in control of her domain, for example, my father's work clothes would not dirty her washing machine, and ashtrays were emptied and washed by my father, the only smoker in the house. The asymmetry of gender–technology relations is obvious in matters of employment, but it is also relations of heterosexuality, as well as gender, that hold the wage-earner relations of technology in place.

Technology and global/local power relations

In primary school I was always at the top of the class in the arithmetic and problem-solving examinations. Mathematics was an area of interest to my father as he needed to learn and use high level mathematics in setting up jobs at work. When I was learning borrowing and carrying in arithmetic, my father presented his 'quicker and easier' alternative. He thought I should try the method of mental arithmetic that he used at work. It was a rounding up technique that worked with the left over units digits as the last step. I argued that it wasn't easier, but I remember using it in certain situations, for example, to confirm my answers during tests. My father's responses to my mathematics successes usually involved his telling me I should become a nuclear physicist. This was in the mid- to late 1950s, the time of 'the cold war' between the USA and the Soviet Union, when to be a nuclear physicist would have represented a position of great power, signifying creation of a god-like technology that could be used to maintain control over the world (Haraway 1991). My father was engaged in the manufacture of part of this cold war apparatus as some of the work done at the factory was for the military but his was a position of little power, low pay and oppressive working conditions. While I didn't know what a nuclear physicist was or did, I did know it was connected with mathematics and science and that it wasn't a job in a factory. My father was proud of my success and encouraged me to develop more expertise but did not have the resources to guide me towards developing it, a situation common to the working-classes in relation to formal education (Reay 1998).

I never seriously thought about becoming a nuclear physicist, however. At the age of ten or 11 years old, I assumed, along with all my girlfriends that I would get married and not want a job that I would do throughout my adult life, mimicking the heterosexual relations I witnessed between my parents. In the scientific ambition my father had for me, there is his implicit acknowledgement that he thought I could be part of that power base, even though I was female. In order to try to explain his early ambitions for me, I asked, where is the race in this? I realized that perhaps he thought I could be a physicist because we were white, as were the images of scientists and their laboratories, images that ignored the work of black people in science and technology (Johnson 1993).

Technology as situated knowledge

As well as telling us about engine lathe operation, my father also talked about the politics of the work situation. I knew that foremen were one step further away from the machine, one step closer to management, supervising who did what and worrying over specific jobs getting done on time. Usually these same foremen were also the shop stewards. Each year my father reported a sell-out in contract negotiations and, more rarely, when they actually did go on strike, an unsatisfactory settlement. I knew that strikes were not only about changes in hourly rates of pay but also about payment per piece and different rates for different pieces, as the more complex the process required to produce a piece of metal, the longer it took to set up and the greater the disaster when it had to be scrapped. As we were eating, we heard about his co-workers, including those on earlier shifts who did or didn't leave all the 'meat-ball' jobs (lower quality metal and lower rates) for my father when he worked the night shift. We knew about the only job that was worse than being left with a bunch of 'meatballs' was that of working in the foundry, in temperatures over 100 degrees F with no piece rates. He saw the jobs of the foundry workers as being more oppressive and lower-skilled than he perceived his job to be and he made a point of telling us that most of the men in this job were black. This intersection of race and class relations demonstrates the oppressive work conditions and the social hierarchies constituted in the construction of technology.

Technology as necessity

The evidence of my mother's technological skills was around us and on us, as she made many of the clothes my sister and I wore. This making was situated not only in a simple economics context of not having the money to buy the clothes but also in a context encompassing a critical analysis of the clothing that we could afford to buy and how poorly it was made. She would design and make her own patterns, a design and learning by doing negotiation that taught my sister and me expertise in clothes making. As we grew older and became more definitive about what we wanted, we would work together with her in making skirts, trousers, tops, suits and coats. She taught us about bias cutting, interfacing and bound buttonholes. We learned how to recognize good fabrics and would go together to shops that sold high quality fabrics at cheap prices. Sewing falls within practices typically gendered female and my father did not attempt to sew.

My parents did some home-based technologies together, such as hanging wallpaper and trying to fix broken appliances. My father would usually comment that my mother had more expertise than him at these jobs. Cooking was an area in which my father sometimes encroached on my mother's domain. While my mother did the great majority of the cooking, my father was interested in doing it when he had time. He usually cooked Sunday breakfast, our only big breakfast of the week, and if there was time before going to work on Fridays, he would make potato latkes. In what I see now as partially an attempt to reconstitute their positions regarding this domestic technology, my father would always praise my mother's cooking, while she usually critiqued his attempts, for example, he used too much bacon fat when frying eggs and the potato was too finely ground for the latkes. The job of washing the dishes was usually assigned to me and my sister and each item of the varied collection of pots, lids, dishes, glasses, etc., presented a new challenge in how to stack them for drying. On weekends, when he didn't have to go out to work, my father did the dishes while 'the cook', my mother, relaxed and read the newspaper.

There were also the cooking and sewing activities of my Italian grandmother. She would occasionally make pasta and when she did so she would organize my sister and me into an assembly line to form the dough into a shape called cavatelli. She taught us to press our index and middle fingers slowly into a floured, plump circle of dough which made it curl over itself into a cylindrical lip shape, ready for the boiling water. My grandmother, who spent most of her day in a seated position, would use most of the time for crocheting and this process of transforming spools of thick white cotton into intricate lace designs seemed magical when I was very young.

The poor design of some artefacts are linked to my memories of my grandmother, just as the process of tying shoelaces is linked to my father's left-handedness. She had one leg amputated above the knee before she moved in to live with us. One of the technologies she brought with her was a leg prosthesis, her artificial leg. This technology was a failure; my grandmother never found it comfortable enough to wear. After a few attempts to use it, it leaned against the back corner of the cupboard and her crutches and wheelchair and our spatial logistics were the technologies used when she changed location.

It wasn't only my father's, mother's and grandmother's making and doing that helped constitute my knowledge of technology, however. There were the other people on the street like my uncle, a house painter, who was always willing to discuss his craft, from shapes, sizes and quality of brushes to mapping of a room for applying paint. Technology also formed part of daily life with my friends, as well as with adults. We all had bicycles, an essential possession in our neighbourhood. The maintenance of these was our own responsibility and the skills of fixing slipped chains and flat tyres were passed down from the older children. A marker of our changing ages and autonomy was how far we travelled on our bikes, progressing from the length of the block to around the corner, across the street, finally taking cycling trips of a few miles.

Technology as summer landscape

The immediate environment provided a backdrop of technologies. While our neighbourhood was residential, there were factories in the immediate area and an elevated railway line that met the back of some of them. Our house was on a corner, at the end of a block, and a paper factory was right across the street. In the summer, with the windows open as we slept, there was a clanging and chugging sound through the night – that of the continual movement of heavy machinery. The smell of glue was sometimes strong in the hot air as we played outside during the day and evening and came through the open windows at night. Many of the photographs from the years when I was a child and teenager were taken by the side of the house with this factory in the background. Some others were taken on the pavement in front of the house with the railway bridge, rather than our house, in the distance behind us. I cannot remember whether this photographic scenery was intentional or circumstantial, but it was a familiar backdrop to our lives in various ways. The factory walls provided large spaces for us to play ball against. Its rubbish bins were sometimes the source of items for play. It also offered what I saw at the time as a glimpse of a 'countryside' world, a bit of green space and flowers. There was a small area at the back of the factory that had a rectangle of grass in front of it, the only grass in the neighbourhood. It was fenced in so not accessible to us, but the fence itself was covered with morning glory in the summer. I visited it every day, on foot or by bicycle, morning and afternoon, to observe its cycle and knew when it closed up for the day. So while the neighbourhood factories were a site of metal machinery, sweat and noise, they were also a site of play and pleasure.

Technology as formal education

Technological knowledge relations have a history rooted in class as well as gender relations. Paechter (1998) cites Penfold in her discussion of the development of technological education and notes the deep-seated prejudices against practical work and the long history of 'design and technology' subjects being used as agents of social control, especially of the poor. In the system of English education, prior to the setting up of comprehensive schools, this usually was represented as the split between a grammar school elite and largely working-class remainder, with technology deemed a subject aimed at the 'less academic', those who were considered to be more able to deal with concrete things than with ideas (p. 86). This classing of certain forms of technology constitutes the working-class technologist as lacking in intelligence and constitutes technology itself as little more than a routine operation. In schooling before implementation of the National Curriculum, gendering of technology was overt, i.e., as that which boys did while girls did cooking and sewing. Lerman's research on nineteenth-century Philadelphia and education of the white and black working classes (1997) finds that technological knowledge is similarly constituted.

Technology as a more abstract concept and in association with science was not a major part of my formal education that was an education for working-class girls. In the high school I attended an intertwining of gender, class and race relations designated white young women as office workers. Even though I was at the top of the class in algebra and geometry, I was not encouraged to continue with mathematics and the sciences but instead to take up typing and stenography. Most of the students who took this route were white, while in the other non-academic pathway offered to us, that of cooking and sewing, many of the students were black. Here young black women were seen as domestic workers, with my high school practising a hierarchy consistent with my father's factory and, again, with Lerman's research.

Technology and local agency

An early experience that helps make sense of my agency in relation to technology relates to visits to my Lithuanian grandmother that we made until I was about nine years of age. She lived 'upstate' in a

Pennsylvania coal-mining region in her own house. I liked to go there because she was the only person we visited who had a garden, a garden in which she grew vegetables as well as flowers. In her house she had a coal-fueled stove with various compartments and doors that required adjustment throughout the cooking process. Her ability to cook an entire meal in and on this stove by the opening and closing of different windows behind which I could see the pulsating orange heat amazed me. The other aspect of her daily living that made me see my grandmother as extraordinary was the location of her toilet. It was in the cellar, a cellar that held a high bank of coal and, sometimes, as yet uncaught, rats. That my grandmother could walk up and down those stairs, crossing a boundary from a warm, peopled kitchen to a cold and possibly rat-inhabited cellar to both get her coal and use the toilet conferred omnipotence upon her to me as a child. My sister and I, quietly terrified, always went down to the cellar together. Her everyday practice, required for survival, of crossing a boundary I had constructed through a fear related to my lack of familiarity with her locality, may have been one of my earliest introductions to the idea of technological knowledge and skills as being a necessary part of living.

Gender, race and class in the construction of technological identity

In considering the gender, race and class intersections of these relations of technology, I can identify a number of strands as they interweave. Regarding gender, there is the asymmetry of my mother's and father's relation to paid work. Butler (1990) provides an explanation for the constancy of the asymmetries in gender relations. She argues that they are held in place or constituted through practices based on heterosexuality. I see the employment constraint upon my mother as grounded in the dynamics of heterosexuality: my father did not want her to be in paid work and, in order to maintain the relationship with him, she was required to comply with this. Explanations of the gendering of technology tend to see through heterosexual relations rather than comment upon them, reproducing these relations as transparent in discussions of gender (Stepulevage 1997).

My high school's construction of young women's opportunities for their futures, as secretaries to male managers, provided a solid grounding in the communications and negotiation skills needed to perform work that is clearly situated within male-dominated domains, domains in which women's technological knowledge is usually essentialized as women's work. Outside of formal education, however, I found a solid grounding in technology as an everyday part of life, part of learning to question, to take care of ourselves and to create, echoing Fourez's aspects of technological literacy concerning autonomy, communications, coping and negotiating (1997). My mother's skills and knowledge in sewing, cooking, wallpaper application, etc., were clearly acknowledged and valued. My father's encroachment on her domain of cooking, in fact, can be seen to enhance its value as a technology, just as his vulnerabilities in relation to engine lathe work can be seen to devalue 'masculine' technologies.

In studies concerned with young black women in the English education system, an active engagement with technology is evident. Mirza (1992: 133–7) notes differences between black, mostly working-class, girls' choice of career as compared to their white, mostly middle-class peers. The black girls choose courses leading to traditional, often male-dominated professions, such as computing while the white girls opted for those associated with females such as languages. As Mirza (1997) points out, however, there are many constraints imposed upon black pupils in schools in relation to career choice. These constraints are evident in my experience story on formal education. White privilege is a facet of social relations in my experience stories, and the character of my relationship with technology was constituted through my white identity. Race relations of technology meant that the education and jobs of black people were constructed to be of less value than those of white people. While the black people I knew had more oppressive jobs and more restricted formal education, the context in which I witnessed this, such as reports of challenges to segregation and the friendships I had with black young women in high school, enabled me to make sense of why – that it was not due to black people's lack of knowledge and skills but rather their situations within domains claimed by white people.

I focus on the working class from a perspective that recognizes class as one of many subject positions rather than a fixed polarization or unified category (Maynard 1994). The complexity of class positioning is evident in my relation to the painter of my ceiling. I was 'taught' about painting as a working-class child, probably with the understanding that I would be doing my own, not hiring a painter. Today, working in a middle-class profession, I am hiring a painter even though I think I should paint the ceiling myself. Lack of time and having enough money to pay for it constitute a situation in which it makes sense to hire someone else to do the painting.

A number of powerful accounts of being brought up working class explore disadvantage (for example, see Walsh 1997) but my childhood stories explore working-class life in a way that reveals other aspects. The people in my stories shared their technologies of sewing, painting, engine lathe operation, etc., with me as a discursive process, a sharing that recognizes that as working-class children, we needed to learn skills that would help us get on in life. It enabled a shift in focus from imposition of technology to engagement with it. The learning of these technologies was intertwined with explanations that helped develop an understanding of technologies as part of a larger world, one in which working-class children needed to be able to cope with situations and negotiate for 'a better life'.

Through these stories of experience, I have constructed a view of technology that is about learning, playing, pleasure, pain, exploration and exclusion. Technology does not always have a distinct presence; it is interwoven into everyday life and involves continuous engagement. I hope to show through these selections of my remembered experiences and some commentary on them that in reflecting upon our everyday engagements with ICTs, we can identify spaces for agency and debate. Recognition of the interweaving of technology in everyday life enables relations to be better understood and also constitutes means through which we develop knowledge about the world and use technologies as we negotiate transformations and changes in our lives. Reflection on our experiences can provide grounds for exploring a new construction of technology, a construction that crosses a boundary of broad social and more individual personal relations; otherwise, for many people technology may continue to be considered only in its most powerful political contexts, those of global corporate networks, government data banks, weaponry, etc., and be considered as something which we might as well not attempt to challenge and transform.

Acknowledgements

With thanks to my mother and sister for their enthusiastic responses to my stories, to Nod Miller for suggesting autobiography as a way to explore gender–technology relations and to colleagues in our autobiographies group for comments on the first draft.

References

Adam, A. (1998) *Artificial Knowing: Gender and the Thinking Machine*, London: Routledge.
Aune, M. (1996) 'The computer in everyday life: patterns of domestication of a new technology' in M. Lie and K. Sorensen (eds) *Making Technology*

Our Own? Domesticating Technology into Everyday Life, Oslo: Scandinavian University Press: 92–120.

Balka, E. (1997) 'Sometimes texts speak louder than users: locating work through textual analysis' in A. F. Grundy, D. Kohler, V. Oechtering and U. Petersen (eds) *Women, Work and Computerization: Spinning a Web from Past to Future*, Berlin: Springer-Verlag: 163–75.

Brewer, S. (1996) 'The political is personal: father–daughter relationships and working-class consciousness', *Feminism and Psychology*, 6 (3): 401–10.

Butler, J. (1990) 'Gender trouble, feminist theory and psychoanalytic discourse' in L. Nicholson (ed.) *Feminism/Postmodernism*, New York: Routledge: 324–40.

Clement, A. (1991) 'Designing without designers: more hidden skill in office computerization?' in I. V. Eriksson, B. A. Kitchenham and K. G. Tijdens (eds) *Women, Work and Computerization: Understanding and Overcoming Bias in Work and Education*, Amsterdam: Elsevier Science: 15–32.

Cockburn, C. and Ormrod, S. (1993) *Gender and Technology in the Making*, London: Sage.

Dixon, C. (1998) 'Action, embodiment and gender in the design and technology classroom' in A. Clark and E. Millard (eds) *Gender in the Secondary Curriculum*, London: Routledge.

Ehn, P. (1993) 'Scandinavian design: on participation and skill' in D. Schuler and A. Namioka (eds) *Participatory Design: Principles and Practices*, Hillsdale: Lawrence Erlbaum Associates: 41–77.

Elkjaer, B. (1992) 'Girls and information technology in Denmark: an account of a socially constructed problem', *Gender and Education*, 4 (1/2): 25–40.

Fourez, G. (1997) 'Scientific and technological literacy as a social practice', *Social Studies of Science*, 27: 903–36.

Glenn, E. N. (1997) 'Looking back in anger? Re-remembering my sociological career' in B. Laslett and B. Thorne (eds) *Feminist Sociology: Life Histories of a Movement*, New Brunswick: Rutgers University Press: 73–102.

Green, E. et al. (eds) (1993) *Gendered By Design? Information Technology and Office Systems*, London: Taylor and Francis.

Hakken, D. and Andrews, B. (1993) *Computing Myths, Class Realities: An Ethnography of Technology and Working People in Sheffield, England*, Boulder, CO: Westview Press.

Haraway, D. (1991) 'Situated knowledges: the science question in feminism and the privilege of partial perspective' in D. Haraway (ed.) *Simians, Cyborgs, and Women: The Re-invention of Nature*, London: Free Association Books: 183–201.

Holtgrewe, U. (1994) 'Everyday experts? Professionals' women assistants and information technology' in A. Adam, J. Emms, E. Green and J. Owen (eds) *Women, Work and Computerization: Breaking Old Boundaries, Building New Forms*, Amsterdam: Elsevier: 121–8.

Jarvis, T. and Rennie, L. (1996) 'Perceptions about technology held by primary teachers in England', *Research in Science and Technological Education*, 14 (1): 43–54.

Johnson, R. (1993) 'Science, technology and black community development' in S. Harding (ed.) *The 'Racial' Economy of Science*, Bloomington: Indiana University Press: 458–71.

Lerman, N. E. (1997) 'Preparing for the duties and practical business of life: technological knowledge and social structure in mid-nineteenth-century Philadelphia', *Technology and Culture*, 38 (1): 21–59.

Maynard, M. (1994) 'Race, gender and the concept of "difference" in feminist thought' in H. Afshhar and M. Maynard (eds) *The Dynamics of 'Race' and Gender*, London: Taylor and Francis: 9–25.

Mirza, H. S. (1992) *Young, Female and Black*, London: Routledge.

Mirza, H. S. (1997) 'Black women in education: a collective movement for social change' in H. S. Mirza (ed.) *Black British Feminism: A Reader*, London: Routledge: 269–77.

Paechter, C. (1998) *Educating the Other: Gender, Power and Schooling*, London: Falmer Press.

Ramsay, H., Panteli, A. and Beirne, M. (1997) 'Empowerment and disempowerment: active agency, structural constraint and women computer users' in R. Lander and A. Adam (eds) *Women in Computing*, Exeter: Intellect Books: 84–93.

Rasmussen, B. (1997) 'Girls and computer science: "It's not me, I'm not interested in sitting behind a machine all day"' in A. F. Grundy, D. Kohler, V. Oechtering and U. Petersen (eds) *Women, Work and Computerization: Spinning a Web from Past to Future*, Berlin: Springer-Verlag: 379–86.

Reay, D. (1998) 'Classifying feminist research: exploring the psychological impact of social class on mothers' involvement in children's schooling', *Feminism and Psychology*, 8 (2): 155–71.

Saljo, R. (1999) 'Learning as the use of tools: a sociocultural perspective on the human-technology link' in K. Littleton and P. Light (eds) *Learning with Computers: Analysing Productive Interaction*, London: Routledge: 144–61.

Smith, V. (1998) *Not Just Race, Not Just Gender*, New York: Routledge.

Stanley, L. (1992) *The Auto/biographical I*, Manchester: Manchester University Press.

Star, S. L. (1991) 'Invisible work and silenced dialogues in knowledge representation' in I. V. Eriksson, B. A. Kitchenham and K. G. Tijdens (eds) *Women, Work and Computerization: Understanding and Overcoming Bias in Work and Education*, Amsterdam: Elsevier Science: 81–92.

Stepulevage, L. (1997) 'Sexuality and computing: transparent relations' in G. Griffin and S. Andermahr (eds) *Straight Studies Modified: Lesbian Interventions in the Academy*, London: Cassell: 197–211.

Suchman, L. (1994) 'Supporting articulation work: aspects of a feminist practice of technology production' in A. Adam, J. Emms, E. Green and J. Owen (eds) *Women, Work and Computerization: Breaking Old Boundaries, Building New Forms*, Amsterdam: Elsevier: 7–21.

Swindells, J. (ed.) (1995) *The Uses of Autobiography*, London: Taylor and Francis.

Volman, M. (1997) 'Care, computers and the playground: gender and identity in education', *Discourse Studies in the Cultural Politics of Education*, 18 (2): 229–39.

Wajcman, J. (1991) *Feminism Confronts Technology*, Cambridge: Polity Press.

Walkerdine, V. (1996) 'Editorial introduction: subjectivity and social class: new directions for feminist psychology', *Feminism and Psychology*, 6 (3): 355–60.

Walsh, V. (1997) 'Interpreting class: auto/biographical imaginations and social change' in P. Mahony and C. Zmroczek (eds) *Class Matters: Working-Class Women's Perspectives on Social Class*, London: Taylor and Francis: 152–74.

Weber, L., Higginbotham, E. and Dill, B. T. (1997) 'Sisterhood as collaboration: building the centre for research on women at the University of Memphis' in B. Laslett and B. Thorne (eds) *Feminist Sociology: Life Histories of a Movement*, New Brunswick: Rutgers University Press: 229–56.

Webster, J. (1996) *Shaping Women's Work: Gender, Employment and Information Technology*, Harlow: Addison Wesley Longman.

Widerberg, K. (1998) 'Teaching gender through writing "experience stories"', *Women's Studies International Forum*, 21 (2): 193–8.

Yoon, S. (1996) 'Power online: a poststructuralist perspective on CMC' in C. Ess (ed.) *Philosophical Perspectives on Computer-Mediated Communication*, Albany: State University of New York Press: 171–96.

Chapter 5

Theoretical reflections on networking in practice

The case of women on the Net

Gillian Youngs

Introduction

This chapter explores the nature of virtual communication and its links to reconceptualizing international politics. The bases for the discussion are rooted in the author's participation in the UNESCO/Society for International Development Women on the Net (WoN) project (Harcourt 1999; see also websites). The points it raises can therefore be regarded as reflections on conceptual and theoretical issues associated with expanding forms of virtual experience drawn directly from the sphere of practice. One of its premises is that the Internet and the new intensified communicative engagements it offers are placing fresh political emphases on the realm of practice, including its power to inform our theorizing effectively. The Internet and the complex and intricate webs of interactions it incorporates draws our attention to the meanings of processes of communication and their implications in the short and long term (see, for example, Brin 1998; Shapiro 1999; Tomlinson 1999).

In a world of growing 'technosociality' (Escobar 1996: 112) we are drawn to focus on the interconnectedness between social relations and technology, to consider those relations in the context of the information and communications technologies (ICTs) by which they are mediated and to develop sensitivities to the specificities of the nature of those mediations. 'Context' is an interesting and important concept in this regard because it signals a number of things about the ways in which we can begin to think about the connections between ICTs and social relations. The cross-boundary qualities of the Internet as a communications medium can lead us all too easily to view it as a blank, neutral and open space, to slide towards a kind of technohomogeneity in our vision of cyber-relations. The virtual qualities of the Internet can similarly lead us to too detached a view of it as a communicative sphere, and fail to focus sufficiently on the sense of it as a social space related to other forms of social space and thus reflect and inform their diverse influences.

This chapter examines such issues from the practice of the WoN project and thereby aims to demonstrate the key role of new cyber-practices in the honing of cybertheories. It moves between practice and theory and it includes sharing of what I, as one participant in the project, feel I have learned from it, as well as my analytical assessments of what I judge can be drawn from it for further broader thinking about the potential, as well as the actual, achievements of cyberactivities. The background to what follows is my sense of such activities as, at least in part, theory in the making or perhaps this would be better expressed as activities oriented towards the possibility for bringing theory and the everyday or moment-by-moment experience into closer connection (Shields 1996: 8).

The chapter is divided into two parts. The first describes the WoN project and its particular characteristics and offers some investigation of how these are influential in shaping its communicative context. Among these are its overtly 'international' nature. I unpack elements of what this means with regard to WoN. The second part considers factors surrounding the relationships between traditionally conceived international space(s) and virtual space(s). It argues that projects like WoN signal the degree to which standard approaches to 'international (international) relations' need to be reconfigured to incorporate awareness of political processes, including virtual ones, which disrupt the conceptual constraints of dominant state-centred approaches. We are talking more of 'relating internationally' than international relations in any conventional sense. This part closes with the theme of boundaries; boundaries to be discovered rather than assumed.

WoN and networking as practice

WoN is symbolic of the new forms of adventure in communication and political and cultural exchange which the Internet can facilitate. It aimed from its outset in 1997 for multiple forms of diversity with regard to the individuals and organizations which it involved. Its founding focus was bringing together technicians, researchers, activists and development practitioners to think about and work collectively to contribute to the potential of the Internet for women. It was in the global spirit of much that had already been achieved in association with the UN's Fourth World

Conference on Women in Beijing to familiarize women and their organizations with ICTs and to get them online to work towards harnessing the full potential of the Internet (Farwell et al. 1999). But in that spirit it also clearly identified the Internet as a means by which new collective spaces could be opened up for thinking through new political possibilities and strategies.

There is a strong sense of the Net as a space of discovery in the words of co-originator of the project, Lourdes Arizpe (1999: xii), about the early stages of WoN:

> When Wendy [Harcourt] and I decided to throw a women's project into the Net-future, we did not expect such a prolific, image-filled outburst of enthusiasm and expertise. Magic: over one hundred women, and men, re-materialized through virtual space saying, yes, we will create this new mythology of cyberspace with you . . .

The beginnings of the project in this way highlight the potential of virtual space for seeking out connections of interest and for testing the collective possibilities around sets of ideas. There are senses in which an individual, a group or a project can launch into that space without knowing precisely what is there or what may result. It is an encouragement to political experimentation. Accepting the unknown is part of the practice. Networks within networks can generate connections with ongoing and unexpected results. Information and ideas may flow through these channels with the knowledge of impacts or continuations not necessarily ever flowing directly back through to the original point or points of departure. 'The non-place of cyberspacetime contains innumerable networks resting on logical lattices abstracted from unthinkably complex data fields that unfold across an endless virtual void' (Nguyen and Alexander 1996: 102). Setting out on a political journey in such circumstances is an uncertain thing; it may have elements of quest, curiosity, hope and fear all mixed up together. For often we are strangers when we meet in cyberspace so there is a politics of encounter to be incorporated into the many other kinds of political endeavours on the Internet. This was certainly the case with aspects of the WoN project as it developed, not least because of its aims to contest and breach multiple boundaries at one and the same time.

WoN aimed to cut across national, cultural and social as well as political and economic boundaries. Equally importantly, it set out to breach north/south and theory/practice divides and promote communication across areas of specialist knowledge which can all too frequently operate in their own spheres. These included theoretical and policy-oriented research, development practice and advocacy, grassroots politics, technical and training work. It was clear as the project developed that the complexity of the communicative challenges it incorporated could only be fully appreciated in the experience of them. This was new terrain. It was happening in part because ICTs made it possible but the technological capacities only provided the means for the networks to be built and operated. These capacities were relevant to the meanings generated but still these predominantly lay with the participants, how they interacted together and the results that occurred. There were clear priorities of a general nature:

> WoN had several aims. First, to encourage women, particularly in the south and in marginal groups in the north (and Central and East Europe), to use the Internet more easily as *their* [my emphasis] space, thereby empowering women to use technology as a political tool. Second, to open up and contribute to the new culture that was being set up on the Internet from a gender perspective at once local and global. Third, to bring together individual women and men working from different institutional bases (women's NGOs, information technology networks, academe, women activists) to explore a transnational women's movement agenda in response to and shaping evolving telecommunication policies. And fourth, to create a resource (community and support) base which could be tapped into by different women's groups in terms of analysis, knowledge and skills in navigating the Internet.
>
> (Harcourt 1999: 1)

It was clear to me from the early stages that the issue of women using the Internet as their space was at the heart of the project. This was a question of habit as well as habitability: it was about knowledge of, access to and ease with the technology, as well as predispositions to be politically active and imaginative about how it might be used effectively towards specific goals. So WoN itself was creating a space within virtual space in which such questions could be explored and acted on. It was as much about how those taking part felt about the technology and the different kinds of communication and action it facilitated, as the shared political and cultural perspectives and aims to which it could contribute. WoN created a space in which a group of individuals from diverse contexts encountered one another. Many already knew one another from working together, at the Beijing conference in 1995 and the Global Knowledge Conference in Canada in 1997 and in other settings and projects associated with women and development, activism and advocacy (Gittler 1999; Huyer 1999).

It was therefore important not to consider WoN in isolation but to recognize its place in an expanding contemporary history of global women's networking, especially around development issues and the strategic role played within these processes of ICT-oriented organizations, such as the Association for Progressive Communications whose Women's Programme (see websites) played a key role in facilitating the computer networking around the Beijing process and beyond (Gittler 1996; Farwell et al. 1999). WoN was a network in a history of women's international networking which was based on the increasingly effective use of a whole range of communications technologies from the more traditional, such as newsletters, to fax and phone and now the different dimensions of the Internet, listserv discussion, webpages, email and so on.

> One of the outstanding features of women's communications and media . . . has been the weaving together of many different media forms and formats in response to very diverse constituencies, organizational forms and working styles. Sharing the daily struggles and victories associated with the practicalities of using electronic networking, whether in training workshops or on-line forums, has been and continues to be a critical part of the learning process. Underlying much of women's electronic networking is the notion that the value of the computer and electronic communications is not in the value of the technologies themselves, but in the ability of the tools to improve, support, protect and enhance women's full and equal participation in all aspects of society.
>
> (Gittler 1999: 100)

WoN's multiple boundary-crossing remit gave it a particular role in the women's networking learning curve. One could wonder what would be the result of attempting to bring together such diverse interests? How could it work? What would be the outcomes? Many participants knew from a little to a great deal about some other colleagues involved in the project, some were much less familiar with most of those involved, their organizations or their work. The scope of the work and interests of the individuals and organizations ranged, for example, across post-Beijing processes of various kinds, community-building for migrant women, capacity-building for civil society, the theory and practice of virtual peace across north and south, grassroots organizing and international strategizing for indigenous peoples, rural women's access to interactive communications technologies; global networking among women scientists and technologists; and much more. The geographical reach of those taking part included the Americas, Africa, Europe, Asia, Canada and Australia (Harcourt 1997).

WoN has combined face-to-face meetings with workshops and presentations and has woven its cyberactivities around those. After the initial meeting in Santiago de Compostela, Spain, in mid-1997 extensive exchanges took place on an email discussion list. Over 2,000 messages were sent and received between the Santiago event and a second meeting at the University of California, Berkeley, where the group also presented the WoN project at a Gender and Globalization Conference in March 1998 (Harcourt 1999: 1–2). The book, *Women@Internet* (Harcourt 1999), was one of the major outcomes of these discussions. An Internet guide (Harcourt 1997) and a digital handbook for first-time users, *Women in the Digital Age* (1998), were other outputs.

The second phase of the project included two Internet workshops that I helped to lead in Zanzibar, Tanzania, and Nairobi, Kenya, in September 1999. The workshops were run in conjunction with local partners and designed to meet a range of needs from introduction to the Internet, its different forms of communication, the web and navigation skills, to the conceptualization, development and organization of webpages and advanced ideas relating to webpage structure. The participants had varied experience of the Net, some not having used computers at all before, some totally unfamiliar with the Net, some working for organizations where they used the Net in particular ways and some with basic and more advanced webpages. Those involved included teachers, community, grassroots and political workers and representatives of various kinds of organizations focused on women's issues.

The actual structure and work of the WoN project signals the degree to which it is important to view virtual activity in the context of its overall social settings. Therein lies the fabric of local-global connections and dynamics that root the Internet activity of different forms in other kinds of social activity. The virtual work which is undertaken on the Net is woven into the networking and strategizing of more familiar concrete social spaces and places. Far from being detached from them, it flows out of them and to them. It may travel via circuitous roots and it may be enhanced or changed by the scope of the virtual connections which the Net's cross-boundary qualities makes possible, but it is firmly grounded in the embodied lives and communities of those involved (Youngs 2000b). WoN's cyberdiscussions, face-to-face meetings and workshops have emphasized the local in the virtual and the local in the global. Over a period of time members of the project have come to know something of each other's perspectives and work and to see some of the detail of contrasting 'local' settings through the virtual and global connections encouraged by WoN. The project is best understood as part of wider processes as, for instance, demonstrated by the hosting of the Zanzibar workshop as the launch event of the Zanzibar Information Technology Center (see websites) formed to foster Net access and ICT use by the local community as part of the work of the Sustainable Advancement of Zanzibar (SAZ), an NGO founded and run by young people.

> While we insist upon the multiple histories of the Internet, it is also imperative to recognize the multiple agencies exercised through it. Internet is a network, linking interactants across space and time, not a 'thing' or a set of computers communicating autonomously without human actors. It is essential to foreground the human in the Net. This resets the Internet as a phenomenon of social and political interest, not just a bright technical toy for engineers.
>
> (Shields 1996: 8)

WoN and 'relating internationally'

In the context of 'the human in the Net', I want to turn now to some of the implications for thinking about the politics of projects such as WoN. The geographical scope of the Net makes it logical to think of such politics as 'international' but their very nature is in many ways fundamentally disruptive of traditional notions of international (inter-national) politics. The socio-spatial reach of the Net actually and potentially confounds the rigid constraints that have dominated conceptualizations of international politics. The Net and the kinds of networks and politics it facilitates signal that it is useful to think beyond inter-national relations, to think more openly in terms of the implications of 'relating internationally'. There are two main areas I wish to discuss. The first is a general point relating to spatial approaches to politics. The second focuses more closely on women and feminist perspectives in this context.

A number of influential critical works in the study of international relations and beyond have linked its limited concerns with politics directly to its limited spatial concepts (in particular, Walker 1993; Agnew and Corbridge 1995). These are argued to be state-centred and atomistic, focusing on a bounded notion of states as actors rather than on the complex of political (and other social) processes within and across state boundaries (Scholte 1993; Youngs 1999b). These traditional conceptualizations feature a sense of political space as territory that extends little if at all beyond expressions of the boundedness of states. Politics is primarily defined via the concept of the state and the mutually reinforcing dualisms of 'inside/outside', order/anarchy (Walker 1993; Youngs 1999b). The state becomes the definer of order (inside) as opposed to anarchy (outside). Anarchy in this respect has a specific meaning: a collection of sovereign states with no overarching system of control. Political meaning is vested in the boundary that divides inside and outside, order and anarchy.

Rob Walker (1993: 9) has drawn attention to the importance of 'sovereign identity' in this 'inside/outside' picture of order/anarchy. There is not space to do justice to the detail of his arguments here but some key implications can be drawn out that are relevant to this discussion. He explains how the abstract notion of the state retains a timeless quality (as opposed to governments which come and go) to which sovereign identity and being (collectively and by association individually) is attached (Ashley 1989). Political community retains its sovereign identity on the spatial basis of bounded territory and a sense of history and future through the timeless category of the state. These are the kinds of bases on which the state has remained too much a particularistic and assumed category in the mainstream study of international relations with regard to political time and space (in particular, pp. 125–40; see also Agnew and Corbridge 1995: 78–100; Youngs 1999b: 28–30). Part of the problem is that 'state territories have been reified as set or fixed units of sovereign space' (Agnew and Corbridge 1995: 83), as if it were freezing them analytically into an eternal rather than a dynamic presence, resulting in a predominantly static sense of them rather than an open and changing one.

Feminists have offered varied insights into the socio-spatial and gendered constraints surrounding this conceptual approach to politics and political (sovereign) identity (man). They have stressed the degree to which women are absent from this strictly configured 'public' denotation of state-centred inter-national relations. It is a masculinist world where the lives of women do not generally appear in any active sense; they are forced into the background and remain a largely assumed, and thus implicitly passive, backdrop to this version of international reality.

Cynthia Enloe (for example, 1990 and 1993) is among those who have done most to disrupt the theoretical and practical orientations of this world without women perspective (also, for example: Peterson 1992a 1992b; Tickner 1992; Marchand and Runyan 2000). The following depiction from over a decade ago remains pertinent:

> So far feminist analysis has had little impact on international politics. Foreign-policy commentators and decision-makers seem particularly confident in dismissing feminist ideas. Rare is the professional commentator on international politics who takes women's experiences seriously. Women's experiences – of war, marriage, trade, travel, factory work – are relegated to the 'human interest' column. Women's roles in creating and sustaining [my emphasis] international politics have been treated as if they were 'natural' and thus not worthy of investigation.
>
> (Enloe 1990: 3–4)

Projects like WoN are sites in which we can see aspects of the roles women are playing in creating and sustaining new forms of international politics – experimental processes of 'relating internationally'. They also contribute to writing new histories of such relating because they overtly build on what has gone before, on the networking achievements and the associated informational and political structures that have been created. WoN is one of the windows on the hidden agency of women in international politics and it highlights different ways in which the Internet facilitates women-to-women connections across boundaries – national, socio-economic, cultural, political and so on (Youngs 1999c). This can be regarded as a potential sea change in the nature of those politics because, to some extent, it cuts across the masculinist lines of traditional international relations and contributes to contesting the state-centred mediation of politics internationally as 'public' and masculine rather than 'public' and 'private' and as intrinsically about women (and children) as well as about men and about social relations of power among other things.

The growth of women's cyberpolitics signals the need to recognize women as 'actively' present in the processes of international politics, broadly and critically defined. These developments link strongly to the diverse arguments in support of complex and embodied approaches to political and economic space which I and others have put forward (in particular: Massey 1994, 1995; Gibson-Graham 1996; Youngs 1999b, 2000a, 2000b). One of the main analytical starting points in this respect is the long-standing feminist emphasis on private–public dynamics which seeks to get beyond masculinist frames of politics, economics and culture, as defined in primary terms by public domains abstracted from the private (and traditionally feminized) domains of family, domesticity and social reproduction. These masculinist frames include a reductionist stance towards political and economic agency as captured by the public realm rather than public–private social relations (Peterson 1992b; Hooper 1999). Political and economic individuals or agents are in this 'hegemonic' mode defined as rational, acting, public and, crucially, masculine entities (Hooper 1999; also Hooper 1998). The spatial emphases of contrasting feminist insistences on understandings of gendered social relations of power as intrinsically involving public–private linkages, and associated questions about the nature of agency, are coming increasingly to the fore. I have argued, for example, that 'gendered imperatives' are vital to attempts towards 'radicalizing spatial understanding of the local' in studies of processes of globalization (Youngs 1999b: 108; also Youngs 2000a).

In the contemporary communications era such points about local and global, public and private, have growing purchase, not least because our understandings of social spatiality itself are pressed in the direction of new analytical sensitivities towards diverse material and the virtual spaces and connections between them. Communications are overtly spatially pervasive. Political and economic activities and relations are increasingly conducted through the virtual spaces of the Net as well as in the more familiar and apparently more concrete settings of state and market, polity and economy. Increasing numbers of people, groups and organizations are operating across virtual and other forms of social space and, influentially, creating new links between them (Sardar 1996; Deibert 1997). This has implications for new thinking about agency because the precise ways in which we occupy and utilize social spaces and our being within them are aspects of the kinds of relative power we possess as well as the possibilities we envisage for social and individual transformations (Youngs 1999a).

In this respect, one particularly interesting aspect of WoN's virtual exchanges was the extent to which they starkly contrasted with the assumptions of conventional international relations: assumptions that we know which boundaries count, that neither they nor their political meanings are out there to be discovered. WoN's conversations and deliberations signalled just the reverse: that in the information age of networking much of our political work will be concentrated on the boundaries we encounter in new forms of communication across lines of expertise, cultures, nations, interest, different forms of 'public' and 'private' and their interactions in social relations of power and so on. These boundaries, understanding what they are based on and the different ways in which they might be mutually negotiated are at the heart of Net-based virtual experience. Openness, interest and sensitivity are positive qualities in negotiating such virtual politics, or at least that is one of the major lessons I began to learn in great detail in the practice of WoN.

'Mediating borders' (Harcourt 1999: 3) may have featured among the aims of the project but it also, interestingly, became central to the project's own problematics. The experience of such more challenging aspects of the internal dynamics of WoN has been sometimes far from comfortable. One soon learned that this was no place for assumptions and that one simply did not know necessarily when or how a 'boundary' of one kind or another might be encountered and what the result of the exchanges in such circumstances might be. For example, in the lead up to the Berkeley meeting, language became a point of intense debate: 'The group began . . . to question quite seriously its use of language, the sense of inclusion and exclusion and the possibility of opening up a new way of dialoguing that could allow for diversity while building solidarity and identity' (Harcourt 1999: 7).

This excerpt from a contribution from Kekula Bray-Crawford, an indigenous woman activist with a technical and lobbying background, indicates how such an exploration could touch as deeply on historical questions of power as on the immediate dynamics of Net conversations:

> I need messages loaded with academic terminology when it is thick to [be interpreted] for me in my own poetic language so I can understand where the discussion or people themselves are coming from. This does give life, appreciation and light to a world I thought was without.
>
> The general concern I speak of is the boundaries academia has presented throughout the colonial period of our existence as indigenous peoples. It was our very first encounter across the board with colonial settlers which were missionaries. Their Bible was the academic imposition (because it was taught like a classroom) upon traditional spirituality, practices and belief systems, coupled with a new language. These impositions created a negative IQ upon native thinking and immediately what were ancient astronomers became

heathen and unintelligent. That is the origin of the thought and becomes the neocolonial framework today upon which a western system is built.

On the same timeline now we have encountered Internet technology which creates the very first window to escape that imposition. My own thoughts only. Where thinkers meet scholars, actors activists and indigenous, Western level communication, creating a new level to the political, social, economic and cultural framework – now crossing regions.

(Harcourt 1999: 8–9; also Bray-Crawford 1999)

Such exchanges have demonstrated for me how embodied our experience of cybercommunications can be, through the sharing of the detail of our histories, their local specificities, their global connections. We are literally bringing those things (our 'real lives') to bear in smaller and larger ways through our 'virtual voices' (Youngs 1999c). Thinking about the potential roles of the Net in forming new kinds of politics, far from representing some kind of futuristic escape from the present or the past, they offer fresh possibilities for revisiting them and critically exploring them, working towards new (potentially shared) understandings. In certain ways therefore WoN has been an experiment in multiple forms of contextualization as well as communication. It is fascinating to me that this is a politics of unravelling; in some senses, a process of working towards the detailing of the challenges which cybercommunications presents. One of the main things I have learned from my participation in WoN is that these challenges will have to be discovered, they cannot simply be assumed or minimized because that works against the logic of the cross-boundary character of the Net, as well as against the possibilities for thinking and working through its full political potential. Another WoN participant, Laura Agustín, posed what to me seem enduring questions about the tensions of trying to work effectively on the Net:

> Obviously we can't all speak or understand the same way, I hope we are not dreaming about a Utopian 'unity'. On the other hand I don't like being in the position of having to ask 'What does that mean?' over and over. My heart seems to go somewhere else while I read such things. If I say that, will some people feel they need to 'silence' themselves?
>
> (Harcourt 1999: 9; also Agustín 1999)

Conclusion

This discussion has ranged from the specifics of the WoN project to wider questions about Net-based politics and the ways they are testing traditional conceptualizations of international relations and its processes. I have argued that projects such as WoN help to demonstrate the urgency of moving beyond conventional state-centred interpretations of international politics to a concern with political processes within and across state boundaries, processes which are about 'relating internationally'. Two powerful implications are highlighted.

The first contributes to transcending the invisibility of women in international politics which has plagued dominant conceptualizations dependent on masculinist and 'public' models of politics and political agency, In the detail of the WoN project, the WoN process or processes, we can identify women as agents, bringing embodied, place-based and historically-grounded senses of politics to the international sphere. Equally importantly, we can identify the links of these virtual activities with the wider political engagements and earlier achievements of individuals and groups involved, included in the more familiar substantive arenas of local, national and international politics. WoN demonstrates how integral virtual and other forms of politics can be considered to be.

Secondly, my assessment of WoN focuses on its critical realization and negotiation of 'boundaries'. I have argued that the WoN experience locates the discovery of boundaries and their problematics as central to virtual politics. This is far distant from, and deeply transgressive of, the assumptions about boundaries which have been characteristic of state-centred approaches to international relations. The spatial reach of the Net means that its politics are shaped by boundary-crossing of various kinds and the critical issues this raises are fundamental to the challenges, as well as the possibilities, it presents. I have argued, too, that this contests notions of the Net as a communicative space primarily locked into the present and the future. WoN's work has shown how new forms of communication on the Net open fresh opportunities for revisiting historical processes that have shaped the present and for reflecting in new shared circumstances on their meanings, and the political implications of these, included for the future.

As we entered this century the Net remained predominantly an elitist sphere with only 2 per cent of people worldwide online and more than 90 per cent of users concentrated in the rich OECD countries (UNDP 1999). In these circumstances, projects such as WoN offer useful early indicators of problems and opportunities that will be shared by more and more people and groups as the rapid spread of Net access continues.

Acknowledgements

I am grateful to UNESCO and SID and other participants for my involvement in the WoN project and to the Social Sciences Faculty of Leicester University, UK, for a grant which helped to support this research work.

References

Agnew, J. and Corbridge, S. (1995) *Mastering Space, Hegemony, Territory and International Political Economy*, London: Routledge.

Agustín, L. (1999) 'They speak, but who listens?' in W. Harcourt (ed.) *Women@Internet*, London: Zed Books.

Arizpe, L. (1999) 'Freedom to create: women's agenda for cyberspace' in W. Harcourt (ed.) *Women@Internet*, London: Zed Books.

Ashley, R. K. (1989) 'Living on border lines: man, poststructuralism, and war' in J. Der Derian and M. Shapiro (eds) *International/Intertextual Relations: Postmodern Readings of World Politics*, New York: Lexington.

Bray-Crawford, K. P. (1999) 'The Ho'okele netwarriors in the liquid continent' in W. Harcourt (ed.) *Women@Internet*, London: Zed Books.

Brin, D. (1998) *The Transparent Society*, Perseus Books: Reading, MA.

Deibert, R. J. (1997) *Parchment, Printing, and Hypermedia: Communication in World Order Transformation*, New York: Columbia University Press.

Enloe, C. (1990) *Bananas, Beaches and Bases: Making Feminist Sense of International Politics*, London: Pandora.

Enloe, C. (1993) *The Morning After: Sexual Politics at the End of the Cold War*, Berkeley: University of California Press.

Escobar, A. (1996) 'Welcome to Cyberia: notes on the anthropology of cyberculture' in Z. Sardar and R. Ravetz (eds) *Cyberfutures: Culture and Politics on the Information Highway*, London: Pluto Press.

Farwell, E. et al. (1999) 'Global networking for change: experiences from the APC women's programme' in W. Harcourt (ed.) *Women@Internet*, London: Zed Books.

Gibson-Graham, J. K. (1996) *The End of Capitalism (As We Knew It): A Feminist Critique of Political Economy*, Oxford: Blackwell.

Gittler, A. M. (1996) 'Taking hold of electronic communications: women making a difference', *Journal of International Communication* 3, 1: 85–101.

Gittler, A. M. (1999) 'Mapping women's global communications and networking' in W. Harcourt (ed.) *Women@Internet*, London: Zed Books.

Harcourt, W. (1997) *An International Annotated Guide to Women Working on the Net*, Revised version, Rome: UNESCO/Society for International Development.

Harcourt, W. (ed.) (1999) *Women@Internet*, London: Zed Books.

Hooper, C. (1998) 'Masculinist practices and gender politics: the operation of multiple masculinities in international relations' in M. Zalewski and J. Parpart (eds) *The 'Man' Question in International Relations*, Oxford: Westview.

Hooper, C. (1999) 'Disembodiment, embodiment and the construction of hegemonic masculinity' in G. Youngs (ed.) *International Relations in a Global Age: A Conceptual Challenge*, Cambridge: Polity Press.

Huyer, S. (1999) 'Shifting agendas at GK97: women and international policy on information and communication technologies' in W. Harcourt (ed.) *Women@Internet*, London: Zed Books.

Marchand, M. H. and Runyan, A. S. (eds) (2000) *Gender and Global Restructuring: Sightings, Sites and Resistances*, London: Routledge.

Massey, D. (1994) *Space, Place and Gender*, Cambridge: Polity Press.

Massey, D. (1995) *Spatial Divisions of Labour: Social Structures and the Geography of Production*, second edition, London: Macmillan.

Nguyen, D. T. and Alexander, J. (1996) 'The coming of cyberspacetime and the end of the polity' in R. Shields (ed.) (1996) *Cultures of Internet: Virtual Spaces, Real Histories, Living Bodies*, London: Sage.

Peterson, V. S. (1992a) *Gendered States: (Re)visions of International Relations Theory*, Boulder, CO.: Lynne Rienner.

Peterson, V. S. (1992b) 'Transgressing boundaries: theories of knowledge, gender, and international relations', *Millennium: Journal of International Studies*, 21: 183–206.

Sardar, Z. (1996) 'alt.civilizations.faq: cyberspace as the darker side of the west' in Z. Sardar and R. Ravetz (eds) *Cyberfutures: Culture and Politics on the Information Highway*, London: Pluto Press.

Scholte, J. A. (1993) *International Relations of Social Change*, Buckingham: Open University Press.

Shapiro, A. (1999) *The Control Revolution: How the Internet is Putting Individuals in Charge and Changing the World We Know*, New York: PublicAffairs.

Shields, R. (ed.) (1996) *Cultures of Internet: Virtual Spaces, Real Histories, Living Bodies*, London: Sage.

Tickner, A. (1992) *Gender in International Relations: Feminist Perspectives on Achieving Global Security*, New York: Columbia University Press.

Tomlinson, J. (1999) *Globalization and Culture*, Cambridge: Polity Press.

United Nations Development Programme (UNDP) (1999) *Human Development Report*, New York: Oxford University Press.

Walker, R. B. J. (1993) *Inside/Outside: International Relations as Political Theory*, Cambridge: Cambridge University Press.

Women in the Digital Age (1998) a Society for International Development and UNESCO publication.

Youngs, G. (1999a) 'Boundary breaking and cyberspace', paper presented at the International Studies Assocation Annual Convention, Washington DC, February: 16–20.

Youngs, G. (1999b) *International Relations in a Global Age: A Conceptual Challenge*, Cambridge: Polity Press.

Youngs, G. (1999c) 'Virtual voices: real lives' in W. Harcourt (ed.) *Women@Internet*, London: Zed Books.

Youngs, G. (2000a) 'Breaking patriarchal boundaries: demythologizing the public/private' in M. H. Marchand and A. S. Runyan (eds) *Gender and Global Restructuring: Sightings, Sites and Resistances*, London: Routledge.
Youngs, G. (ed.) (2000b) *Political Economy, Power and the Body: Global Perspectives*, London: Macmillan.

Websites
Association for Progressive Communications Women's Programme – http:www.apc.org/women
Women on the Net – http://www.waw.be/sid/won/won.htm
Zanzibar Information Technology Center (ZITeC) – http://www.zitec.org

Part II

Leisure, pleasure and consumption

Chapter 6

Understanding computer game cultures

A situated approach

Simeon J. Yates and Karen Littleton

Abstract

This chapter uses data and theory from psychological and sociological sources in order to examine computer gamers' engagement with computer games. The chapter employs data from studies of gender difference in computer game interactions in order to open up theoretically the rich diversity of gamers' interactions with games. The theoretical discussion employs a mix of psychological ideas, especially those of affordances, effectivities and attunement, with ideas from cultural studies, especially those of subject positions and preferred readings. The chapter argues that gaming needs to be viewed as an activity taking place in cultural niches that arise in the complex interaction between games, gamers and gaming cultures.

Introduction

Be it hand-held Nintendo GameBoys™ or networked multi-player sessions of Unreal™ or Rockett's World™, computer games pervade contemporary popular culture. Gaming technologies and the gaming industry are growing at a rapid pace and are converging with existing media production – notably film and video. Despite this, current theorizing about computer gaming has not matched the growing empirical literature. Moreover, the conceptualization of use and engagement with computer games has lagged behind contemporary theorizing of ICT use in work and education. In this chapter we bring together evidence and theory from both sociology and psychology to develop a deeper understanding of computer gaming and gaming cultures. We are specifically interested in using the relationship between gender and computer gaming as a means of opening up and understanding general notions of 'engagement' between gamers and computer games.

Computer gaming involves the use of ICTs for leisure purposes, but, as a number of writers have already noted, leisure use of ICTs is not restricted to computer gaming. Leisure activities also include the use of computer-mediated communications and the World Wide Web. There is evidence that gender differences exist in the use of ICTs for leisure purposes (Green and Adam 1998) and that computer gaming is a male-dominated activity. Work on gender and computer gaming has therefore traditionally focused upon women and girls' exclusion from gaming and gaming cultures. By focusing on their absence from gaming culture such research ignores the voices of those women and girls who do engage with computer games. There is a growing number – if still a minority – of women and girls who actively use computer games. In a recent survey, for instance, Roe and Muijus found that girls accounted for 23.2 per cent of 'heavy users' of computer games (1998). This chapter does not deny the male domination of the production and consumption of computer games, nor does it deny that computer games often contain very sexist or male-orientated content (Dietz 1998). Rather gender difference is used as a means of theorizing the rich diversity of ways in which gamers engage with computer games – and often have to negotiate the various 'preferred readings' of computer games. That is the subject position to which the text is orientated.

Our conceptualization of engagement with computer games and the role of gender in such engagements is based upon two assertions. First, what counts as computer gaming is not fixed but relative and, second, the motivations for computer gaming are dependent upon a set of relative engagements with games software. In both cases the term 'relative' is used to indicate that definitions of, and engagement with, computer games is highly dependent upon a range of elements within the life worlds of the gamers. It is important to note that we are not using gender as a simple explanatory variable – as has often been the case in other studies of computer gaming – but rather we wish to use gender as a means of exploring some of the rich detail in gamers definitions of, and engagement with, computer games in the context of their social lives and leisure practices. In doing this, this chapter attempts to deconstruct what it means to play and engage with computer games.

Current research context

The existing research into gender and computer games has tended to focus on the absence of girls and women from computer culture or upon the need to engage girls and women with computers. There is a large psychological literature investigating the relationship between gender and electronic game playing (Griffiths 1991; Griffiths 1996) which typically presents males as having considerably more computer game experience than females (Subrahmanyam and Greenfield 1994; Greenfield 1995). Moreover, women and girls are presented as being alienated from computer game culture (Stutz 1996). There is a parallel more limited literature in sociology and media studies, mostly echoing the 'media effects debate' (Dominick 1984; Funk and Buchman 1996b). Other sociological literature focuses upon the 'negative' portrayal and absence of women characters in many games (Dietz 1998).

Many of the interventions based upon such research have implicitly assumed that the 'problem' is a 'problem of women and girls' relationship with technology'. As men and boys engage with computers it is girls' lack of engagement with the technology that is defined as the problem to be tackled. Recently the gaming industry itself has attempted to respond to these issues by generating games software designed to engage women and girls. Brenda Laurel, one of the leading figures in the Girls' Games Movement in the USA and founder of Purple Moon software, has stated that:

> Boys tend to have an advantage with computers because they achieve a certain comfort level with the technology by virtue of being motivated by video games to put their hands on it. . . . Girls weren't getting that chance to the same degree because they didn't have things that motivated them in the same way that video games motivated boys.
>
> (Laurel 1998)

Such goals are clearly important and the development of girl-orientated software at Purple Moon and similar organizations has been quite successful. Purple Moon products such as Rockett's World are based on extensive social research into girls' attitudes and interests. There are two problems with this position that prevent such results providing a deeper sociological and psychological understanding of 'why' girls find Rockett's World more engaging than Doom™ or Unreal. Firstly, buried in the arguments made by many in the Girls' Games Movement are a number of implicit essentialist assumptions. The fact that girls and boys have different preferences is assumed and the question is one of catering to them rather than of challenging them. Secondly, there are women gamers who are quite vocal in their opposition to some elements of the Girls' Games Movement. The criticisms made by these women gamers are directed at the ideological positions and definitions of female subjectivities which they see in the products and statements of the Girls' Games Movement. As Nikki Douglas, a Grrl Gamer forcefully stated in response to Sherry Turkle's (1984, 1996) assertion that girls and women prefer community building and non-violent activities:

> Yawwwwnnn. Community and collaboration are what women bring to the table? God, that is so 1950s, so retro, so family and hearth and Donna Reed . . . We don't ever really do anything ground breaking, just create nice little places to live and work and raise our babies! . . . If we work together we can all be friends. Well, screw that! I don't want to be friends! I want to be King! That's right, King, Hail to the King, baby! . . . Not very community driven and collaborative, am I? . . . Maybe it's a problem, Sherry, that little girls DON'T like to play games that slaughter entire planets. Maybe that is why we are still underpaid, still struggling, still fighting for our rights. Maybe if we had the mettle to take on an entire planet, we could fight some of the smaller battles we face every day. Women are not Men and Men are not Women, but all Women are not members of the doily of the month club either.
>
> (N. Douglas, quoted in Jenkins 1998)

Any full understanding of girls' and women's engagement with games software must be able to encompass both the success of enterprises such as Purple Moon[1] and the presence of women who actively engage with existing games software.

First, we need to address the question: what are 'girls and women' or 'boys and men' actually a shorthand for in this debate? We can begin to answer this by exploring how gender positions and roles are constructed in relation to games software. Secondly, by viewing gaming as a socially constructed activity we can begin to explore the set of practices that gamers themselves define as gaming and which in turn they see as defining themselves as gamers. We therefore believe that both positions, that of the Girls' Games Movement and that of Grrl Gamers, can be theoretically encompassed and understood if computer gaming is viewed as a contextually situated and socially constructed activity that draws heavily upon the cultural position of the gamers themselves. We therefore view computer gaming as something that is constructed out of the set of practices that computer gamers engage in. In taking this position this chapter maintains that computer games cannot be viewed from the simple human–computer interaction (HCI) framework that has dominated much previous research. Though all computer games require a person to interact with a computer, defining computer gaming in such a simple and nominalist fashion ignores the range of practices that gamers themselves define as gaming. In the following sections the 'relational conception of computer games and computer gaming' will be developed in two stages. First, the issue of interaction and engagement with the software itself will be addressed and the need to place such engagement in its social and cultural context will be pointed out. Second, the social and cultural context of gaming by viewing gaming from the perspective of media consumption rather than human computer interaction will be considered.

Data sources

This chapter makes use of two main sources of empirical data. First, it draws upon a body of psychological research (Littleton et al. 1998; Littleton et al. in press) which has explored various aspects of children's engagement with computer software as well as their affective responses to computer use and gaming. Second, the chapter draws upon a participant observation ethnographic study of a group of adult computer game-players. This data includes separate focus group discussions with the men and women gamers within this group. The group itself consists of young professionals in the age range 20–35, mostly with experience of computing or managerial work. One important feature of the group is the role played by computer gaming, specifically networked computer gaming, in a number of their social leisure activities. In making use of these two data sources we recognize that we are bringing together very diverse approaches to understanding issues surrounding gender and computer games. This data is not intended to be exhaustive nor, especially in the case of the focus group material, representative of other groups, but we believe that it provides the basis for new theoretical insights.

Women and girl's engagement with games

In order to explore the specific differences in players' engagement with computer games we will draw upon psychological theories of engagement with technologies through the use of the concept of 'affordances'. Though originally developed in the context of psychological theories of perception (Gibson 1977) the relational nature of the concept of affordances provides a useful tool in explaining the situated interaction among actors or between actors and objects. When an actor interacts with some other 'system' the conditions that enable that interaction include properties of both the actor and the system. Interactions can therefore be seen to have two important elements. First, the contributing properties of the system and overall environment provide the 'affordances'. Second, the actor(s) contribute specific 'abilities' or 'effectivities' that allow them to make use of the available affordances (Shaw et al. 1982; Greeno 1994). Such a model is useful when considering the use of technologies as it provides a framework for exploring the richness of the interaction without recourse to polarized debates over 'technological-determinism'. Understanding the available affordances and effectivities provides the basis for understanding 'constraints' upon the type of interaction taking place. One of the key parts of this process is that of understanding which and what type of affordance the actor can perceive as being available to them, and which of their 'abilities' or 'effectivities' they can deploy. As Greeno notes in a discussion of Gibson's work:

> He proposed that a mailbox provides an affordance for the posting of letters, and it surely does that. It seems likely that for most people, in most if not all circumstances, the processes of cognizing that affordance includes classifying the physical object as a mail box.
>
> (Greeno 1994)

This therefore implies that a key part of the process of perceiving affordances involves the use of existing conceptual systems. This provides the opportunity of linking the situated interaction of user and technology to the wider social and cultural context which provide the conceptual systems upon which that interaction is based. The 'tuning of particular persons to the particular demands and opportunities of a situation, thus resides in the combination of person-in-situation, not "in the mind" alone' (Snow 1994). Moreover, if the person-in-situation becomes key then we need to understand more about how people come to be 'tuned' and how and why they perceive particular affordances in a situation. Situations are also cultural and psychological spaces as well as physical spaces and therefore require 'attunement to the attunement of others' (Rommetveit 1992). 'Attunement' therefore depends upon a person's reading of the technology in relation to both the interpersonal and the cultural context. From a sociological perspective how we read the technology and the social context depends upon the manner in which we have been positioned by the discourses tied to the technology and to the situation. We can therefore view the manner in which the affordances of games software are read as being dependent upon the discourses in which the user is situated. At the same time the user must interpret the effectivities they can bring to bear. The effectivities they bring will depend upon the affordances they have read and upon the cultural practices and resources that their discursive position provides.

By combining arguments from both sociological and psychological theory we can view the 'person-in situation' as a 'cultural niche' within which the often conflicting demands of various discourses and practices define the reading of affordances and the application of effectivities. The conception of abilities, or effectivities, as linked to affordances emphasizes the importance of the 'attunement' between person and situation. It is unlikely therefore that players will engage with a game unless their cultural and discursive position make it possible for the affordances of the game and their effectivities to work together. In the discussions that follow we will deploy the results of studying gender differences in understanding players' readings of affordances and their own effectivities and therefore their level and type of engagement with computer games.

Girls, engagement and software design

In this section an overview of the results of a number of socio-psychological studies are given which have highlighted the importance of both context and content in understanding children's interaction with software. These studies also make clear that differences in boys' and girls' interactions with software are not the product of differences in innate physical or psychological abilities.

As noted previously, affordances are not just read off from objects, they are also signalled by the broader social and cultural context within which the object is set. The importance of this was demonstrated by Littleton et al. in a study of children's interaction with a software 'game/task' (Littleton et al. in press). In this study the context of a computer-based task was varied without making any changes at all to the software itself. For this study a piece of software modelled on a physical game was produced. The physical version of the game involves manoeuvring a metal ring around a bent wire in such a way as not to touch the wire. If the ring touches the wire, it closes a circuit and makes a buzz. The software version of this 'game/task' involves a mouse-controlled cursor that represents a section through the metal ring and a deformed angular line representing the wire. The parameters of the task were set so that 11-year-olds would suffer at least a few collisions, despite their best efforts. In the study the software was represented either as a game (called Electric Eel) or as a skills test. Analyses performed on the frequency of collisions revealed that when the software was introduced to the children as a test there was no gender difference in performance. By contrast, where exactly the same task was introduced as a game, the boys' and girls' performance diverged to a point where there was a significant gender difference, favouring the boys. So even with a single, standard piece of software (tapping, on the face of it, basic sensory motor skills) children's performance can be significantly affected by the way in which that software is presented and therefore read.

This study emphasizes the importance of social and cultural context on the readings made of software. At the same time it also seems to imply that girls have problems engaging with games. In a different set of studies, however, Littleton et al. (1998) demonstrated that the issue is not simply one of games versus tasks but rather the type and content of games.

Two structurally isomorphic versions of a problem solving 'adventure game' were produced. The first, named 'King and Crown', consisted of a quest to recover a king's missing crown without encountering pirates and other obstacles. The second, called 'Honeybears', consisted of a quest to recover the bears' missing honey while trying to avoid honey monsters. Both games required the same solution strategy. Each game had characters with specific roles such as Pilot, Driver and Captain in the King and Crown; Airbear, Ponybear and Waterbear in the Honeybears. The representation of the bears in 'Honeybears' was as gender neutral as possible whereas the King and Crown contained more overtly male characters.

Littleton et al. conducted a series of studies that made direct comparisons between the performance – as measured by successful moves – of 11 to 12-year-old girls and boys working with the two versions. They found that the girls' performance was substantially affected by the version of the software in use, it being far superior for 'Honeybears'. On the other hand the boys' performance was little affected by the version of the software they were using. Such a result highlights the importance of content upon users' reading of software. Despite the constraints and demands of the task being identical in both versions of the software, the images and metaphors used to 'carry' the task had a crucial bearing on girls' interaction with the software. These results are viewed as evidence that the engagement of the children with the software was highly dependent upon their discursively constructed subject positions. The different metaphors and representations in the software provide the different possible readings of the software made by the children. Following Hall (1980, 1997), such readings are viewed as constructing a range of possible 'subject positions'. These subject positions, and therefore the read affordances, allow the children to interpret the effectivities they can bring to bear. These two sets of studies make clear that explanations of girls' engagement with games must focus on practices and activities situated in particular social and cultural contexts. These studies also highlight the weakness of arguments based upon claims about innate skills or preferences.

Women, engagement and software design

The interaction of the children with both the context and content of software can be viewed in terms of the preferred readings of a text. In the case of the children, both the content ('Honeybears' versus 'Kings and Crown') or the context (game versus work-related skills) allow them to take up subject positions from which they can read the game's affordances and therefore attune themselves to the task. In making this argument we are viewing games and computing technology as a medium to be read like any other media text or technology. There has been considerable research into the gender readings of soap operas and related television programming (Brunsdon 1982; Modleski 1982; Ang 1985). More specifically a number of writers have focused upon the manner in which soap operas are orientated towards gendered preferred readings that draw upon the cultural competencies of women rather than men; that is they draw upon the 'learned interpretative frameworks and reading skills employed by different social groups . . . to decode signs and representations' (Gledhill 1997). For most computer games the case is inverted with the preferred readings being orientated to male subject positions and cultural competencies.

In interviews with adult gamers for this chapter, this issue of engagement and the negotiation of readings and subject positions was explored. As part of the focus group interview the participants were asked to discuss those elements of the games they played which they found most engaging. This was achieved by asking a number of questions about what first drew them to gaming, what elements they liked most about the games they currently played and by asking them to think up an 'ideal' game. The women highlighted a number of different elements they found engaging: these included exploring, problem-solving, planning, graphics and gender representations. Each of the women had their own clearly articulated favoured combination of these elements. For one woman the chance to explore 'new worlds' was most important:

DWF   I like the exploring, I like . . . Almost as if you were in a place you had never been before you sort of looking round the next corner going through doors and finding what's in the next room and discovering things . . . second after that is puzzle solving.

For another the problem-solving element was key:

IVA   It's definitely the problem solving side be it working out for Day of the Tentacle or Discworld that I need this, this and this in this order or be it I know I have to take three steps a running jump and a back flip . . . it's all problem solving.

For another it was the strategy and planning elements:

EMI   I like planning. I think the nice thing about strategy things is that you're responsible for what happens. It's all played out for you without you really being affected.

Such a diversity within one small group of women gamers implies, as does the Honeybears result, that what makes games 'boring' (Laurel 1998) or 'exciting' for girls and women is not the underlying structure of the game but the content through which this is activated. At the same time their engagements were negotiated in terms of other elements of their personal life, such as work or other leisure interests. Two of the women noted that much of the planning and strategy elements were akin to their day-to-day work practices:

EMI   In my situation it's not dissimilar to work but it's a really nice safe environment in which to do it.
INT   So when the monsters eat all your troops and you've lost it does not matter.
EMI   [Laughter] Yes, there you go.
DWF   I wish real life was like that where you could save at a point, try something.
IVA   Exactly, if it goes to pot, [laughter] go back and try something different.
EMI   It's a bit of a fantasy there – if only life was like that.

Another noted that 'driving games' fitted elements of her own self-conception:

IVA   I like the driving as well. I haven't played the driving game for a while but I think I'm a girl racer and I like that. It simulates the speed type thing.

All of the above can be viewed in terms of the women selecting and negotiating subject positions – drawn from their own life worlds – that allow them to engage with games software through the employment of specific cultural competencies. The women, however, clearly articulated some of the problems faced in negotiating and countering the male-gendered preferred readings within the games. When asked to describe their perfect game one woman replied:

IVA   Like Tomb Raider only instead of having scantily clad women who would I have? Have Mel Gibson! [Laughter]

She later went on to qualify this statement in the following way:

IVA   Actually thinking about it, going back to Tomb Raider thing and me saying scantily clad men, actually probably I wouldn't because I know that there are a lot of sad muppets out there who that go for large . . . you know fellas because she's a scantily clad woman and so on, but I actually like it being a woman albeit she's not too way out like some of the new ones because I'm a woman and that's my skill, so I . . . it's more visualization of myself on the character. Whereas if it was a man I think it would be much more not me, if you see what I mean.

The problem faced here is one of fighting the male readings of Tomb Raider™. Tomb Raider sets up a classic male subject position for the player that reflects those provided in other media such as film and television in which the female (in this case Lara Croft) is passively watched rather than actively watched. Yet at the same time Lara Croft is the hero of the game and the most active character in it. This provides the opportunity for a reading of the game in which the women can take a proactive subject position. Despite this the women disliked the male readings that Lara Croft's physical appearance were orientated towards:

IVA   I don't like the ones that they've started to bring out, they've all coming out with these Lara Croft clones, but if you look at them a lot of them are very erm, I mean okay, Lara Croft, I mean nobody, nobody with that chest size could run like that. [Laughter] . . . I mean some of the new ones they are bringing out are really, really stupid. Now I guess that appeals to the fellas more but from my point of view that's just . . . stupid . . . At least she's wearing the sort of outfit you can just about imagine, okay, but you could just about imagine somebody that was doing that kind of discovery would actually wear that kind of get-up. So it's sort of that one does seem like you're playing it yourself, so I take it back about the Mel Gibson look alike [Laughter]

In analysing this and similar interactions it becomes clear that when discussing the elements of games with which they engage, women are distinguishing between structural elements (for example, problem-solving and strategy) with the representational elements (for example, characters and graphics). In making these distinctions the women made use of game genres in order to distinguish between general game types. Such genres included 'first-person-shoot-em-ups', 'god-games', 'strategy-games', 'networked games', 'driving games', 'fighting games' and so forth. These distinctions worked by focusing on structural or content elements or combinations of both, making it possible for games to be both a strategy and a networked game. Game genres are clearly a resource that gamers employ in their reading of games and provide the basis for expectations about the structure, content and affordances provided by a game. The flexibility and interactivity of digital media may in fact place a greater reliance on genre as a way into the reading of texts and technologies (Yates and Sumner 1997).

The men made similar distinctions and their perfect game had a number of similar structural elements to that of the women. It involved a multi-player strategy and planning game with one person controlling the overall activity of several others, each having their own role. There were a number of important differences in the nature of their discussion, as compared to the women. The men, for instance, spent a considerable amount of time discussing specific structural details of the games and their engagement with these. Such discussions included consideration of whether or not a character could swim or leave footprints in a specific 'first-person-shoot-em-up' (Doom™). The men's use of game genre was far more extensive than the women's and involved finer grain distinctions. What is most notably lacking in the men's discussion is any need to contest the dominant or preferred readings of the games.

It is clear that the gamers studied here employed complex and diverse readings of the games. More specifically in relation to the concepts of affordances and effectivities, the ability to read affordances and therefore employ effectivities is dependent upon the users' interaction with both the content and the context of the games they are playing. These readings and interactions are themselves made possible by the subject positions that the gamers take up. These subject positions provide the basis upon which the gamers can attune their effectivities to the game's affordances through the cultural competencies that they bring to the gaming context.

In the case of the women gamers, it is clear that elements from other areas of their life and worlds provide the competencies for reading and engaging with the software. At the same time as playing, they are actively negotiating and resisting some of the preferred readings and subject positions inherent in the games, something which the men do not do. From this position both the success of Girls' Games products and the oppositional positions of some Grrl Gamers can be explained. First, Girls' Games products succeed by allowing girls to attune their effectives to the affordances of the games through the use of structural and content elements that set up girl orientated preferred readings and subject positions. Just as soap operas can be seen as having preferred readings based in female cultural competencies (Brunsdon 1982), so can successful 'girl-orientated' games. At the same time, the Grrl Gamers who make criticisms of such software (mostly adults) are able to negotiate the male-orientated preferred readings inherent in contemporary games. In doing this, a number of Grrl Gamers have taken up subject positions which are critical of some of the ideological positions that they perceive in the Girls' Games Movement. These ideological positions derive from the ways in which Girls' Games draw upon and reflect society's current dominant discourses and ideologies of femininity.

Gaming and being a gamer in context

In order to complete our analysis of gendered engagement with computer games we need to consider two issues. First, the assertion that games need to be viewed as media texts has implications for how we view and theorize gamers. Second, how gamers view 'gaming' needs to be considered. It is interesting to note that players of computer games are still conceptualized as 'individuals' in a one-to-one relationship with the medium, while television viewers form 'audiences'. At the same time a number of research projects have sought to identify the common social and cultural characteristics of these individuals – in essence viewing them as an atomized mass. This conceptualization has to be challenged on two grounds. First, given the current prevalence of networked games – in addition to changes in the overall patterns of media consumption to include interactive and Internet-based media – gamers form very large and highly connected communities. Second, such a conceptualization reflects some of the initial models of television and radio audiences. More recent work has focused upon the differentiated and negotiated character of media consumption and audience membership. As Thompson notes in criticism of the idea of a mass audience:

> the messages transmitted by the mass media are received by specific individuals in definite social–historical contexts. These individuals . . . actively interpret and make sense of these messages and relate them to other aspects of their lives. This ongoing appropriation of media messages is an inherently critical and socially differentiated process . . . there are systematic variations . . . which are linked to socially structured differences in the audience.
>
> (Thompson 1988: 365–6)

Support for such a claim about the 'audience' for games can be seen in the previous discussion of men and women's engagement with games. Having said this, a central part of actively interpreting and appropriating media lies in constructing a subject position of being part of an audience and, in the case of television, of being a viewer. This is also the case for games and gaming. One possible gender difference between male and female engagement with games might arise from the willingness or not to assume the subject position of a gamer.

Costs of being a gamer

The authors' recent work (Littleton et al. in press), which involves the in-depth interviewing of girls and boys about their use of computers, reveals that there are social costs to taking up a gaming or active computer-user subject position. In the interviews children talked about the penalties associated with being characterized as a 'boff', a 'geek' or a 'jonah' (loner). Similarly, in the focus group discussions with adult gamers the men were overtly aware of this. As one man noted in response to the rest of the group's enthusiastic descriptions of their first encounters with computer games:

MD   When I started playing games everyone who played computer games were just complete geekoid nerds . . . something I didn't want to admit, kept it really quiet.

A number of researchers have noted that various media can carry cultural stigmas through being 'socially disvalued'; consequently such media are then viewed as markers of delinquent or socially disparaged behaviour (Creasey and Myers 1986; Roe 1995; Funk and Buchman 1996a). In the same manner that being an active fan of soap operas has at times been socially stigmatized, so has being an active computer game player. This perception of computer games reflects some of the academic and public discourses on gaming which have tended to focus on issues such as 'addiction', 'social isolation' and 'impaired social skills'. These same discourses have been appropriated into popular culture and are reflected in the children and adults' statements about 'being a gamer'. As the quote from MD implies, gamers are therefore required to negotiate their gaming subject position in relation to the other subject positions they have to take up in other areas of their life.

Women and being a gamer

Contained within the writings of a number of social scientists (Turkle 1984, 1996; Hoyles 1988) and the Girls' Games Movement (Laurel 1998), are claims that girls and women are more concerned than boys and men about the role and use of ICTs in social relationships and social perceptions. If this is the case, then the social stigma of taking up the subject position of being a gamer is likely to have more of an impact upon women and girls than on men and boys. Evidence for this might be found in the 'Electric Eel' study by Littleton et al. (1998) where the boys appeared to take on the gamer role and view the activity as a game more readily than the girls. It is interesting to note that the women gamers we interviewed seemed constantly to be negotiating complex subject positions for themselves, positions in which they 'were but were not' active game players. This negotiation is interesting for a number of reasons. First, their knowledge of games was as detailed, if not more so, than male games players known to the interviewer who actively expressed their interest in computer games. Second, the extent to which the women individually negotiated their position clearly differed from the males. When asked, for instance, if they ever held women-only gaming sessions, the women provided a mixed answer:

DWF   We don't play games without setting up with the blokes, we don't play games together.
EMI/IVA   [inaudible]
DWF   We've used computers together, you and I do, but we don't play games, we use them for designing web pages and doing our [IVA: Needlework] cross-stitch patterns . . . Not game playing.
EMI   Although when you've been away we've been down and played.
DWF   Oh right . . .
EMI   Because that's when I did that Starcraft, Starcraft. But we've never done a just girls, a girl's thing.
IVA   Didn't we play Whacky Wheelers? I've forgotten about Whacky Wheelers.
DWF   I remember but it was just the two of us there and we hap-pened to have the two PCs but we never organized it . . .
IVA   No, we've never organized a meeting and stuff . . .

In this interaction it is clear that the women are stressing the fact that they do not organize their own gaming sessions. At the same time, both here and in the rest of the discussion, they acknowledge their exten-sive and active use of computers and the range of games that they have played. In the above interaction DWF appears to construct a position of having knowledge of games but not being an active gamer. This posi-tion is partly negated by the assertions of IVA and EMI that they have played games. Here, and elsewhere in the discussion, the women set up games as being fun leisure activities, especially when played as part of a social group, but they are not central to their personal or social leisure activities. This often led to a discussion of the relationship between the women's and men's social gaming activity. The women did not see their social gaming as being 'tagged on to' the men's activity:

IVA   I wouldn't say tagged on but involves them. We don't . . . It's not something we do as a choice separate from them, it's something we do as a choice jointly with them.
DWF   Part of the social event [EMI: Yes] rather than seen as means to an end. [EMI/IVA: Umm] They get together to play games

we get together as a social event [*EMI*: Yes] and the game play-ing happens to be part [*IVA*: Yes] of it and we take part.

As part of this discussion the women commented upon various elements of such events that they viewed as enjoyable leisure time. This included different levels of interaction with the game and game playing. IVA, for instance, described how she found watching the men playing a net-worked game enjoyable in itself: 'you do get involved with it, I do enjoy watching them play not just watching the game, I enjoy watching the comments, some of the comments are hilarious.'

This aspect of game-playing being part of a relationship with male friends and partners was a recurring theme. When asked how they started playing games, one of the women stated:

IVA   I think it was, well for me it was playing, it was something I could be doing on the computer the same time as Shaun because again if he's sitting in front of the computer it can be very isolating. So we got into playing Day of the Tentacle because it's something we could sit and do together. I think Tomb Raider was the first game I really started playing on my own. Every other game has been as part of a thing so that we could play together. Do something of an evening apart from watching the television. [Laughter] Although quite how different it is watch-ing a computer than watching the television, I don't know [Laughter] . . .

The implication that one of the routes into gaming was through rela-tionships with male partners also reflects the role of the PC within the household. Despite the fact that the households represented in the group were those of dual-working, young, mostly computing professionals, many of the same gender roles adopted in relation to the computer mirrored those related to domestic technology (Cockburn 1992; Wheelock 1992). The women perceived the computer initially as something for work rather than leisure. Although the women then noted how this changed as they re-evaluated the computer and computer gaming in the light of their use of other media:

DWF   I thought they were a waste of time until you expressed the way that one wasted a lot of time watching TV, which is again when he plays games. [*EMI*: Yes] I must admit just recently

TV starts to bore me. I do, especially if he is out [*EMI*: Yes] I'll go and play games.

In comparing the statements made by both women and men it is clear that both are aware of the possible social stigma of being viewed as a gamer. In the case of the men, this was directly addressed. In the case of the women, addressing this issue involved the negotiation of a number of other subject positions, including those connected with other forms of ICT use in the home, with work, with relationships with male friends and partners and possibly with other media use.

Conclusion

Throughout, this chapter has presented evidence and arguments that stress the importance of viewing computer gaming from a social and cultural perspective. In doing this, the chapter rejects the nominalist and HCI-based approach that underlies many previous studies. It has been argued that if we are to understand gamers' engagement with computer games, both empirically and theoretically, the following must be explored:

- the affordances inherent to games – both technological and cultural;
- the effectivities of gamers – derived from their life experiences;
- games as media texts which therefore carry preferred readings;
- gamers as having cultural competencies through which to read games;
- how the reading of games foregrounds certain affordances;
- how the reading of games sets up subject positions for gamers;
- how subject positions mobilize gamers' effectivities.

Taking all these elements together we view gaming as taking place in 'cultural niches' which arise in the complex interaction between games, gamers and gaming cultures. Understanding the engagements of men and women and girls and boys with games therefore requires an understanding of the cultural niches in which such interactions take place. An important part of this process is taking up the subject position of being an active gamer. The discursive achievement of 'gamer' is very complex since it requires the negotiation of both the preferred readings inherent to games and the current, often disparaging, discourses about gaming. In the context of the current rapid development of both games technology and the games industry, the empirical and theoretical exploration of the elements set out above constitute a challenging and exciting way forward.

Note

1 It is interesting to note that, as this chapter was being written, Purple Moon was taken over by its main competitor, Mattel, whose girl games software, based around 'Barbie'™ dolls, lack the feminist elements of Purple Moon's products.

References

Ang, I. (1985) *Watching Dallas: Soap Opera and the Melodramatic Imagination*, New York: Methuen.

Brunsdon, C. (1982) 'Crossroads: notes on soap opera', *Screen*, 22 (4): 32–7.

Cockburn, C. (1992) 'The circuit of technology: gender, identity and power' in R. Silverstone and E. Hirsch (eds) *Consuming Technologies: Media and Information in Domestic Spaces*, London: Routledge.

Creasey, G. L. and Myers, B. J. (1986) 'Video games and children: effects on leisure activities, schoolwork, and peer involvement', *Merrill-Palmer Quarterly*, 32 (3): 251–62.

Dietz, T. L. (1998) 'An examination of violence and gender role portrayals in video games: implications for gender socialisation and aggressive behaviour', *Sex Roles*, 38 (5/6): 425–42.

Dominick, J. R. (1984) 'Video games, television violence and aggression in teenagers', *Journal of Communication*, 34: 136–47.

Funk, J. B. and Buchman, D. D. (1996a) 'Children's perception of gender differences in approval for playing electronic games', *Sex Roles*, 35 (3/4): 219–31.

Funk, J. B. and Buchman, D. D. (1996b) 'Playing violent video and computer games and adolescent self-concept', *Journal of Communication*, 46: 19–32.

Gibson, J. J. (1977) 'The theory of affordances' in R. Shaw and J. Bransford (eds) *Perceiving, Acting and Knowing: Toward an Ecological Psychology*, Hilsdale: Erlbaum.

Gledhill, C. (1997) 'Genre and gender: the case of soap opera' in S. Hall (ed.) *Representation: Cultural Representations and Signifying Practices*, London: Sage in association with the Open University.

Green, E. and Adam, A. (1998) 'On-line leisure: gender and ICTs in the home', *Information, Communication and Society*, 1 (3): 291–312.

Greenfield, T. (1995) 'Sex differences in science museum exhibit attraction', *Journal of Research in Science Teaching*, 32: 925–38.

Greeno, J. G. (1994) 'Gibson's affordances', *Psychological Review*, 101 (2): 336–42.

Griffiths, M. (1991) 'Amusement machine playing in childhood and adolescence: a comparative analysis of video games and fruit machines', *Journal of Adolescence*, 14: 53–73.

Griffiths, M. (1996) 'Computer game-playing in children and adolescents: a review of the literature' in T. Gill (ed.) *Electronic Children: How Children are*

Responding to the Information Revolution, London: National Children's Bureau.

Hall, S. (1980) 'Encoding/decoding' in CFCC Studies (ed.) *Culture, Media, Language*, London: Hutchinson.

Hall, S. (1997) 'The work of representation' in S. Hall (ed.) *Representation: Cultural Representations and Signifying Practices*, London: Sage in association with the Open University.

Hoyles, C. (ed.) (1988) *Girls and Computers*, Bedford Way Papers 34, London: Institute of Education.

Jenkins, H. (1998) 'Voices from the combat zone: Game Grrlz talk back' in J. Cassell and H. Jenkins (eds) *From Barbie to Mortal Kombat: Gender and Computer Games*, London: MIT Press.

Laurel, B. (1998) 'An interview with Brenda Laurel (Purple Moon)' in J. Cassell and H. Jenkins (eds) *From Barbie to Mortal Kombat: Gender and Computer Games*, London: MIT Press.

Littleton, K., Light, P., Joiner, R., Messer, D. and Barnes, P. (1998) 'Gender, task scenarios and children's and children's computer-based problem solving', *Educational Psychology*, 18 (3): 327–40.

Littleton, K., Ashman, H., Light, P., Artis, J., Roberts, T. and Oosterwegel, A. (in press) 'Gender, task contexts and children's performance on a computer-based task', *European Journal of Psychology of Education*.

Modleski, T. (1982) *Loving with a Vengeance: Mass-Produced Fantasies for Women*, New York: Methuen.

Roe, K. (1995) 'Adolescents' use of socially disvalued media: towards a theory of media delinquency', *Journal of Youth and Adolescence*, 24 (5): 617–31.

Roe, K. and Muijus, D. (1998) 'Children and computer games', *European Journal of Communication*, 13 (2): 181–200.

Rommetveit, R. (1992) 'Outlines of a dialogically based social-cognitive approach to human cognition and communication' in A. Wold (ed.) *The Dialogical Alternative: Towards a Theory of Language and Mind*, Oslo: Scandinavian Press.

Shaw, R., Turvey, M. T. and Mace, W. (1982) 'Ecological psychology: the consequences of a commitment to realism' in W. Weimer and D. Palermo (eds) *Cognition and the Symbolic Processes II*, Hillsdale: Erlbaum.

Snow, R. (1994) 'Abilities in academic tasks' in R. Sternberg and R. Wagner (eds) *Mind in Context: Interactionist Perspectives on Human Intelligence*, Cambridge: Cambridge University Press.

Stutz, E. (1996) 'Is electronic entertainment hindering children's play and social development?' in T. Gill (ed.) *Electronic Children: How Children are Responding to the Information Revolution*, London: National Children's Bureau.

Subrahmanyam, K. and Greenfield, P. (1994) 'Effect of video-game practice on spatial skills in girls and boys', *Journal of Applied Developmental Psychology*, 15: 13–32.

Thompson, J. (1988) 'Mass communication and modern culture: contribution to a critical theory of ideology', *Sociology*, 22 (3): 359–83.

Turkle, S. (1984) *The Second Self: Computers and Human Spirit*, New York: Simon and Schuster.

Turkle, S. (1996) *Life on the Screen*, New York: Simon and Schuster.

Wheelock, J. (1992) 'Personal computers, gender and an institutional model of the household' in R. Silverstone and E. Hirsch (eds) *Consuming Technologies: Media and Information in Domestic Spaces*, London: Routledge.

Yates, S. J. and Sumner, T. (1997) 'Digital genres and the new burden of fixity, paper presented at the Hawaii International Conference on System Sciences, Maui, Hawaii.

Chapter 7

Visual pleasure in textual places

Gazing in multi-user object-oriented worlds

Michèle White

Abstract

This chapter relates the textual processes of looking and gazing on MOOs (multi-user object-oriented worlds) to feminist theories of the gaze. The gaze and look are privileged terms in these chat oriented settings because of the programming decision to associate information inquiries with the typed command to 'look <character or object name>'. The use of the look command makes it seem that physiognomy-oriented character descriptions and architecturally familiar room types can be seen. Many users want to believe that character descriptions offer a view that is like the 'real' body of the user. The constructed nature of the character, literally produced by text, is partially concealed by the insistence that the metaphorical sight of the look is the equivalent of truth. A series of other commands, such as @watch, @peruse, @kgb, @fbi, @scope, @glance, @peep, @gawk and @see, also emphasize sight so that the textual setting is made over into a visual space. The names of these commands, and the detailed sets of information that they supply, make users aware of the transparent structure of the MOO and its surveillant aspects. The virtual look of certain characters, penetrating into any 'space' in order to examine other characters and determine their gender, renders an empowered gaze. The mastering gaze of characters and the voyeuristic terminology of MOO commands perpetuate a series of limiting identity constructs. This chapter establishes some preliminary ways to interrogate these identity processes and advocates further critical considerations of the ways that bodies, spaces and objects are constructed online.

Introduction

This chapter describes how textual forms of looking and gazing function on MOOs, like LambdaMOO, work. Feminist theories about the gaze are employed in order to interrogate the MOO's construction of virtual sight. There is a wealth of feminist and gender scholarship that considers how the gaze, which can be defined as a form of power-laden staring, produces and enforces gendered positions but the gaze of the Internet user remains largely unconsidered. Gazing must be radically rethought in online settings because the traditional relationship between subject and object is problematized by the loss of both Cartesian space and the unitary self. Any critical consideration of the ways that bodies, spaces and objects are constructed online must contend with the specific aspects of each interface. The wide variety of online technologies, which include the World Wide Web, usenet, gopher, CU-SeeME and MUDs (which different users have defined as multi-user dungeons, domains or dimensions), provide vastly different experiences that cannot be explained adequately by a singular theory of the gaze.

This chapter provides some preliminary tools for critiquing looking relations in MOO settings, which can be revised in order to examine other interfaces. For instance, this consideration of the virtual look on MOOs could be amended to consider other text-based chat spaces, including MUDs, which also employ the virtual look. This study begins with a description of MOOs and an outline of some of the essential scholarship on the gaze. An appendix provides a compendium of the basic MOO terms and commands that are discussed in this chapter. A close reading of the MOO setting is employed in order to demonstrate the ways that looking and gazing produce a version of the material body online and regulate virtual characters.[1]

MOOs

MOOs are a form of MUDs. MUDs are a 'class of multi-player interactive game, accessible via the Internet or a modem' (*Free On-Line Dictionary of Computing*, 1998). LambdaMOO is the oldest MOO and probably has the largest population. LambdaMOO has been Internet accessible since October 1990 (Curtis 1992) and currently has 5,526 characters (LambdaMOO 1999a). Xerox originally ran LambdaMOO as part of a research project to design online settings in which scientists could communicate (Curtis 1993). Stanford University and Placeware Incorporated now support the MOO.

LambdaMOO is described as 'a new kind of society, where thousands of people voluntarily come together from all over the world' (LambdaMOO 1999b). Users can participate in a real time setting because MOOs facilitate multiple simultaneous connections. When users log in to the host's computer they see an initial welcoming screen that provides some information about the system and advice on how to behave in this virtual setting. Individuals can connect either as a named character, which they have previously constructed, or as a guest. While named characters have a more stable identity within the system, all characters have a unique name and number. MOOs have specific rules and codes that the participants must consent to in order to log in. On LambdaMOO these codes are outlined in a 'help manners' document that is available to the general community (anyone who has logged in). Some users find it difficult to adjust to the idea of speaking about these structures as communities. There is no physically embodied interaction between people online and there is no specific 'real' space in which interactions take place. These virtual settings are completely text based. All communication on the MOO is accomplished through descriptions that appear on the screen.

Most of the material in this chapter will be based on LambdaMOO and its programming language. The MOO's object-oriented programming, which is similar to the C++ and Java computer languages, allows users to change the structure by designing such objects as rooms, manipulable things and characters. This programming is also used, sometimes in a less elaborate form, on other MOOs. The MOO presents a particularly useful first case study for an examination of the virtual gaze because of the accessibility of the MOO's programming language and its detailed help system that provides online documentation for many of the MOO's most common aspects. A variety of MOO commands, such as @show, @list, @verbs and @examine, allow users to gain additional information about objects, including the way that they were programmed. This means that the MOO's programmed code is available for analysis and critique. The 'help' for individual interactive objects, which often includes the programmer's comments, also provides insight into the ways that the system contextualizes texts.

The look and the gaze

An initial consideration of MOOs with their textual base may make a consideration of looking relations and a theory of the gaze an unlikely project. Users virtually look in order to navigate their characters through

the system because of the programming decision to associate information inquiries with the 'look' verb or the user's consistent typed commands to look at other characters, rooms and objects. So, the user initiates
a command to look and the user and character presumably sees when
the system generates a description. The experience of reading text is
supplanted by a doctrine of looking and seeing. It is perhaps not surprising, considering the vernacular of these systems, that participants
often comment that they 'haven't read anything lately'.[2]

The MOO's visual vernacular and optical processes allow users to
preserve the presumed naturalness of the material body and its accom-
panying technologies online. To look is after all 'to ascertain by the
use of one's eyes' (*Merriam Webster Dictionary*, 1998). It is associated
with the gaze because to look is 'to exercise the power of vision upon'
someone or something. The look could be associated with the MOO's
process of information inquiries because it also means 'to make sure'.
This suggests that the term 'look' might be employed on MOOs
because of the ubiquity of visual metaphors in the English language.
The term 'look' may mean a number of different things on MOOs but
it evokes sight even when it isn't explicitly about the process of seeing.
In these cases, the primacy of vision is still an underlying ideology. The
following passage simultaneously performs and critiques the ways
that the visual has permeated our linguistic practices. It suggests that
an examination of the MOO's vernacular can allow us to disable its
more limiting terms.

> Even a rapid glance at the language we commonly use will demon-
> strate the ubiquity of visual metaphors . . . Depending, of course,
> on one's outlook or point of view, the prevalence of such
> metaphors will be counted an obstacle or an aid to our knowledge
> of reality. It is, however, no idle speculation or figment of imagi-
> nation to claim that if blinded to their importance, we will dam-
> age our ability to inspect the world outside and inspect the world
> within. And our prospects for escaping their thrall, if indeed that
> is ever our foreseeable goal, will be greatly dimmed.
>
> (Jay 1994: 1)

Jay's passage suggests that the employment of visual metaphors
produces significant effects. On MOOs the visual vernacular recreates
parts of the physical world in order to structure a particular kind of
reality. The virtual look, because it seems to provide access to 'real'
bodies, is often employed as part of a conservative tendency to resist

gender transgressions (cross-dressing, defying gender characteristics and discrepancies between the character's set gender and typed pronouns). The constructed nature of the body, literally produced by text, is partially concealed by the insistence that the metaphorical sight of the look is the equivalent of truth.

A common dictionary definition of the gaze is 'to fix the eyes in a steady and intent look and often with eagerness or studious attention' (*Merriam Webster Dictionary*, 1998). Salecel and Zizek describe the gaze as 'the medium of control (in the guise of the inspecting gaze) as well as of the fascination that entices the other into submission (in the guise of the subject's gaze bewitched by the spectacle of power)' (1996: 3).

The overlap in the meaning of the look and gaze, both in dictionary definitions and in academic scholarship, suggests a similar conflation of these terms on MOOs. There is a direct relationship between virtually looking and gazing but not all MOO looks are equally related to the feminist psychoanalytical criticism that has produced some of the most significant contemporary theories of the gaze. Mulvey (1986) describes a deeply gendered process of looking and being looked at in 'visual pleasure and narrative cinema'. This chapter, which was originally published in the Autumn 1975 issue of *Screen*, presented a ground-breaking analysis of the classical narrative cinema. Mulvey argues that the cinema spectator gains a sense of agency by identifying with the active male protagonist. She 'attributed the polarity of gender, of masculinity versus femininity, to the very structures of identification in the classical cinema' (Mayne 1994: 48). The subject of the gaze is male, assisted by an implicit association with the camera's viewpoint, while its object is female:

> In a world ordered by sexual imbalance, pleasure in looking has been split between an active/male and passive/female. The determining male gaze projects its fantasy onto the female figure, which is styled accordingly. In their traditional exhibitionist role women are simultaneously looked at and displayed, with their appearance coded for strong visual and erotic impact so that they can be said to connote to-be-looked-at-ness.

(Mulvey 1986: 203)

Mulvey associates identification, voyeurism and fetishism with the gaze. The concept of an empowered male gaze, theorized by Mulvey (1986), Metz (1982) and others, is a reduction of Lacan's (1981) theory in which the gaze is not associated with a unified subject or desire. Doane describes the reasons that feminist film theory has made the gaze more subjective. 'Lacan's gaze cannot be used to analyse sexual difference because it allows no differential analysis of mastery and subjection – everyone is subjected to a gaze which is outside' (Doane 1991: 86). A number of scholars, including Mulvey (1981), have reconsidered the early feminist film theory that describes the gaze as a totalizing and purely patriarchal structure. Doane's theory of a female gaze – which employs masquerade as a way of flaunting femininity and thus holding it at a distance – may provide an alternative model for discussing the ways that some characters and users look. Mayne suggests that a 'major task for all feminist critics is to rethink dualism itself', a process that Kaplan describes as the need to move beyond those 'long-held cultural and linguistic patterns of oppositions' (Mayne 1994: 50). On MOOs this rethinking of such oppositions as male and female must include the availability of ten genders (neuter, male, female, splat, Spivak which is named after a programmer, royal, plural, second, either and egotistical), gender transgressions and masquerades. Despite such challenges to traditional oppositions and the appearance of new theoretical work on spectatorship and the gaze, Mulvey's thesis does describe the deeply gendered and voyeuristic virtual looking that happens on MOOs.

This chapter employs the term 'gaze', as it is used in feminist film theory, to describe looking relationships in which voyeurism, an empowered panoptic stare and/or an erotic perusal are employed. Foucault (1995) describes such forms of looking as part of a system of social regulation that is engaged through surveillance. In Foucault's discussion of the panopticon, which was designed by Jeremy Bentham, the architectural layout of the building allows guards, officials or citizens to perform a surreptitious surveillance. Prisoners know that they can be watched but they don't know when they are being observed and they can't see or identify the people who are looking at them. Anyone subjected to the panopticon's field of visibility, or its gaze, learns to regulate their own behaviour because of this effect. On MOOs, as well as in other settings, this type of social regulation is implemented through a series of effects that act as a reminder of the larger surveillant forces at work:

> Power has its principle not so much in a person as in a certain concerted distribution of bodies, surfaces, lights, gazes . . . He who is subjected to a field of visibility, and who knows it, assumes responsibility for the constraints of power; he makes them play spontaneously upon himself; he inscribes in himself the power relation in

which he simultaneously plays both roles; he becomes the principle of his own subjection.

(Foucault 1995: 202–3)

This chapter considers the high level of visibility that all characters experience on MOOs and argues that gazing works as part of a panoptic
system of power that regulates virtual bodies and maintains binary
gender.[3]

Character creation and attributes on MOOs

A slim 5′ 9″ fellow who enjoys biking, golf and Windows programming. So go ahead and ask: 'What do you do for fun?'
(hmm) I enjoy watching Dave, and try not to get mugged when
waiting for tickets . . . He is awake, but has been staring off into
space for 4 minutes.

(Abraxas 1998)

Lavender_Guest: Jeff, 23, 5ft 10, low 200, brown/blue . . . He is
awake and looks alert.

(LambdaMOO, 14 December 1998)

Green_Guest: Karen. 31, 5 ft 8. Slender, brown eyes, round face,
wide mouth, very dark brown hair. I am the secretary to the owner
of a local retail store . . . She is awake and looks alert.

(LambdaMOO, 24 December 1998)

The first thing that someone creates on the MOO is a character. The
attributes of a character, including the character's description, gender,
the objects it carries and the messages that appear when a character
navigates the virtual setting can be adjusted and readjusted at will.
The text that contextualizes the character is known as the character's
'description' because it is set by typing '@describe <object> as
<description>' (LambdaMOO 1999c). Guests can and often do use
@describe as a way of personalizing their more temporary virtual bodies.
Some members of the MOO community render their virtual bodies and
read other characters as the equivalent of physical individuals despite,
or perhaps because, characters can rewrite their descriptions and
have more than one description through a process called 'morphing'.
Character descriptions often include such physical traits as age, height,
weight, body type, eye colour, hair colour and type of clothes.[4] This

practice may have been encouraged by the help text example for @describe. 'Munchkin types this: @describe me as a "very fine fellow, if a bit on the short side"' (LambdaMOO 1999c). The @describe help text suggests that community conventions require this kind of character description. It also encourages capitalization that makes the character's alias into a proper name. The differences between character and user, which can often be quite extreme, are hidden by what appears to be the 'truth' of these physiognomy-oriented character descriptions.

LambdaMOO's policy, outlined under 'help character' (LambdaMOO 1999c), maintains the direct correspondence between user and character because it generally expects 'only one character per person'. Defining characters as 'objects' on MOOs also contributes to the belief that there is a direct physiognomic correlation between the user and their character. 'Objects are the fundamental building blocks of the MOO. Every object has a unique number, a name, an owner, a location, and various other properties' (LambdaMOO 1999c). This means that all things on the MOO, including rooms, characters and manipulable things, are objects. The relationship between subjects and objects in physical environments, and even feminist critiques of the gaze, may be problematized by the terminology that is employed in these virtual domains.

While MOOing, there is a cinematic-like segregation of space between user and character. The continued perceptual collapse of user and character, however, is quite different than descriptions of cinematic spectatorship as a passive form of identification with the apparatus and the actors on the screen.

It is often difficult to differentiate between user and character, to describe the self that has the agency and undergoes the experiences, when talking about the MOO setting. These forms of identification are related to the participatory structures that fan cultures produce. Fans and characters literally can speak the parts from their favourite films, books, comics and television shows (Jenkins 1992). Users can never become their character even though they have a higher level of control over the performance of their character than fans. MOO characters have a relationship with virtual objects that users cannot attain because users exist outside the virtual setting and are held back by the screen. For instance, characters can pick up virtual objects, touch other characters and record or even participate in events when the user is not online. It is difficult to describe characters as subjects, even though the character 'acts' while outside the user's control, because of the continued perceptual conflation of user and character by many system participants.

The employment of gender online also assists in the collapse of character and user because it supports the illusion that character descriptions depict 'real' bodies. Most users choose to depict themselves as either male or female despite the other gender choices. A fairly typical breakdown of the gender of characters on LambdaMOO was '92 males (52 per cent), 65 females (36 per cent) and 19 others (10 per cent)' (Stetson 1999). All characters must have a gender which they usually select but features such as race, the age of the user and the user's socio-economic class need not be chosen or indicated in the character's description.[5] The system provides information on gender when a character accesses another character's description. Gender is also highlighted when one character pages another: a pre-programmed message appears followed by the statement 'she (he, it, . . .) pages, <message>'. When asked why the system constructs gendered characters by employing pronouns, many programmers argue that the system's generation of texts, such as the one just quoted, 'require' pronouns to facilitate natural language parsing. This contention seems to be supported by the high occurrence of pronouns, which match the set gender of the character, in the messages that are triggered when characters interact with the MOO. But obviously, with some textual awkwardness, the character's name could be substituted for all pronominal markers.

The construction of gendered positions is one of the many ways that a detailed architecture of belief, or a uniform community outlook, is supported on MOOs. The architecture of belief is maintained because the bodies, settings, and objects that users programme are available as part of the system even when the user is not online. A significant part of the setting is the employment of social and architectural vernaculars from the physical world. Some members of MOOs construct textual versions of familiar architectural types so that visitors will not become disoriented when employing such unfamiliar types of movement as 'teleporting'. Characters can move through this MOO setting in two basic ways. They can 'walk' by typing such compass directions as north, south, south-east, as well as other directions like up and out. They can also teleport into 'unlocked rooms' by typing '@go <room number>'. Describing separate chat spaces as 'rooms' allows users to conceive of the MOO setting as an ordered space.[6] The core of LambdaMOO is even laid out like the 'archwizard' and programmer Pavel Curtis' house in Palo Alto, complete with living room, kitchen and deck. This representation is reinforced by a series of diagrammatic ASCII maps that use the characters on the standard keyboard to visualize the MOO as a gridded plan in which most room walls meet at right angles. These maps and other spatializing devices make the MOO into a kind of visual space that can be viewed.

The look and the gaze on MOOs

The look is a privileged term in MOO systems even though characters communicate and comprehend the MOO setting by reading and writing texts. Characters need to virtually look in order to navigate this textual system because of the programming decision to associate typed information inquiries with the look command.[7] The read and @read commands, which relate the MOO to textual narratives, are only employed when specific MOO documents are meant to stand in for written texts. According to 'help read', read <note> 'prints the text written on the named object, usually a note or letter' (LambdaMOO 1999c). The @read command allows characters to read specific listserv-like MOO mailing lists and to examine their personal MOO mail (the in-system version of email). The read and @read commands compliment the visual and object-oriented nature of the system by suggesting that there are multiple levels to the environment that include tangible objects that can be read. Some of these objects are supposed to be visual and dimensional, yet produced through text, and others are meant to be purely textual. The general understanding of MOO objects as tangible is produced by the community's understanding of the term 'reading', the overwhelming use of descriptions and MOO programming that requires characters to virtually pick up and thus conceptually 'touch' and 'hold' many MOO objects in order to manipulate them.

The most common way to access information about MOO objects, which includes characters, is by typing 'look <character or object name>'. The importance of the look command is underlined by its inclusion in the introductory help text for LambdaMOO as one of 'the first five kinds of commands you'll want to know' (LambdaMOO 1999c). This list, in the order that the items appear in the help text is: look, say, @wwho, movement and @quit. The look command provides a consistent set of information to users. When characters virtually look at a room they receive the room's name, description and contents (a list of objects and characters in that room). Characters that virtually look at another character receive the character's name, description, log in status (the character is described as 'awake' or 'sleeping') and the level of activity if the character is online (the character is described as 'alert' or idle for a certain amount of time). This form of character information retrieval works in the same virtual room with 'look

<character name>' and works from any MOO setting with 'look
~<character name>'. One of the reasons that this 'near' (characters in
the same room) or 'far' (characters in different MOO rooms) form
of information access is usually associated with looking is because,
through the 'look_detect option', the system informs characters that
'<character name> looks you over'. The look_detect option notifies
characters when their description is being accessed and codifies this
information retrieval as a 'look'. The character's gender is also rein-
scribed in this series of MOO looks and system notifications because
pronouns are used to describe the character's log in status. When characters virtually look at another character, the message reads 'She (he,
it) is awake and looks alert'. The look command and look_detect
feature work together to form a setting in which characters clearly gaze
at gendered virtual bodies.

This rendering of the gaze is consistently supported by the terminology of MOO systems. The look_detect notification text, which informs
characters when another character is virtually looking at them, is called
the '@watched' message. The character also has a setting called the
'@owatched' me message that can be set to notify everyone in the room
when the character is being virtually looked at by another character.
Such public evidence can lead to long bouts where participants virtually look at a particular character. The weight of such MOO looks
is underlined by the distressed way that certain characters respond to
being observed. The transformation of the look command into an
empowered gaze is suggested by one guest's description: 'Headless.
Somebody bit it off. Ahh, the blood, the blood!! They oughtta put a
warning on the look command, nobody told me it was socially unac-
ceptable to use it' (Stetson 1999). As this guest description suggests,
some characters demand that the community stops looking at them.
The system provides a number of complex tools to patrol individual
characters despite the aversion that some characters have to being watched.
For instance, users can patrol a particular character with the '@watch
<character name>' command. This command provides notification
when the specified character stops idling. The user is provided with
a heightened awareness of the transparent and panoptic functions of
the system by such command names as @watch, @watched me and
@owatched me. The MOO is recontextualized when requests for information, or a reading of a text, are understood and described by the
community as 'looking' and 'watching'. The names of these messages
clearly link information inquiries with the more disturbing message,

sometimes literally sent by the system, that you are being looked at. These aspects of the MOO, which can be understood as a series of gazes, make information retrieval into the kind of regulatory and surveillant mechanism that Foucault describes:

> The enclosed, segmented space, observed at every point, in which the individuals are inserted in a fixed place, in which the slightest movements are supervised, in which all events are recorded, in which an uninterrupted work of writing links the centre and the periphery . . . all this constitutes a compact model of the disciplinary mechanism.
>
> (Foucault 1995: 197)

All the ramifications of this eerie version of being watched and disciplinary mechanism aren't apparent. Information about the user's life isn't readily available but the panoptic aspects of the system make online information about characters easily accessible. Everything in the virtual community is clocked, dated and catalogued. Each 'individual is constantly located' and 'examined' (Foucault 1995: 197). Characters, for instance, can form a database and then access the object number, amount of time connected, idle time and present location for all currently logged in characters that they find 'interesting' by inputting '@wwho'. Typing '@crowd <character name or room number>' provides a list of the characters in a room, their 'sex', the amount of time they have been idle, and the room name and object number. The command '@spy <character name>' provides the character's status (is the character awake or asleep) and object number, present room and room description, a list of objects and characters in that room, and a map of the surrounding rooms. The inclusion of the map suggests that characters may use these commands to track other characters. However commands often supply information that the user wasn't specifically seeking.

The amount of time which users spend in the system and the characters that they associate with are known by all their virtual acquaintances. There are few discreet ways of logging a character into a virtual setting. On some MOOs, notification is provided when characters log in to the system. Users can also be informed immediately when characters on their 'interesting list' log in. These forms of information inquiry make the community into a transparent structure. Users support the panoptic effects of the system when they employ these commands to move their character through the MOO.

A panoptic effect is also produced by @peruse, @kgb, @fbi, @scope, @glance, @peep, @gawk, @see, @dossier, @report, @whois and @examine.[8] These forms of information inquiry are commonly thought of as a form of looking even though they don't all trigger the character's @watch message and provide notice of the virtual look. The character Rusty's comments about @kgb and @fbi suggest that virtual looking can endow characters with a scopic power. 'Life on the cutting edge! What does it all boil down to? WHO'S GOT INFO AND WHO DOESN'T! Those who @add-feature this baby are smugly in the former category' (Rusty 1999). Rusty's @kgb command provides one of the most detailed sets of information about a character. The command lists the character's name, object number, last log out, amount of time logged out for, last log in, amount of time logged in for, amount of time idling, current time, MOO age, seniority among all MOO characters, real life timezone (if set by the user) and time in that zone, gender, name of player, class (each player class provides the character with a slightly different set of capabilities), programmer status (characters must request to be programmers), number of feature objects used (features can be added in order to increase the character's functionality), MOO home, current location and list of other characters in that room, shortest alias or other names for the character, number and names of morphs (other names, genders, and descriptions that the character can change into), current description, online club memberships, currently held objects, total amount of quota (the amount of database space that the character can use to do such things as write descriptions, copy objects from pre-existing programs, or program), total quota currently used, quota still available and relationship to the character (this may show that the character lists them as a 'pal' or uses their feature objects). These commands may seem to be textual because they provide detailed tabulations but they continue to reinscribe the MOO's visual discourse. @kgb, for example, refers to characters' descriptions as their 'appearance'. The user of @report accesses the character's description and is then informed 'this is from eye-witness reports <character name> may be wearing different clothes at this time'. The help file for the @report command states that it 'calls up an X-File about anyone in the MOO' (GreyDruid 1999). These descriptions highlight the ways that individual characters can be documented and analysed. Even the names of many of these commands, which clearly are meant to evoke voyeurism, link textual visual pleasure to power by making the MOO system into a scopic regime.

Gendered gazing on MOOs

Yes I'm a guy, but hey this is cyberspace, right. You can be whatever you want, I'm Cindy. I love pantyhose, nylons and especially the hot lace body stocking I probably have on right now.

(Hammer 1998)

Teal_Guest: A pretty little cumslut, on her knees, dress tugged up over the lace of her stockings. She looks up at you and you can see that her face, dress and hair are streaked and spattered with cum.

(LambdaMOO 1998)[9]

Red_Guest: Eyes downcast, blushing faintly . . . She is awake and looks alert.

(LambdaMOO 1999)

Olive_Guest: A hot sexy babe in her late teens, 19 to be exact. She has long brown hair and big brown eyes. She's wearing shorts and a tight tank top that shows off her belly. She's feeling extra happy tonight.

(LambdaMOO 1998)

Mulvey argues that 'cinematic codes create a gaze, a world, and an object, thereby producing an illusion cut to the measure of desire' (1986: 208). According to Mulvey, such structures as the cinema create an architecture of belief in which a particular kind of desire is fulfilled. MOOs create a similar set of seemingly real illusions through the construction of an architecture of belief that includes particular kinds of character descriptions. It is perhaps not surprising that this series of illusions provide a number of fantasy structures for individual users. Within this fantasy context, male guests are often provided with such attributes as 'tall and muscular' or the 'strong, silent type' (LambdaMOO, 6 December 1998). Female guests have 'huge breasts', narrow waists, and are often half clad in a 'short skirt' (LambdaMOO, 6 December 1998). The construction of this limited set of bodies where men are strong and women connote 'to-be-looked-at-ness', like Teal_Guest looking up in order to be looked at, seems to support Mulvey's split of the gaze into active/male and passive/female. The production of such stereotyped bodies may be in reaction to the ways that this formula of looking is sometimes disrupted.

All characters connote 'to-be-looked-at-ness' because users write descriptions so that other characters will look at them. In this sense, all characters are the object of the gaze. Every character's position as the object of the virtual look is an important and as yet unexplored aspect of MOO culture. Silverman suggests that feminists should consider the ways that men also perform as objects of the gaze. She argues that we 'have at times assumed that dominant cinema's scopic regime could be overturned by "giving" woman the gaze, rather than by exposing the impossibility of anyone ever owning that visual agency, or of him or herself escaping specularity' (Silverman 1992: 152). Male identified characters don't escape the kind of virtual looks that provide other characters with detailed information.

Overtly sexual male descriptions, which are more common among guests, may disturb the presumed naturalness of match-ups between male and female characters and attract the erotic gaze of other male characters. It would seem that male guests are often 'hard and horny' with a '$10\frac{1}{2}$-inch cock [that] stands fully erect' (Purple_Guest 1999). Male characters with a more stable identity in the system may list 'their' height and eye colour but they almost never describe genital attributes. The almost complete absence of hypersexual male character descriptions on most MOOs suggests that these descriptions don't represent an appropriate masculinity, offer an identity that users are willing to sustain with less anonymity or attract a desired gaze.[10] This gaze may either be encouraged or resisted with provisos like 'I am straight' (Rosy_Guest 1999) and descriptions of the kinds of chats that the character is seeking. There are also a variety of reasons, along with the character's set gender, that make characters the object of the look and the gaze. Characters are sometimes looked at because they have a name that other characters find interesting. Users communicate with a character that doesn't recognize them, express an interesting or provocative statement while in the same room as other characters, gain notoriety from what they post to public MOO mail lists or dispute with other characters or have had their private sexual chat reposted to a public MOO mail list. This suggests that the look can be part of a shared communication between characters or be turned into a more regulatory gaze when characters engage in some behaviour that the community finds suspect.

These forms of virtual looking can become invasive. Consistent and inexplicable bouts of being virtually looked at suggest that character attributes are being tabulated and patrolled by the larger community. The virtual look of certain characters, penetrating into any space in order to examine other characters, renders a panoptic form of gazing.

This may suggest a difference between the position that all characters have as the object of the look and the position that some characters, particularly female ones, are consistently culturally scripted into as the object of the gaze. It is possible to gain an equally detailed amount of information by virtually looking back. However, a returned virtual look is sometimes understood as an acceptance of an implicit request for erotic chat because characters do use long distance virtual looking as a way to find appropriate Net sex partners. The character Renfair's feature object, for instance, includes a gaze verb that 'discreetly tells another [player] that you find them especially interesting' (Renfair 1999).

No one escapes specularity on MOOs but a version of the classic cinematic-looking relationship is still perpetuated. Virtually looking and gazing are too often the terrain of male-identified characters. There is a disproportionately high number of male characters that 'own' the feature objects that make long distance looking commands available to the general MOO community. Female characters, because of their gender setting, are more likely to be the object of the virtual look. Frequent @owatched messages from female characters that are being virtually looked at and discussions about this topic in public rooms and MOO mailing lists make the community aware of the different ways that male and female characters are viewed. Ironic descriptions – 'I have gigantic breasts. Please hit on me relentlessly' (Technicolor_Guest 1999) – also demonstrate the different ways that male and female characters are treated on MOOs. Some women have chosen to identify themselves as another gender online in order to remove themselves from this dynamic. However, intergender characters also experience a disproportionate number of looks from male characters and are often presumed to be female.[11]

Female characters and female users could employ the online processes of gazing in a proactive way in order to destabilize the male look. Of course, the relationship between female characters and users would remain largely unverified by the general community. Online conversations with female users suggest that any subversion of the gaze by virtually looking back is not always easy for women who have been scripted as the object of the gaze in other settings. Female identified characters quickly learn that gazing back at male characters is likely to generate responses like 'Do you like what you see?' (Tman 1998). Such responses underscore the deeply ingrained visual vernacular of these systems and the use of virtual looks as a way to find appropriate Net sex partners.

Looking back can mean something very different than the initial process of gazing. Doane has written about the inherent problems in the female cinema viewer's appropriation of the gaze:

[E]ven if it is admitted that the woman is frequently the object of the voyeuristic or fetishistic gaze in the cinema, what is there to prevent her from reversing the relation and appropriating the gaze for her own pleasure? Precisely the fact that the reversal itself remains locked within the same logic. The male striptease – the gigolo – both inevitably signify the mechanism of reversal itself, constituting themselves as aberrations whose acknowledgement simply reinforces the dominant system of aligning sexual difference with a subject/object dichotomy.

(Doane 1991: 20–1)

On LambdaMoo a similar reversal is revealed in this quote:

Plaid_Guest: A really submissive guy, and he's really fun. Please page him if you want to.

(LambdaMOO, 27 December 1998)

The female viewer's appropriation of the gaze reinscribes the male position by acknowledging it as the dominant model. As Doane suggests, the representation of passive men may structure their continued scopic power in normative situations. Visions of male striptease have become a common phenomenon online. It unfortunately appears that such 'men', if we presume that they are identified as such outside of the MOO space, can play with these representations while still assuming their right to power in other environments and their ability to choose to be submissive. Reading these characters as women might suggest some quite different possibilities, which would be based on a performative drag masquerade, but there is little evidence for such a supposition. There is a great deal of evidence and cybercultural lore, however, to support the idea that men often perform as women online.

Mulvey's division of gazing along binary gender lines doesn't provide a full explanation of looking on MOOs. The objectifying look of male users at available female characters is disturbed by the community's acknowledgement, represented by Cindy's character description, that men often construct the overtly sexual and available female characters. The binary relation between active/male and passive/female is also disordered by the existence of ten 'standard' genders on LambdaMOO. There are a variety of ways that the MOO community represses these alternative identities and gazes. Cross-identified characters, for instance, don't necessarily classify themselves as intergender. A guest character description that reads 'some fat white guy claiming to be a woman' is gendered as female (Beige_Guest 1999). Some members of the community insist that binary gender labels should be attached to alternative genders. An addition to an online MOO newsgroup reproduces a commonly shared belief about intergender identification. 'Periwinkle_Guest [to Plaid_ Guest]: So, r u a male it, or a female it?' (Periwinkle_Guest 1995). The Spivak frequently asked questions (see Appendix), which provides answers to frequently asked questions about intergender identification, is ironically subtitled 'r u m or f?' (Phaedrus 1999). Users construct binary identity on top of liminal gender positions through such devices. Characters also sometimes examine morph names and aliases in order to find clues that will indicate a user's 'real' gender. These virtual looks suggest a regulatory attempt to inscribe gender on to unattributed bodies and to determine real gender through a series of 'codes'.

Gazes at intergender characters are often followed by requests, hysterical demands and even harassment that seeks to determine the user's 'real' gender. The following exchange with all its real-time typing mistakes, which was posted to the MOO mailing list 'GrrlTalk', points to the ridiculous methods that users try to employ in order to determine 'real' gender:

You sense that Infrared_Guest is looking for you in The Coat Closet.
It pages   'you are a girl, your name is too feminine.'
page infrared   feminine like bobby and tony?
Your message has been sent.
You sense that Infrared_Guest is looking for you in The Coat Closet.
It pages   'Will you reveal your sex to me?'
page infrared   I'm spivak
You sense that Infrared_Guest is looking for you in The Coat Closet.
It pages   'Would you say hello or Hi?'
page infrared   i don't know. would you?
You sense that Infrared_Guest is looking for you in The Coat Closet.
It pages   'It is obvious to me now that you are male, I am studying Psdychology'.

(Lemi 1997)

This post illustrates a desire among certain system users for scientific methods, reason and facts: the kinds of truths that it seems can be verified by looking. Ideological disagreements between participants over the ways that MOOs represent characters may explain a number of recent gender related disputes on LambdaMOO. These gender disputes – like the one in which the character Ibid was harassed by Downtime and other characters for having an intergender identity – often lead to users having their physical whereabouts and 'real' attributes identified. These gender 'problems' allow the 'real' binary of male and female to become 'fictional' online genders. In many ways, the MOO's multiple and not always clear gender positions lead to a yearning for the material body. Virtual kitchens and bathrooms, for example, provide a setting for the body's corporeal functions. The virtual bodies and objects of deceased users have also been preserved.

This nostalgia for the material body is also evoked by the appearance of mirrors and mirroring gazes (the virtual look is reprogrammed so that the character accesses their own description when they look at another character). Mirrors help to make lists of characters and textual descriptions into a three-dimensional space in which objects appear to have a particular position within an environment. When you virtually look at 'a useless mirror hung in the middle of the curve of the west wall', for example, you see the virtual reflection of the corridor (Rog 1999). This powder room mirror suggests that each character has a particular position and point of view within the 'landscape' of the MOO. The mirroring gaze of characters produce a similar spatial effect. Characters that look at Bewitch, for example, receive her description and the message that 'Bewitch eyes you suspiciously', then they see their own description 'in Bewitch's eyes' (1998). Characters seem to have a spatial relationship to Bewitch because they can see 'themselves' reflected in her eyes: the mirror 'forms images by reflection' (*Merriam Webster Dictionary*, 1998). It consolidates or forms character descriptions into bodies by 'reflecting' the MOO's spatial narratives and suggesting complex arrangements of objects.

The use of mirrors, as well as the whole relationship between user and character, could be read as a reinvocation of Lacan's mirror stage (1977). At this stage, the child first acquires a sense of self and discovers the agency of its body through a series of imaginary identifications that are caused by an initial sense of difference. Metz's employment of the mirror stage as a way of analysing the cinema viewer's identification with the ideal image on the screen (1982) can also be applied to the user's identification with the character, although it must be noted that Metz privileges the viewer's identification with the camera. Doane questions the assurances that identification with the screen offers because it provides 'a guarantee of the untroubled centrality and unity of the subject' (1980: 28). The use of the look and the gaze on MOOs can offer users a similar rendering of the empowered subject.

Conclusion

Film identification can provide the spectator with a view into coherent identity. However, spectators may also be able to take up multiple points of identification. It would seem that such options as the ability to use morphing as a way of creating different versions of the character and the tendency to have different characters simultaneously logged into other MOOs would present users with multiple points of identification rather than satisfying unity. While this is certainly possible, a number of the MOO's features, which include the look and the gaze, offer users the ability to make their MOO character into an ideal image. In addition, many of the MOO's fragmenting tendencies also provide unifying possibilities. Characters often use the same name on different MOO systems as a way of maintaining coherent identity and morphs are always contained under the character's singular object number. MOO programming not only offers users the ability to form their virtual body-construct into an ideal image but also contains some elements and community behaviours that prevent the design of body-constructs from highlighting fragmentation and inadequacy.

The ability to 'look' at character descriptions which have detailed physiognomic attributes produces a kind of visual terrain in text-based settings. The prevalence of these sights suggests that the unitary material body exists even online. There are, of course, other types of character representations but the use of the look as a verifying tendency persists despite these anomalies. The look supports material representations and has been used to 'determine' the binary gender of inter-gender characters because seeing has long been equated with truth. Male users who announce that they are female guests still include female descriptions that connote 'to-be-looked-at-ness'. These descriptions perpetuate the dominant cinema's scripting of male subjects who control and look upon female objects. A troubling part of the MOO system is that empowered gazes are often met with 'sleep in her eyes' (Matte_Guest 1999), 'an innocent look' (Copper_Guest 1999) or downcast eyes. This suggests that the mastering gaze also forms a corollary passive female model. The fascination with the 'spectacle of power' and with being visual rather than having visual pleasure can entice 'the other into submission' (Salecel and Zizek 1996: 3). These lures enable the mastering gaze of certain characters and the voyeuristic terminology of MOO commands to perpetuate a series of limiting identity constructs.

Notes

1 In this chapter, the term 'user' describes the physical person who sits in front of the computer screen and types commands. The term 'character' describes the virtual avatar, with all of its programmed attributes, that is maintained by the host computer. There are many times, however, that these two terms commingle. It is easy to describe the user performing all functions since the corporeal person usually maintains the agency in this relationship.

2 The idea that characters are unread is ironically performed in the following guest character description. 'Hi! My name's Tiffany. I read a book once. It was pretty cool, full of words n stuff' (Loki 1998).

3 In the work of contemporary theorists, including Bennett (1995) and Cartwright (1995), Foucault's model of the panopticon is altered to include panoptic social regulation by community surveillance. In other words, community codes are maintained by a mutual understanding of social standards and the knowledge that the community itself is or could be watching.

4 There are a number of ways that guests can also be used to establish a fixed identity. Some guest users choose to employ the same description every time that they log in as a guest. Other users simply label the guest with a name, such as Sue or Ben, which makes it seem as if this is their 'real' name.

5 Users who don't set their character's gender by typing '@gender <gender>' will have their gender remain as 'neuter'. If a character sets their gender to something other than the one of the ten gender choices then the system uses 'neuter' pronouns. A few characters have circumvented the neuter pronominal markers by programming their own set of gender pronouns.

6 Of course this representation is disabled by conflicting representations but unfortunately I don't have time to talk about these incongruities or opposing forces in this chapter.

7 It is possible that users could employ the '@examine <object name or number>'. However most users, at least when they access information about other characters, use the 'look' command. I have determined this by using a program to record all the times that characters look at me as well as the type of command that they employ. (My thanks to John Bump for writing this program for me.)

8 The user must add the appropriate feature object before most of these commands will function.

9 The existence of salacious guest descriptions has become such a regular part of MOO systems that a MOO mailing list was formed for users to post these descriptions. It is my belief that some of these descriptions are written by characters solely for the entertainment of the list readers. This position was performed by Plaid_Guest's description: 'Hi! I am Loki. I logged on as a guest and entered a goofy description just so I could post it here for all to see! Thanks!' (LambdaMOO, 7 December 1998).

10 There is a higher proportion of both male and female erotic descriptions on some small adult-oriented MOOs.

11 A number of intergender characters – including the character Irradiate – have shared their experiences on this topic with me. An informal study supports these claims. My intergender character was looked at 22 times by male characters, ten times by female characters and four times by intergender characters between 3 March 1999 and 1 June 1999.

References

Abraxas (1998) character description, type 'look ~Abraxas'. Available online via telnet: lambda.moo.mud.org8888 (21 December 1998).

Bennett, T. (1995) *The Birth of the Museum: History, Theory, Politics*, New York: Routledge.

Bewitch (1998) character description, type 'look~Bewitch'. Available online via telnet: lambda.moo.mud.org8888 (21 December 1998).

Cartwright, L. (1995) *Screening the Body: Tracing Medicine's Visual Culture*, Minneapolis: University of Minnesota Press.

Curtis, P. (1992) 'Mudding: social phenomena in text-based virtual realities', presented at the conference on Directions and Implications of Advanced Computing, sponsored by Computer Professionals for Social Responsibility. Available online: ftp://parcftp.xerox.com/pub/moo/papers/DIAC92 (27 November 1998).

Curtis, P. (1993) 'Muds grow up', presented at the Third International Conference on Cyberspace, May 1993. Available online: ftp://parcftp.xerox.com/pub/moo/papers (27 November 1998).

Doane, M. A. (1980) 'Misrecognition and identity', *Cine-Tracts*, 11 (3): 25–32.

Doane, M. A. (1991) *Femmes Fatales: Feminism, Film Theory, Psychoanalysis*, New York: Routledge.

Foucault, M. (1995) *Discipline and Punish: The Birth of the Prison*, New York: Vintage Books.

Free On-Line Dictionary of Computing (1998) 'Multi-user dimension from FOLDOC'. Available online: http://wombat.doc.ic.ac.uk/foldoc/foldoc.cgi?MUD (27 November 1998).

GreyDruid (1999) type 'help#49074'. Available online via telnet: lambda.moo.mud.org8888 (2 January 1999).

Hammer (1998) '*Silly/Stupid/Salacious-Guest-Descriptions'. Available online via telnet: lambda.moo.mud.org8888 (6 December 1998)

Jay, M. (1994) *Downcast Eyes: The Denigration of Vision in Twentieth-Century French Thought*, Berkeley: University of California Press.

Jenkins, H. (1992) *Textual Poachers: Television Fans and Participatory Culture*, New York: Routledge.

Lacan, J. (1977) *Écrits: A Selection*, trans. A. Sheridan, New York: W. W. Norton.

Lacan, J. (1981) *The Four Fundamental Concepts of Psycho-Analysis*, trans. A. Sheridan, New York: W. W. Norton.

LambdaMOO (1999a) 'type "length(players)" ' after becoming a programmer. Available online via telnet: lambda.moo.mud.org8888 (2 January 1999).

LambdaMOO (1999b) log on screen. Available online via telnet: lambda.moo.mud.org8888 (2 January 1999).

LambdaMOO (1999c) 'type "help <topic>"'. Available online via telnet: lambda.moo.mud.org8888 (2 January 1999).

Lemi (1997) '*best-of-the-lists'. Available online via telnet: lambda.moo.mud.org8888 (13 January 1997).

Loki (1998) '*Silly/Stupid/Salacious-Guest-Descriptions'. Available online via telnet: lambda.moo.mud.org8888 (6 December 1998).

Mayne, J. (1994) 'Feminist film theory and criticism' in D. Carson, L. Dittmar and J. R. Welsch (eds) *Multiple Voices in Feminist Film Criticism*, Minneapolis: University of Minnesota Press.

Merriam Webster Dictionary (1998) 'WWWebster Dictionary – search screen'. Available online: http://www.m-w.com/cgi-bin/netdict (2 January 1999).

Metz, C. (1982) *The Imaginary Signifier: Psychoanalysis and the Cinema*, Bloomington: Indiana University Press.

Mulvey, L. (1981) 'Afterthoughts on "visual pleasure and narrative cinema" inspired by Duel in the Sun', *Framework*, 15–17: 12–15.

Mulvey, L. (1986) 'Visual pleasure and narrative cinema' in P. Rosen (ed.) *Narrative, Apparatus, Ideology: A Film Theory Reader*, New York: Columbia University Press.

Periwinkle_Guest (1995) 'Quoted-Out-Of-Context'. Available online via telnet: lambda.moo.mud.org8888 (10 August 1995).

Phaedrus (1999) 'The-Official-Spivak-FAQ'. Available online: http://www.jacksonville.net/~phaedrus/spivak.html (1 June 1999).

Renfair (1999) 'type "help #67671"'. Available online via telnet: lambda.moo.mud.org8888 (2 January 1999).

Rog (1999) 'type "@go #116", "look useless mirror"'. Available online via telnet: lambda.moo.mud.org8888 (8 June 1999).

Rusty (1999) 'type "help #24262"'. Available online via telnet: lambda.moo.mud.org8888 (2 January 1999).

Salecel, R. and Zizek, S. (1996) *Gaze and Voice as Love Objects*, Durham, NC: Duke University Press.

Silverman, K. (1992) *Male Subjectivity at the Margins*, New York: Routledge.

Stetson (1999) 'feature object, type "genwho"'. Available online via telnet: lambda.moo.mud.org8888 (1 June 1999).

Tman (1998) 'paged comment'. Available online via telnet: LambdaMOO, lambda.moo.mud.org8888 (2 January 1999).

Appendix

This appendix describes most of the basic MOO terms and commands that are employed in this chapter. Most of the commands listed are available on all MOOs but a few of the commands are only available on LambdaMOO.

command   These terms are typed by the user in order to manipulate the character through the MOO setting. Commands allow characters to 'speak', 'move', 'look' and access information and interact with other characters in a variety of ways.

@crowd   This command provides information on all the characters that are in a room. It lists the room name and object number, the character's 'sex' and the amount of time that characters have been idle. '@crowd character name or room number>' can be used from any room in the MOO.

@describe   This command is used to narrate or portray the character. It also allows the character to describe any object that they own. Characters' descriptions can be accessed with commands like 'look', '@examine', or '@kgb'.

@examine   This command identifies the object's full name, aliases, object number, description, contents, obvious commands and the object's owner.

@fbi   This command is part of a feature object (see below). It provides a detailed set of information about a character, including the character's description.

feature object   Features can be added in order to increase the character's functionality.

@go   This command allows the character to 'teleport' or to move directly to any 'unlocked' room.

help <term>   This is used to access the help system which provides online documentation for many of the MOO's most common aspects.

@kgb   This command is part of a feature object. It provides a detailed set of information about a character, including the character's description.

look   This command shows a description of any object that is in the same room as the character. Characters can type 'look' and access a description of the room that they are in and a list of the objects in that room. Characters can use 'look <character name>' to access a description of any character in the same room or 'look ~<char­acter name>' to access other character descriptions. Objects can also be looked at from anywhere in the MOO with the command 'look <object number>'.

look_detect   This is an option that notifies characters when another character 'looks' at them or accesses their description. This option can be turned on and off.

MOO   This acronym stands for multi-user object-oriented world. MOOs are text-based chat spaces where users can either connect as a guest or as a character that has a more stable identity in the system. The MOO's object-oriented programming, which is similar to the Java and the C++ computer languages, allows users to change the structure by designing such objects as rooms, manipulable things and characters.

morphing Characters can morph or change into different names, descriptions, and genders. Characters may morph into a different body-construct but they always have the same object number.

object number Everything on the MOO, including characters, rooms and articles is an object. Each object has a unique object number.

read This command allows characters to access the text written on certain objects such as a 'note' or 'letter'.

@read This command works with different objects than read. It allows characters to read specific listserv-like MOO mailing lists and to examine their personal MOO mail (the in-system version of email).

@report This command is part of a feature object. It provides a detailed set of information about a character, including the character's description.

Spivak The Spivak gender is named after Michael Spivak because of the extensive work that 'e' has done with pronouns. The Spivak pronouns are 'e' (subjective), 'em' (objective), 'eir' (possessive – adjective), 'eirs' (possessive – noun) and 'emself' (reflexive). LambdaMOO users can obtain a definition of the Spivak gender and a list of pronouns by typing 'help Spivak'. The characters Velvet and Nosredna have worked on this definition. The other intergender categories remain undefined.

@spy This command is part of a feature object. Using '@spy <character name>' provides the character's status (is the character awake or asleep?) and object number, present room and room description, a list of objects and characters in that room, and a map of the surrounding rooms.

teleport Characters can use the command '@go <room number>' and move directly into any unlocked room.

@watch This is a command that characters can use to receive notification when another character stops idling.

@watched me This command sets a message. The @watched message provides notification when the character's description has been accessed. The character can leave this message in the default setting or can customize it.

@owatched me This command sets a message. The @owatched me message notifies everyone in the room when another character accesses the character's description. The character can leave this message in the default setting or can customize it.

@wwho   This command is part of the 'log in watcher' feature object. It allows users to find out additional information about other characters that they find 'interesting', including the characters' object number, amount of time connected, idle time and present location. Characters are added to an 'interesting list' with the command '@interesting <character name>'.

Chapter 8

Strange yet stylish headgear

Virtual reality consumption and the construction of gender

Nicola Green

Abstract

This chapter analyses the ways in which gender is important in studies of virtual reality (VR) technologies. Gender is inscribed in virtual subjects. Virtual reality systems become embedded in 'everyday life' through leisure and consumption. Previous studies have tended to polarize the vision of bodily transcendence in cyberspace against the reproduction of social and cultural inequalities hence the specific sites, in which the social relations of virtual reality are enacted, have tended to be neglected.

A multi-sited ethnographic study of immersive virtual reality systems is the basis for discussion of how virtual reality technologies produce gender in specific sites. Virtual systems are positioned and used differently in various locales, such as arcades, art galleries, bars, theme parks and cafés. The chapter discusses the practices of consumption which (re)produce and maintain conventional bodily and subjective boundaries. What relationships are becoming institutionalized? Are new conventions of gender created in these consumption relationships? The construction of spectacle and space and the specific bodily disciplines required for participation in virtual realities in locations of consumption are particularly important in the formation of gender dynamics. Multiple subject positions are offered through competing technical, economic and cultural practices in diverse sites. These positions can establish new conventions of virtual identities and experiences, but also remain shot through with familiar operational categories of gendered identities and bodily practices. This chapter argues that immersive virtual reality technologies cannot be understood without some consideration of the locales in which they are embedded and the social identities they make possible or constrain. A local, reflexive and feminist orientation assists in understanding the gendered dynamics associated with 'becoming virtual'.

Introduction

This chapter examines how gender is inscribed and reproduced in the processes of consuming virtual reality technologies. The focus is on how virtual reality systems become embedded in everyday life through leisure and consumption and how the spectacles and disciplines associated with such consumption produce specifically gendered virtual subjects.

Studies of new communications technologies have tended to polarize a vision of bodily transcendence through virtual systems (Benedikt 1991; McCaffrey 1991; Biocca 1992; Plant 1996) and the critique of such visions from social theorists who focus on the reproduction of social and cultural inequalities in digital space (Brook and Boal 1995; Kramerae 1995). These approaches tend to focus on 'cyberspaces' at the expense of the specific social locales in which they are embedded. It is only recently that local studies which draw on ethnographic and empirical work (for example, Schroeder 1996) have emerged. The focus on locating cyberspaces with immersive virtual reality systems in specific sites, so far neglected, forms the focus of this chapter.

According to Menser and Aronowitz (1996: 13), we can 'chart the manners in which a technocultural entity or apparatus takes on different functions or produces different effects when it changes milieu'. By examining how virtual technologies and the realities they produce are differentially positioned and used across sites it is argued that the practices of consumption which produce gendered virtual persons are multiple and sometimes contradictory. In particular, questions are asked about how conventional bodily and subjective boundaries are played out, reproduced and maintained in contexts where virtual systems are available and used. Are new conventions of gender created in these consumption relationships? Are dominant gender relationships reworked? What new relationships are institutionalized?

This chapter draws on my ethnographic study of immersive virtual reality systems as the basis for discussion. The aim is to explore the particular practices through which virtual systems are institutionalized in specific forms. How virtual reality technologies become embedded in diverse sites through spectacles and disciplines that organize gendered cultures of consumption will be examined. My purpose is to consider how the construction, regulation and negotiation of virtual bodies and identities are played out in sites that enable and institutionalize some forms of gendered virtual subjectivity and constrain others.

Researching virtual reality technologies

Immersive virtual realities attempt to simulate immersion in digital or 'cyber' space – the 'space' created by information. Human perception is linked to computer graphic simulations of virtual worlds through head-mounted displays, data gloves or other navigation devices such as 3D joysticks. The head-mounted display consists of computer graphics run through stereoscopic video screens that are viewed by the user as three-dimensional images. Aural stimulation is provided by stereo headphones which provide computer-generated sound in three dimensions. Data gloves (or other input devices) provide a sense of touch when moving in virtual space. Data gloves, through attached 'trackers', input information to the computer as to the orientation of body parts and simultaneously provide tactile feedback of objects in the virtual world.

It was interesting to see how these technologies were becoming embedded in 'everyday life' (Terry and Calvert 1997). Of those virtual reality systems that are publicly available (rather than those found in public or private research labs), the chapter focuses on entertainment, art and 'garage' virtual reality. Having identified specific virtual systems to study, participant observation and interviewing were conducted in a variety of different venues including arcades, art galleries, bars, theme parks, cafés and education centres. The research was conducted across Australasia, North America and Europe over the course of two years and included the study of 13 different sites of entertainment and art consumption. Twenty ethnographic interviews and two months of participation and observation provided the research materials for the analysis of consumption.

The discussion here focuses on two major cases. The first is one of the most widely distributed immersive games systems in location-based entertainment markets, manufactured by Virtuality® Entertainment Ltd.[1] Its most popular game is Dactyl Nightmare™ in the 'action' genre. By way of contrast, OSMOSE©, an interactive piece of artwork by Char Davies of Softimage, Canada, uses an immersive virtual reality system to construct a world with 12 different 'dimensions' (Davies 1995). This was a one-off project at Softimage that was designed for gallery installation. It has been exhibited at four different galleries in North America and Europe.

In both these cases, attention is paid as to how the technologies produce gender as a mode of embodiment and subjectivity in different locations. Participation in virtual worlds entails moving between the digital spaces of virtual worlds and the non-programmed spaces of consumption sites. Shifting practices of gender are involved in these transitional practices.

Consuming worlds – the digital enactment of gender

There seems little doubt that new computing and communications technologies are implicated in the reproduction and maintenance of gender in various ways, whether in the gendered production of computing technologies (Ullman 1995; Stone 1996), the gendered consumption of ICTs (Haddon 1992; Sofia 1993) or the gender politics of domestic ICT use (Silverstone and Haddon 1996). Virtual reality technologies too, have been the subject of such analyses. Kramarae (1995), for example, provided comment on the role of women in producing virtual reality and the kinds of virtual worlds produced. Sofia (1992) similarly explored the psychoanalytic dimensions of virtual world spaces and their implications for producing gender. More recently, Balsamo (1996) and Hayles (1996) have investigated virtual reality technologies in use and what these processes of use might mean for the production of gendered bodies and gendered persons.

Certainly such digital genderings were apparent in the digital worlds researched here. The most popular game encountered in the reconnaissance of entertainment sites was Dactyl Nightmare, played in Virtuality Ltd's virtual reality system. In Dactyl Nightmare, the objective of the game is to score points by 'shooting' other characters. The participants play across a game board suspended in space – five fields that are connected on two different levels via staircases. A recurrent threat is a pterodactyl which attempts to pick up and drop (thereby 'killing') the players in the game.

The digitized bodies – 'avatars' – which all players are assigned take the form of a 'generic' human figure, a chunky body with squarish outlines of arms and legs, having blue legs, a white torso, and a dark upper head (culturally endowed with jeans, T-shirt and short dark hair). Such cultural markers are clearly masculine in the western context. The general shape is consistent with the construction of 'the body', the historically constructed western individualist subject whom Grosz (1994) suggests is a historical abstraction because it evokes sameness, similarity and continuity. As Robins (1996) notes in the case of virtual systems, one potential outcome of 'becoming digital' is that if previously exclusionary categories of difference are disrupted by the malleability of digital bodies and spaces, all identities can be rendered as one of these 'universal' (masculine) digital identities, thus suppressing the material effects of difference in digital interaction.

In other games such as Legend Quest™, differences are inscribed in/on the digital bodies of participants (Schroeder 1996). Legend Quest adds the metaphors of 'fantasy' to Virtuality's 'action' genres. The game is played in a series of rooms and the creatures which a participant encounters as they move through the game include skeletons, wolves, bats and 'maidens'. Participants can become a number of characters, including warriors, elves, dwarves, wizards and humans. A number of personal characteristics, such as hair colour or markers of gender, can be selected (Schroeder 1996). These bodies present other kinds of problems than those of the 'universal' digital body. As Kramarae (1995) argues, the representations of some material bodies are generally privileged at the expense of others in digital worlds as elsewhere. Just as the cultural codings of masculinity are generalized in 'generic' digital bodies, the coding of difference in 'customized' digital bodies (re)inscribe conventional markers to represent stereotypical categories of personhood already overly familiar.

Doane (1989: 163) asserts that 'when technology intersects with the body in the realm of representation, the question of sexual difference is inevitably involved'. Indeed, sexual difference bears heightened significance where other categories of difference – real/unreal, human/machine – are called into question (Bergstrom 1991). Such is the case with popular film depictions of bodies in near future virtual realities. In *The Lawnmower Man*, for example, the two central characters enter virtual reality. As they do so, the central male character tells his (heterosexual) lover that in virtual worlds 'we can be whatever we want to be'. What they become is illustrated in Figure 8.1. The virtual bodies assume shape and contour which exaggerate the morphological sexual differences between women and men. Moreover, 'his' virtual body is represented in blue, whereas 'her' virtual body is coloured pink.

In contrast to Dactyl Nightmare and Legend Quest, some digital worlds do not represent a body for a participant. Rather, embodiment is signalled entirely through the construction of a 'point of view' (POV). In OSMOSE, for example, a POV is constructed entirely through a free-floating gaze as a point of consciousness, drawing on the conventions of first person visual perspective. OSMOSE is not one

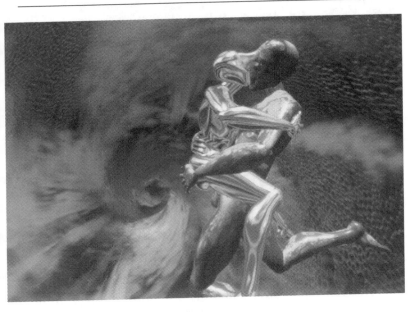

Figure 8.1 Bodies from *The Lawnmower Man*

world, but rather an assemblage of multiple worlds – including text, cloud, clearing, tree, leaf, forest, subterranean earth, pond, abyss, code, Cartesian grid and lifeworld – that seek to explore the connections between technology, nature and embodiment. Most of these dozen world spaces are presented as 'archetypal' elements of nature, framed through 'referential' worlds: the Cartesian grid for initial orientation, the textual 'superstratum' (excerpts of poetic/philosophical writing on nature–technology relations), the code 'substratum' (comprised of some of the code used to generate the worlds in OSMOSE) and the 'lifeworld' which draws the participant out of the experience. These worlds are interrelated and overlapping. It is possible to move through them, but also to hover between them, and to experience different elements of each world simultaneously (see Morse 1997; Heim 1998 for discussions of OSMOSE).

The techniques used in OSMOSE nevertheless construct a POV familiar from other media (including entertainment software). The development of perspectival representation enabled particular kinds of perception and interpretation, and constrained others. As Berger (1974: 10) notes, 'every image embodies a way of seeing', and the very perception of images shifts historically in relation to the ways in which images are socially produced and situated. In western societies, the Renaissance produced a shift to the conventions of perspective in image making which

> centres everything on the eye of the beholder . . . The conventions called those appearances *reality*. Perspective makes the single eye the centre of the visible world. Everything converges on to the eye as to the vanishing point of infinity. The visible world is arranged for the spectator as the universe was once thought to be arranged for God. According to the convention of perspective there is no visual reciprocity.
>
> (Berger 1974: 16, emphasis in original)

Relations of the visible are culturally specific (Grosz 1994) and contextual (Merleau-Ponty 1962), and western histories have privileged the visual (Crary 1990; Nast and Kobayashi 1996) historically associated with masculinity (Classon 1997).

How participants take up gendered identities in digital spaces is, however, rather more fraught than a simple mapping of digital gender on to organic bodies or point of view on to 'consciousness'. Gender is not a product but rather a process. There is no 'fixed' meaning to digital representations, nor is there a single way those signs are interpreted. As Balsamo argues '[i]f we think of . . . embodiment as an effect . . . we can begin to ask questions about how the body is staged differently in different realities' (1996: 131). On the one hand, being 'dispossessed' of a body offers possibilities for ambiguity in the construction of self and bodily experience. On the other hand, digitally-coded bodily attributes become markers available for participants to negotiate as already materially-embodied beings with biographies and histories (Grosz 1994). The shape and form of a digital body, coding clothing, skin colour or hairstyle, points to the ways these markers of difference are explicitly constructed and therefore open up performative possibilities. While the bodies, for example, in Dactyl Nightmare bear unmistakable western cultural codes of masculinity, participants coded generic bodies as the more 'everyday', performative genders of themselves and other participants. Women can and do experience the 'generic' digital representation of their body in Dactyl Nightmare as 'feminine':

> I mean I went as a woman and I was a woman in the thing . . . You were on a . . . floating platform in space with stairs . . . And . . . definitely, you know. I was a woman in virtual reality, as I am

in real life. It made a difference in the sense that it seemed more real, like if I was a bloke, a man in the game [grimace]. But I was a curvaceous woman and I played it to suit me.

(Interview, Cate, Auckland, March 1996)

Considering the specificity of bodily form and action in digital worlds, and asking questions about the identities and investments of participants, therefore suggest a fraught and contradictory field of investments in gender across programmed and non-programmed worlds. If the histories and biographies of participants are important in the construction of virtual engendering, the histories and biographies of the machines are equally so, including the material sites in which the machines are embedded. Crucially, the worlds discussed here are situated in sites of consumption of various sorts. The practices of consumption have important effects in what it means to 'become virtual' and how gender is enacted in that process.

Consuming technologies: gender in sites of consumption

As I encountered sites of virtual reality consumption, I became aware of the diversity of contexts in which virtual reality technologies are sold and consumed as public activities. It seems that the places where virtual reality technologies are situated offer various contexts through which to situate gendering as a practice and a process of 'becoming virtual'. What kinds of sites 'locate' the worlds described above? What opportunities for consumption are there, and how are they taken up/ enacted?

In the sites explored virtual experiences are positioned as pleasurable leisure practices through which participants are invited to situate themselves as consumers of virtual experiences. Hawkins suggests that consumption should be considered as 'a practice marked by the cultural relations and processes which consumers bring to a commodity *and the conditions under which they use it*. The meanings and pleasure of leisure emerge in the relationship between leisure commodities and their consumers . . .' (1990: 215, emphasis in original).

The consumption of virtual realities is where a range of technical systems, publics, audiences, leisure centre operators and virtual reality producers come together in specific sites. These locations are embedded in networks of capital industry deployed for the production and profit associated with the construction of pleasurable experiences.

Meaning circulates here through representational techniques, but so do money and networks of business organization, so do publics and their relationships with each other. What is sold and consumed in virtual reality sites are not tangible objects, but rather a series of effects: pleasure, entertainment and spectacle (Hawkins 1990: 210–11). What makes these effects compelling is the opportunity to rework embodiment and subjectivity through the collapse of distinctions between body and technology in sites that encourage these boundary crossings.

Technologies in these sites of consumption often serve to alter bodily states, thus constructing alternative bodily spaces, activities and experiences. As Bennett notes, what is done through the consumption of bodily pleasures – danger, thrills and the achievement of otherwise impossible states – is to rearrange bodily boundaries temporarily: 'suspending the physical laws that normally restrict its movement, breaking the social codes that normally regulate its conduct, inverting the usual relations between the body and machinery and generally inscribing the body in relations different from those in which it is caught and held in everyday life' (1983: 147). It is not so much that virtual reality provides an 'escape' from reality, but that it provides a temporarily alternative reality (Springer 1996: 81) among a number of such alternatives that are embedded in everyday life but are also resistant to it (Cohen and Taylor 1992).

The locales visited employed various techniques to produce the effects of pleasure in sites coded for the consumption of experiences as commodities. Virtual reality technologies become integrated into the social worlds of cafés, arcades and galleries, but are positioned differently in each of those sites. Arcades were a common place to find Virtuality systems among more familiar video games. Video arcades are packed with machines in every available space and are filled with light and sound effects; signals that the machines are at work, therefore consumers are having 'fun'. The audiences for the pleasures of arcades are predominantly young men (Shuker 1995) and game scenarios which focus on physical/bodily mastery both reflect and construct this audience. The opportunities for men to play out qualities of masculinity (such as 'competitiveness' or 'aggression') in these public spaces seems to prompt some staff, operators and consumers to agree that virtual reality has its highest appeal with men because it requires/allows exactly this kind of bodily movement. This assumption effectively reinscribes already established categories of gender. A staff member in a VR-themed leisure centre assumed that men's 'competitiveness' made virtual realities more attractive to them:

Well during the day our sales are to a lot of business people, corporate people. I can say a lot of women come in but I have a lot of men come in as well and they like it a lot more . . . they will want to be shooting each other. They're competitive.

(Interview, Christina, San Francisco, March 1996)

These spaces combine the pleasures of game mastery and skills, crowds, noise, imagery and spectacle. They are the contemporary worlds of 'carnivalesque':

> Carnival is not a spectacle seen by the people; they live in it, and everyone participates . . . While carnival lasts, there is no other life outside it. During carnival time life is subject only to its laws, that is, the laws of its own freedom . . . Carnival celebrated temporary liberation from the prevailing truth and from the established order . . . it demanded ever changing, playful, undefined forms.
>
> (Bakhtin 1984: 7–11)

The 'danger' often associated with arcades reflects this boundary crossing and at least partly arises from the way the unruliness of interpersonal relationships encourages consumption. The pleasures of playing virtual reality among crowds involves not only the fun of game skill but also the fun provided by competition with significant others. Games involve intense interaction, competition, direct sociality and a symbolic aggression which is out of bounds in other arenas, but which can be acted out safely in spaces 'framed off' from everyday life (Goffman 1972). The 'moral panics' associated with this kind of intensive and competitive interaction have prompted a reorganization of leisure sites towards a more controlled and regulated consumption which finds its most clear and developed expression in the 'theme park'. Accordingly, what were once male-dominated video game arcades in downtown areas of cities are becoming suburban 'family entertainment centres', urban bars and cafés or themed leisure centres. These sites offer pleasures unavailable in arcades with which those who wouldn't participate in arcade life can identify.

Themed virtual reality centres produce environments that encourage ordered crowds and controlled spectacles: they are disciplined pleasures. The prototype of the contemporary theme park is Disneyland. According to Weinstein (1992), Disneyland was created as a family amusement park, a clean and safe (sanitized and beautified) middle-American environment. As one theme centre manager remarked, the 'vision' for the virtual reality store he managed:

> ... was kind of like the Disney store, where you can just walk into any city ... and you'd know exactly what to expect when you came ... They'd be dressed the same, they would have the same uniforms, they'd have similar games, same price structure, and it would be just a new big thing in every major city.
>
> (Interview, Ben, San Francisco, March 1996)

Familiar bodily conventions, activities and regulations are employed to reappropriate 'risk' to make the space of virtual reality consumption mundane and not too fantastic. The conventionality of public leisure spaces underlines the ways that the fantastic is progressively becoming more mundane at the same time as 'everyday life' is, through mediation, becoming mundanely spectacular (Rojek 1993). Such conventions serve to provide spaces where everyday gender identities can be unproblematically assumed, thereby repressing any challenges presented by the potential ambiguities of digital worlds or the unruliness they might 'engender'.

By contrast with arcades and theme centres, art galleries and museums as spaces for consumption share a conventional orientation towards knowledge and aesthetic consumption as the framework for pleasurable experience. In the rise of industrialization, a particularly bourgeois consciousness emerged where 'experience' becomes a form of moral and ethical work, positioned in direct opposition to the play of 'low' culture. The collection of experiences is designed for 'self-realization', self improvement and education. Alongside this vision are the bourgeois institutions of 'high' modernism which act as intermediaries to position virtual realities in the arenas of 'art' and 'culture' (Bourdieu 1979). Audiences here are assumed to be educated, reflexive and critical. It is a captive and spectacular world for consumers but the bodies in the spaces – through muted voices, subtle bodily gestures and the effacement of the technology – generate an alternative consumption environment to that of the arcade or leisure centre.

What these different sites share across the struggle over 'high' and 'low' cultures is a studied organization of physical and social spaces which foreground the pleasures of virtual experiences as experiential commodities. The consumption of virtual reality across different sites follows the familiar ways that technical systems are already embedded in an industrial complex vis-à-vis consumer ICT and media industries. These industries already draw on the stories of digitally mediated selfhood as a rationale for technical research and development.

The relations in consumption sites position subjects as actors in a spectacular consumption designed by culture industries to encourage use and therefore payment. The discourses of technical mastery and progress, and the simulation of selfhood, are both available to consolidate familiar and new/transfigured social activities in the service of an already entrenched consumption of leisure and pleasure (Balsamo 1996).

The consumption of culture tends to be gendered, both in product and process, because the gendered sensibilities of audiences in specific sites are already assumed by the individuals and institutions of the relevant 'culture industries' (Traube 1996). This is certainly the case in spaces where virtual reality technologies are consumed. On the one hand, spaces such as leisure centres remain dominated by men, even when such spaces become controlled and sanitized through the mechanisms of theming. While galleries deploy controlled pleasures that are ostensibly universal, its audiences are deeply implicated in the construction of the gendered subject of enlightenment modernity. In all these spaces, binary oppositions – immanence/transcendence, low/high, nature/technology, body/mind – are associated and articulated with the feminine/masculine gender binary. The association of dominant terms in technology relations – masculine, transcendence and technology – alongside the historical construction of masculine spaces tends to reinforce virtual reality as an enterprise of consumption in which a material body is simultaneously suppressed/erased in a masculinized transcendence and simultaneously called into the immanent service of a digital body in a digital world.

Diverse subject positions are therefore offered through competing technical, economic and cultural practices of virtual reality consumption. Different pleasures – competitive sociality, eating and drinking, buying merchandise, knowledge as pleasure, and mastery and skill – render virtual realities familiar and make them accessible for mass consumption. At the same time, virtual reality configures the consumption of technically mediated experiences in new ways. While 'mass' consumption appropriates the potential ambiguities and boundary crossing of digital spaces, it does not ever finally recoup them. These practices can therefore reinforce familiar ways of being gendered in public spaces of leisure consumption, and can establish new conventions of virtual identities and experiences and offer a number of different spaces for their articulation. One space through which gendering practices are articulated is through the spectacles in virtual reality consumption sites.

Spectacles: gender and relations of looking

The sites explored drew on familiar conventions of spectacular spaces and relations of looking to encourage consumption of virtual reality. Those who do the work of organizing such spaces attempt to generate particular meanings for the use of virtual reality technologies that will incite the desire to consume. Just as the dominant mode of perception and relation in digital worlds is visual, sites of virtual reality consumption are organized around relations of looking (Hillis 1996).

In arcades, images are everywhere. Multiple television monitors are often arranged adjacent to virtual reality machines, and are designed to interpret the digital world and make sense of the 'real life' actions of participants. Monitors display the points of view of any participants in the game at the time, and promotional 'videos' provide ongoing images of what the game looks like, the character the player will 'be' and how the technical objects should be handled and worn. The monitors are accompanied by prominent posters. One advertisement for a VR-themed leisure centre bore the legend:

> Because reality sucks: Here's the deal. Reality has toxic waste spills, transmission overhauls and bad hair days. Virtual Reality has nothing but totally fun games played in strange yet stylish headgear. Which would you prefer?
>
> CyberMind Virtual Reality Centers

The text was accompanied by the image of a woman. Figure 8.2 displays two 'takes' on this image of an older woman in a floral print dress with her hair in curlers. In the first, she has an old hairdryer poised over her head and looks bored. In the second, she has on a head-mounted display. Her mouth is now open in astonishment, her body springing upwards. Williams (in Bukatman 1995: 282) notes that these articulations signal 'a retreat from technology into technology' which incorporates a 'phantasmagoria of progress' which further 'involves a sustained immersion within an artificial environment that suggests technology's own ability to incorporate what it has generally excluded' (Bukatman 1995: 283). This incorporation includes those identities and forms of embodiment historically excluded from connection with advanced computing and communications technologies.

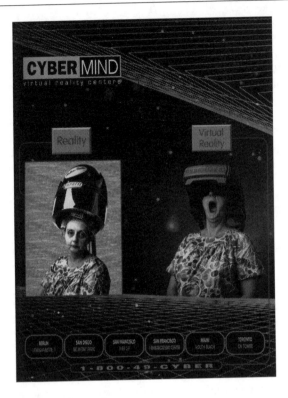

Figure 8.2 Because reality sucks

Promotional images in centres are underscored by spectacles of bodily interaction, prompted by the intensive and competitive sociality among groups of people. People's movement, noise, talk and discussion produces a 'spectacle of voice . . . movement and gesture' (Lynch 1995: 227). Furthermore, sitting and passing time are implicitly but effectively discouraged by the lack of seats: when I visited arcades to do observation, I found there was nowhere to sit down unless I sat on the floor. Standing bodies, clustered around machines, instead invites a reading of intense and spectacular bodily activity, conveyed to the observer through stance and movement. The bodies of other participants become a promise of the pleasures available and act to advertise the excitement of virtual reality consumption.

Bodies in crowds are translated into a digitized informational spectacle when people are used in advertisements for virtual reality. Watching and being watched become licensed and relations of 'the gaze' are inevitably assumed. Rose (1993) has argued that the occupation of public space can be a fraught process for women in particular, given their historical association with private and domestic space (see also Duncan 1996). Yet there are also the pleasures of publicly demonstrating competence in a virtual world projected as entertainment for others. There are pleasures for both women and men in looking and being looked at. While looking is inevitably gendered and sexualized, especially in the ways that the digital and public is associated with the 'disembodied' mind, and femininity with the materiality of the body, these are not stable categories – they shift with context. Kipnis (1993) suggests that there are ways of looking other than the positions outlined by Mulvey (1975) who first asserted that masculine subjects constructed relations of looking which position women as 'objects' in film representation. This alternative looking draws on the space of the city. The scenes of Baudelaire's *flâneur* (Benjamin 1973), the ambiguous dream spaces of Benjamin's 'arcades' (Buck-Morss 1989; Boyer 1996), or Simmel's 'metropolis' (Frisby 1986) are urban sites where the chaotic, the contingent, the ephemeral and the new piled vision upon vision. These spaces both call on and reinforce existing modes of media and leisure consumption such as the spectacles of crowds in shopping centres (Langman 1992).

It is not only the spectacles of interacting bodies that act to 'engender' participants. The form of the virtual reality machines themselves provides imagery symbolic of technological progress as a human (enlightenment) ideal. They can be read as texts that advertise the high-tech science fiction pleasures of virtual realities. Their physical manifestation, their size and their more or less prominent location in specific spaces invoke the ultimate 'seriousness' of virtual reality. The form of artefacts such as Virtuality machines is reminiscent of other discourses of human/machine fusion and invite responses centred in the celebration of the cybernetic interface (Springer 1996). The enclosing pod of black sleek plastic on the Virtuality machines and the head-mounted displays, connect referentially with science fiction texts such as the 'Borg' in *Star Trek: The Next Generation* (Fuchs 1993), signifying technological progress, expansion and the frontiers of human/computer relations where human/machine hybrids are created.

OSMOSE is similarly referential of science fiction texts. In OSMOSE, an immersant's connection with the technologies is projected for an audience through a transparent screen on which the silhouette of the immersant appears via background lighting. The head mount and cables connected to the body are rendered as a poetic element to be viewed by others. While the body of a participant is on view, the audience is given licence to watch and identify with human connection to virtual reality technology.

As Springer (1996) points out, these technically enhanced bodies are those of a technologically mediated dream to master the uncertainties and threats to the various hegemonies of masculine subjectivities at the end of the twentieth century. Expected audiences frame how virtual reality spectacles are constructed in consumption spaces. On the one hand, the diversity of different spectacles, both within and across sites, offers freedom of choice for different ways of understanding what it means to 'become virtual', potentially destabilizing developmental 'trajectories' for virtual reality technologies and the uses of them as technologies of gender (de Lauretis 1987). On the other hand, spectacles such as the elevation of participants' bodies, and the appropriation of interpersonal interaction as advertising, physically produces the 'self-surveilling' subject (Foucault 1973, 1979). In virtual reality technologies, self-surveilling subjects are produced through the identification with available spectacles and its attendant desire to consume. Such identification requires the (willing) discipline of participants' bodies by the machines and the regulation of their performance by their own assumption of an all-encompassing gaze. Consumers' bodies must be disciplined to produce and participate in such spectacles and made to operate in formalized, standardized and often gendered ways for the spectacular effect to take place.

Disciplines: the bodily performance of gender

In order to create consumption spectacles in particular locales, bodies must be encouraged to work both with each other and with technologies. As we have already seen, this work is achieved through the production of the desire to become virtual in various ways and the multiple pleasures of consumption therein. The pleasures of virtual reality interfaces are, however, only achievable through specific bodily disciplines.

The system itself as a technical bio-apparatus participates in the process of regulating consumption behaviour, both organizing 'appropriate' consumption activities and defining which bodies are able to consume. The machines simultaneously define what bodies can participate while encouraging the imaginary that everybody can consume equally. Manufacturers of the products, for example, provide safety guidelines displayed both on the machines and on adjacent signs. A large and prominent sandwich board next to a machine in one site announced:

Warning! Do not play this game if you:

- Are less than 110 cm tall;

- Are pregnant or may be pregnant;

- Are under the influence of alcohol or drugs;

- Have high blood pressure or a heart ailment;

- Have neck or spinal pain;

- Have eye disease;

- Need assistance when walking;

- Have experienced muscle twitches, loss of awareness while watching TV, playing video games or being exposed to strong light stimulation.

Before game

The MVD (Mega Visor Display [the head-mounted display]) is to be used without eyeglasses. This may cause difficulty in focusing for some individuals.

Some hairstyles may keep the MVD from fitting properly.

Please wipe off any perspiration before putting on the MVD.

Please refrain from playing this game without a break.

During game

If you experience dizziness or discomfort while playing this game, immediately discontinue play.

In case of mechanical difficulties, please call a nearby attendant.

After game

If you experience eye fatigue, drying of the eyes, flickering or dizziness after playing this game, be sure to rest until fully recovered.

Do not drive automobiles immediately after playing this game.

Attention! The MVD is a sophisticated piece of machinery. Please do not hit, drop, pull or otherwise damage the MVD.

The signs point out how humans should interact with the machine, including the appropriate use and handling of artefacts. Specific bodily states (such as epilepsy) and particularly gendered states (such as pregnancy) are either excluded or regulated by the bio-apparatus. These transgressive states, outside the categories of 'normal' (Sawicki 1991) are marginalized through their explicit exclusion. When these bodies do participate, they cause uneasiness and challenge the categories defined through normalizing practices at the sites:

> One time this guy came in, and his wife with him, and his wife was very pregnant and she was playing – which, I was concerned about but . . . I kept an eye on her. They got out of the game, [and] his other friend was very upset at him that he kept killing his wife . . . and child . . . shooting his wife and child over and over . . .
>
> (Interview, Kelly, San Francisco, March 1996)

This scene is disturbing in context for participants in the sites, not only because it crosses the boundaries of 'appropriate' consumers, but also because it challenges assumptions about appropriate behaviour for masculine and feminine bodies as defined through specific bodily states and practices. The most disturbing feature for the friend was not the 'physical' risks associated with her pregnancy, but the symbolic significance of the continual shooting. Here, femininity is defined through pregnancy rendering the woman's engagement in digital technology – which might be dangerous to herself and therefore her child's health (although how is not specified) – inappropriate, especially as she is playing a competitive game through it. Masculinity is equally defined by bodily actions and an inappropriate masculinity behaviour is one in which the man 'shoots' his wife – the potential mother – and the potential child. Virtual bodies are obviously not pregnant bodies and it seems that virtual bodies are also highly gendered through the material practices available for them.

These occasions demonstrate how virtual reality technologies produce different disciplinary effects on different bodies. For cyberpunk communities, submission to or penetration by the machine's apparatus might signify the redefinition and expansion of the human body by information technologies. When that body is gendered feminine, however, and acts as a woman's body, such disciplines have inescapable resonance with genres such as pornography. Women's important means of social agency – their ability to see, to speak and to have voice – can be erased by a technical bio-apparatus such as virtual reality which physically closes off the eyes and mouth. The symbolic significance of these disciplines is therefore potentially different for differentially gendered bodies.

The consumption of virtual worlds and technologies is a set of practices that connect representation in programmed and non-programmed worlds with material practices of gender. Virtual reality technologies are implicated in popular representations of digital space and embodiment but are also intimately connected with the ways that virtual systems are already lived 'everyday': prosthetics matter. Consuming the virtual doesn't mean that gender is erased in digitally saturated contexts. Rather, gendered bodily activities are enabled and/or constrained by a range of digital embodiments, commodity spectacles, consumption possibilities and forms of bio-apparatus. Bodies in virtual reality technologies become sites of struggle for competing forms of discipline that operate at the level of, and on, the body as it enacts virtual embodiment and subjectivity.

Conclusions

The connections between representation and practice in sites of consumption are fraught and present contradictory subject positions for women (and men) who want to participate in virtual worlds. This discussion has explored some of the ways in which 'the virtual', its spectacles and disciplines are consumed in a range of local sites. Spaces framed for leisure generate completely 'real' embodied pleasures which are attractive because they are already completely fantastic.

The politics of becoming virtual are not simply related to the subjective possibilities and constraints of cyberspaces. Rather, the politics of 'becoming virtual' are also caught up with how gendered virtual bodies and identities are inscribed and elaborated through the social locations in which virtual reality technologies are used/consumed.

Paying particular attention to spectacle and space in sites of consumption, and the bodily disciplines required for the consumption of virtual realities, draws attention to a range of different consumer pleasures constructed in diverse locations. Various subject positions are offered through competing technical, economic and cultural practices. These subject positions can establish new conventions of virtual identities and experiences, and offer a number of different spaces for their articulation.

Gendered identities and the confusion of them across programmed and non-programmed spaces are possible. In order to understand how virtual realities might rework conventional boundaries of body and identity, we must examine the multiple contexts in which virtual reality technologies come to be consumed. As Balsamo argues however, both programmed and non-programmed worlds are simultaneously cultural and technical constructions, both 'fully saturated by the media and other forms of everyday technologies' (1996: 125). The ways gendered identities and embodiments are taken up remain shot through, albeit unevenly, with familiar operational categories of gendered identities and bodily practices. How technologies become embedded in social spaces impacts significantly on the forms of virtual subjectivity and identity possible. Immersive virtual reality technologies cannot be understood as social artefacts without some consideration of the locales in which they are embedded and the consumption practices on which they draw, deeply implicated as they are in 'culture industries'. A local, reflexive and feminist orientation assists in understanding the gendered dynamics associated with 'becoming virtual'.

Note

1 The names of all games and equipment in this chapter are copyrighted and/or trademarked to the respective authors, artists and/or companies that have developed and produced them.

References

Bakhtin, M. (1984) *Rabelais and His World*, Bloomington: Indiana University Press.
Balsamo, A. (1996) *Technologies of the Gendered Body: Reading Cyborg Women*, Durham, NC: Duke University Press.
Benedikt, M. (1991) *Cyberspace: First Steps*, Cambridge, MA: The MIT Press.
Benjamin, W. (1973) *Charles Baudelaire: A Lyric Poet in the Era of High Capitalism*, trans. H. Zohn, London: New Left Books.
Bennett, T. (1983) *Formations of Pleasure*, London: Routledge and Kegan Paul.
Berger, J. (1974) *Ways of Seeing*, London: BBC and Penguin Books.

Bergstrom, J. (1991) 'Androids and androgyny' in C. Penley, E. Lyon, L. Spigel and J. Bergstrom (eds) *Close Encounters: Film, Feminism and Science Fiction*, Minneapolis: University of Minnesota Press.

Biocca, F. (1992) 'Communication within virtual reality: creating a space for research', *Journal of Communication*, 42 (4): 5–21.

Bourdieu, P. (1979) *Distinction: A Social Critique of the Judgement of Taste*, trans. Richard Nice, Cambridge, MA: Harvard University Press.

Boyer, M. Christine (1996) *Cybercities: Visual Perception in the Age of Electronic Communication*, New York: Princeton Architectural Press.

Brook, J. and Boal, I. A. (eds) (1995) *Resisting the Virtual Life: The Culture and Politics of Information*, San Francisco: City Lights.

Buck-Morss, S. (1989) *The Dialectics of Seeing: Walter Benjamin and the Arcades Project*, Cambridge, MA: The MIT Press.

Bukatman, S. (1995) 'The artificial infinite: on special effects and the sublime' in L. Cooke and P. Wollen (eds) *Visual Display: Culture Beyond Appearances*, Dia Centre for the Arts, Discussions in Contemporary Culture No. 10, Seattle, WA: Bay Press.

Classon, C. (1997) 'Engendering perception: gender ideologies and sensory hierarchies in western history', *Body and Society*, 3 (2): 1–19.

Cohen, S. and Taylor, L. (1992) *Escape Attempts: The Theory and Practice of Resistance to Everyday Life* (second edition), London: Routledge.

Crary, J. (1990) *Techniques of the Observer: On Vision and Modernity in the Nineteenth Century*, Cambridge, MA: The MIT Press.

Davies, C. (1995) *OSMOSE: Fly Through and Interviews*, video recording, Canada: Softimage.

De Lauretis, T. (1987) *Technologies of Gender: Essays on Theory, Film and Fiction*, Indiana University Press: United States.

Doane, M. A. (1989) 'Commentary: cyborgs, origins and subjectivity' in E. Weed (ed.) *Coming to Terms: Feminism, Theory, Politics*, New York: Routledge.

Duncan, N. (1996) 'Renegotiating gender and sexuality in public and private spaces' in N. Duncan (ed.) *BodySpace: Destabilizing Geographies of Gender and Sexuality*, London: Routledge.

Foucault, M. (1973) *The Birth of the Clinic: An Archeology of Medical Perception*, trans. A. M. Sheridan, London: Tavistock.

Foucault, M. (1979) [1977] *Discipline and Punish: The Birth of the Prison*, trans. Alan Sheridan, New York: Vintage Books.

Frisby, D. (1986) *Fragments of Modernity*, Cambridge, MA: The MIT Press.

Fuchs, C. J. (1993) ' "Death is irrelevant": cyborgs, reproduction and the future of male hysteria', *Genders*, 18: 113–33.

Goffman, E. (1972) *Encounters: Two Studies in the Sociology of Interaction*, Harmondsworth: Penguin.

Grosz, E. (1994) *Volatile Bodies: Toward a Corporeal Feminism*, Australia: Allen and Unwin.

Haddon, L. (1992) 'Explaining ICT consumption: the case of the home computer' in R. Silverstone and E. Hirsch (eds) *Consuming Technologies: Media and Information in Domestic Spaces*, London: Routledge.

Hawkins, G. (1990) 'Too much fun: producing and consuming pleasure at Australia's wonderland' in D. Rowe and G. Lawrence (eds) *Sport and Leisure: Trends in Australian Popular Culture*, Sydney: Harcourt Brace Jovanovich.

Hayles, N. K. (1996) 'Embodied virtuality: or how to put bodies back into the picture' in M. A. Moser (ed.) *Immersed in Technology: Art and Virtual Environments*, Cambridge, MA: MIT Press.

Heim, M. (1998) *Virtual Realism*, New York: Oxford University Press.

Hillis, K. (1996) 'A geography of the eye: the technologies of virtual reality' in R. Sheilds (ed.) *Cultures of Internet: Virtual Spaces, Real Histories, Living Bodies*, London: Sage.

Kipnis, L. (1993) *Ecstasy Unlimited: On Sex, Capital, Gender and Aesthetics*, Minneapolis: University of Minnesota Press.

Kramarae, C. (1995) 'A backstage critique of virtual reality' in S. Jones (ed.) *Cybersociety: Computer-mediated Communication and Community*, Thousand Oaks, CA: Sage.

Langman, L. (1992) 'Neon cages: shopping for subjectivity' in R. Sheilds (ed.) *Lifestyle Shopping: The Subject of Consumption*, London: Routledge.

Lynch, M. (1995) 'Laboratory space and the technological complex: an investigation of topical contexture' in S. L. Star (ed.) *Ecologies of Knowledge: Work and Politics in Science and Technology*, Albany: State University of New York Press.

McCaffrey, L. (ed.) (1991) *Storming the Reality Studio: A Casebook of Cyberpunk and Postmodern Science Fiction*, Durham, NC: Duke University Press.

Menser, M. and Aronowitz, S. (1996) 'On cultural studies, science, and technology' in S. Aronowitz, B. Martinson, M. Menser and J. Rich (eds) *Technoscience and Cyberculture*, New York: Routledge.

Merleau-Ponty, M. (1962) *Phenomenology of Perception*, trans. C. Smith, London: Routledge and Kegan Paul.

Morse, M. (1997) *Virtualities: Television, Media Art, Cyberculture*, Bloomington: Indiana University Press.

Mulvey, L. (1975) 'Visual pleasure and narrative cinema', *Screen*, 16 (3): 6–18.

Nast, H. J. and Kobayashi, A. (1996) 'Re-corporealising vision' in N. Duncan (ed.) *BodySpace*, London: Routledge.

Plant, S. (1996) 'Feminizations: reflections on women and virtual reality' in L. Hershman Leeson (ed.) *Clicking In: Hot Links to a Digital Culture*, Seattle, WA: Bay Press.

Robins, K. (1996) 'Cyberspace and the world we live in' in J. Dovey (ed.) *Fractal Dreams: New Media in Social Context*, London: Lawrence and Wishart.

Rojek, C. (1993) *Ways of Escape: Modern Transformations in Leisure and Travel*, London: Macmillan Press.

Rose, G. (1993) *Feminism and Geography: The Limits of Geographical Knowledge*, University of Minnesota Press: Minneapolis.

Sawicki, J. (1991) *Disciplining Foucault: Feminism, Power and the Body*, New York: Routledge.

Schroeder, R. (1996) *Possible Worlds: The Social Dynamic of Virtual Reality Technology*, Boulder, CO: Westview Press.

Shuker, R. (1995) 'Video games: serious fun', *Sites*, 31: 50–70.

Silverstone, R. and Haddon, L. (1996) 'Design and the domestication of information and communication technologies: technical change and everyday life' in R. Mansell and R. Silverstone (eds) *Communication by Design: The Politics of Information and Communication Technologies*, Oxford: Oxford University Press.

Sofia, Z. (1992) 'Virtual corporeality: a feminist view', *Australian Feminist Studies*, 15: 11–24.

Sofia, Z. (1993) *Whose Second Self? Gender and (Ir)Rationality in Computer Culture*, Geelong: Deakin University Press.

Springer, C. (1996) *Electronic Eros: Bodies and Desire in the Post-Industrial Age*, Austin: University of Texas Press.

Stone, A. R. (1996) 'Cyberdämmerung at wellspring systems' in M. A. Moser (ed.) (with D. MacLeod) *Immersed in Technology: Art and Virtual Environments*, Banff Centre for the Arts, Cambridge, MA: The MIT Press.

Terry, J. and Calvert, M. (1997) 'Introduction: machines/lives' in J. Terry and M. Calvert (eds) *Processed Lives: Gender and Technology in Everyday Life*, London and New York: Routledge.

Traube, E. (1996) 'Introduction' in R. Ohmann (ed.) with G. Averill, M. Curtin, D. Shumway and E. Traube *Making and Selling Culture*, Hanover: Wesleyan University Press.

Ullman, E. (1995) 'Out of time: reflections on the programming life' in J. Brook and I. A. Boal (eds) *Resisting the Virtual Life: The Culture and Politics of Information*, San Francisco: City Lights.

Weinstein, R. M. (1992) 'Disneyland and Coney Island: reflections of the evolution of the modern amusement park', *Journal of Popular Culture*, 26 (1): 131–64.

Chapter 9

Technology, leisure and everyday practices

Eileen Green

Introduction

A rapid expansion of information and communication technologies (ICTs) for use in the household over the last decade has generated a corresponding academic interest in the design and use of technologies for domestic consumption, whether for work or leisure purposes. Despite this, empirical research in the area remains limited; especially that which addresses gender issues (Green and Adam 1998; Green 2000). New forms of technology are announced daily, ranging from hand-held mobile phones with Internet connections to interactive, digital television, which promises to deliver multiple services from our living rooms. We know that the number of users online has expanded rapidly, increasing from an estimated 9 per cent of the UK population in 1997 to double that figure by December 1998 (Hamill 2000: 12) and that individuals are using an increasing variety of ICTs for leisure and work in the home. However, we know little about either the economic or social context of such use and the negotiations involved, including the gender dimensions.

Despite educational campaigns to ensure uniform levels of access to school children and public policy initiatives to expand the number of households online, little in-depth research has been conducted into the use of ICTs in the home. Earlier interest in the impact of technology centered upon paid employment generating a raft of workplace studies within the UK and Scandinavia, including feminist-inspired work on the design of computerized office systems in the 1980s and early 1990s (Vehviläinen 1991; Green et al. 1993). However, recent research on IT and gender seems to have shifted away from employment or workplace studies. Occupying centre-stage instead are studies of virtuality, including debates about gender and virtual identity and gendered cyborgs (Balsamo 1996; Green 2000). This emphasis upon the possibilities of virtual environments moves our attention away from empirical projects which highlight structural inequalities in access to and consumption of ICTs, focusing instead upon the individual and highlighting such issues as personal agency and virtual identities. Interesting and important though these debates are, the tendency for inequalities to become inscribed in ever more complex ways still requires our attention.

This chapter argues for the need for more research on access to, and the differential use of, ICTS and the meanings which specific artefacts, such as PCs, assume within everyday life. It explores the potential impact of ICTs upon leisure patterns within the household, suggesting the need for research which asks questions about the extent to which differences such as gender affect the level and type of use of ICTs. Feminist leisure research has long argued for holistic understandings of women's leisure, indicating that shortage of time and opportunities mostly constrain women's leisure choices (Green et al. 1990; Wearing 1998). Are such inequalities replicated within electronic leisure? And do space and time continue to be defining factors? Focusing upon the contribution of research which examines 'the everyday', this chapter suggests the need for more information about the ways in which new ICTS are appropriated and consumed within households. Such data would inform our understanding of the social practices associated with the introduction and use of ICTs in the home and would enable insights into the complex web of social meanings which become embedded in the placing of specific technologies and social interaction around ownership and use.

ICTs and the everyday

The traditional portrayal of technological innovation as an end in itself fails to address the complexity of the interaction between technology, personal consumption and the construction of identity. We need to know more about the ways in which 'ordinary people' appropriate 'ordinary technologies'. The mundane, routine aspects of the everyday, the ordinary, rather than the extraordinary, provide the backdrop for most people's lives; including those of women, as they perform the caring, domestic and organizing roles which keep the fabric of the household together. Researching the ways in which consumers appropriate specific technologies and adapt them within household contexts can also provide important insights into the constantly evolving nature of the gendered social relations which constitute 'normal family life', including the use of leisure or free time. Technological artefacts may be marketed as 'leisure goods' but for an object or a technology to be accepted, it has to be found a space and assume a function; in short, it needs to mesh with the everyday.

Contemporary theorizations of the family (Morgan 1996, 1999) emphasize the centrality of the household as an arena in which family practices, including those of consumption, are located; practices which include the acquisition and use of technologies (Silva 2000). The final meaning and significance of particular technologies is not prescribed but arises instead out of complex processes of social negotiation. Indeed, as has been argued elsewhere, technology is best understood as a social as well as technical process (Silverstone and Haddon 1996; Green and Adam 1998), which blends seamlessly with the everyday. We need, therefore, to examine the relationship between the process of technological innovation and the ways in which various ICTs are consumed and become domesticated. As Stepulevage argues:

> Recognition of the interweaving of technology in everyday life enables relations to be better understood as also constituting means through which we develop knowledge about the world and use technologies as we negotiate transformations in our lives. Reflection upon our experiences can provide grounds for exploring a new construction of technology, a construction that crosses a boundary of broad social and more individual personal relations.
>
> (Stepulevage 1999: 415)

A number of feminists (Silva 2000) among others, have drawn upon Bourdieu's concept of the habitus[1] to analyse the significance of the everyday, including the domestic routines and responsibilities embedded in ordinary family life. Through the concept of habitus, Bourdieu describes ways of doing and being which individuals acquire via a continuous socialization process, the acquisition of which he terms 'practical sense' or 'knowing how' rather than 'knowing that'. This is a form of common sense which includes gendered ways of knowing and being which become an inextricable part of the intimate details of everyday life. However, as Silva comments 'Although Bourdieu has an understanding of the gendered character of dispositions, this is by no means central to his framework. This leads to a neglect of the emotional dimension in accounts of the "habitus"' (2000: 3). It falls to feminist theorists such as Silva, to theorize the gender dimensions of such conceptualization adequately. Interrogating the emotional dimensions provides us with vital insights on the nature of women's role in the construction of 'home life', including their contribution to domestic arrangements and caring regimes within which individual identities and collective belongings are formed. Family relaxation and leisure practices are a key site of such habitus and, as such, as will be argued later, constitute a key site of sociological enquiry.

From technology and women's employment to technologies of the everyday

Perhaps the most well known and often cited work on the gender technology relation is that provided by Cynthia Cockburn (1983, 1985) whose early work focused on the relationship between technological change, deskilling and gender inequalities. Her work and that of Game and Pringle (1983), engaged with Marxist labour process theory inspired work (Braverman 1974) in an effort to bridge the theoretical gap between 'technology as neutral' but misappropriated under capitalism, and the embryonic social constructionist frameworks which adopted a 'social shaping' approach to technology (Mackenzie and Wajcman 1985). Detailed analysis of this debate is beyond the scope of this chapter,[2] but is of interest and relevant to our purposes, as are the reflections of Cockburn (1992) who argues that feminists and social shaping theorists (particularly actor network theorists) are asking different questions. Feminists are concerned with the continuities of gendered social relations which manifest themselves through each successive wave of technological innovation. However, more traditional sociologies of technology assume the key question to be the relationship between technological innovation and social change but ignore the importance of gender relations which make a key contribution to the transformation of everyday living.

At a theoretical level, the shift of intellectual interest from technologies associated with women's employment to those being introduced into the domestic sphere brings together literature from a variety of sources. These sources include the sociology of technology, and feminist-inspired debates on the family, households and the organization of everyday life. This work builds upon a now substantial body of literature emanating from the 'gender and technology' debate (succinctly summarized by Henwood 1993) and includes Cockburn and Ormrod's ground-breaking work on domestic technology (1993) and that of Faulkner and Arnold (1985). This debate draws upon research conducted in the 1980s into the effects of 'new' technologies on women's jobs.

Over the last two decades, this has evolved into a series of linked debates about what is commonly referred to as the gender–technology relation (Wajcman 1991; Grint and Gill 1995). Pertinent questions within these debates include: Is technology inherently masculine? Are technologies implicated in women's oppression or might they provide the means for their liberation? Can we separate theoretical understandings of the gender–technology relation from the empirical contexts within which they are studied? In the 1980s the quest seemed to be to extrapolate the components of a feminist theory of technology from empirically grounded analyses that constituted gender relations as a key focus. Two decades later such 'grand' theorization continues to elude us. However, the key to moving this debate forward may be contained within a closer analysis of gender–technology relations, which are inextricably bound up with everyday practices. Diverting our attention from the everyday in pursuit of 'grand theory' may be misplaced in contexts where those everyday practices are becoming transformed in concert with a bewildering array of newly available 'domesticated' ICTs.

What feminists working in the area come together on is the premise that rather than perceiving technology as having 'social aspects', we need instead to work from a base which represents technology (in this case ICTs) as social. Remembering the dream of the 1980s Utopian 'paperless office', which as Woolgar (2000) comments, still hasn't emerged, we need to resist the temptation to focus primarily upon the potential of new ICTs to achieve the extraordinary. Whether such events occur in the home (24-hour virtual entertainment) or in the office (virtual communication), we need to remember instead that it is the capacity of ICTs to become a routine part of the mundane everyday, which is important. Gender is clearly about social relations and, to understand the multiplicity of ways in which gender and technology interact with and shape each other, we also need to perceive ICTs as social relations (Cockburn and Furst-Dilic 1994).

And back to the sociology of family life

The focus then becomes not the ICTs themselves but the household or family practices within which they take shape and acquire meanings. This takes us away from the gender technology debate as traditionally conceived and back into the home where these practices occur within the gendered politics of a broadly conceived 'family life'. This is the same 'family' which is being targeted as potential consumers of the newest ICTs for education and leisure purposes, as the following extract from

British Telecom's *Future Talk* magazine demonstrates: 'Use new technology to catch up with your kids, stay in touch with your family and shop online' (BT 2000).

Like sociologist David Morgan (1996, 1999), marketing consultants advertising BT's new Internet access are well aware that modern families are more appropriately characterized by what they *do* together than on the nature of some traditional pre-given structure or household. Recent UK statistics from the Office for National Statistics (ONS) confirm a steadily growing trend towards cohabitation over the last two decades. This trend means that an increasing number of children are born outside marriage (four out of ten were born outside marriage in 1999, compared with just one in ten in 1979, Carvel 2000). The normal family of the twenty-first century is increasingly likely to include remarried or cohabiting adults and several sets of children who may or may not be biologically related to those adults and each other. These individuals are also likely to be part of several family and household groupings and routinely spend time in each; a pattern which almost certainly means that key leisure technologies will be regularly in transit between households, and may inhabit different spaces and be invested with different meanings across those households.

At an academic level, some of the most interesting attempts to theorize the use of technologies in the home (Cowan 1983; Silva 1999) have developed interdisciplinary perspectives, drawing upon both the sociology of consumption and contemporary sociologies of the family (Silva and Smart 1999; Smart and Neale 1999).

Such frameworks seem more promising than the more conventional sociology of technology approaches in terms of their potential to elucidate the complexity of everyday family practices of which technological relations form a part. Furthermore, it could be argued that the appropriation, acquisition and use of ICTs in ordinary households are part of the wider project of the pursuit of self and personal identity which some have argued characterizes late modernity (Giddens 1991). A study of the place and meaning of ICTs for leisure and pleasure in reconstituted families and households could make a major contribution to understanding contemporary family life, but more importantly for our purposes, would necessarily include a clear analysis of everyday practices. It seems that we need to return to more mainstream sociological theory to find theoretical frameworks robust enough to analyse the place and meaning of contemporary ICTs. Conceiving of them as everyday practices allows us to begin to explore the ways in which they acquire meaning, becoming embedded in apparently trivial domestic routines which link individual members within and across households and construct 'normal, everyday life'. In the same way that feminists have argued for an understanding of technology as a social process, so the most persuasive approaches which form part of the renaissance of micro-sociologies of the family are those which represent the family as 'an active process rather than a thing-like object of detached social investigation' (Morgan 1999: 16).

Contemporary leisure practices

Postmodern society is characterized as an increasingly 'time pressured' environment within which time itself is the newest commodity (Adam 1995). Time scarcity and the lack of leisure time are central to on-going discussions about the quality of contemporary life (Hothschild 1989; Schor 1991). There is growing evidence that individuals from all areas of life are experiencing a shortage of leisure time, especially women who routinely juggle work, family responsibilities and leisure (Wimbush and Talbot 1988; Bittman and Wajcman 1999). Although data drawn from the Multinational Time Budget Data Archive and the Australian Time Use Survey (Bittman and Wajcman 1999) suggests that men and women have similar amounts of time outside the hours consumed by paid work, it also demonstrates major differences in the use of such time. This confirms earlier UK-based research findings (Green et al. 1990) which portray women's leisure as more interrupted, fragmented and less relaxing than that of men.

Such quantitative data also confirms the fact that mothers, especially those with young children have the least personal leisure. During a period (1971–95) when expenditure on recreation, entertainment and education almost trebled in the UK (Hamill 2000), the amount of free time available to individuals did not increase significantly, nor did the ways in which they spent that free time. UK survey data continues to show that watching television and listening to the radio dominate adults' use of free time (ONS 1999) and aggregated European data confirms a relatively stable 60:40 split between home-based leisure and that enjoyed outside the home. However, it fails to contextualize such activities and conceals significant differences in the quality of home-based leisure between women and men, and between women located in differing circumstances. Quantitative data sets cannot illuminate the different meanings which particular leisure spaces and activities assume for individuals.

Furthermore, recent theorization of women's leisure (Wearing 1992; Le Feuvre 1994) has pointed to the need to beware of assuming heterogeneity. New feminist theories of leisure, including those based upon post-structuralism (Aitchison 2000), have emphasized identity, subjectivity and diversity, rather than focusing upon women's common position. In addition, as Deem comments, more awareness of the significance of wider social theory debates for understanding leisure has helped to draw our attention to 'new aspects of old concepts' (1996: 8). Deem (1996) reminds us that adopting Bourdieu's concept of cultural capital as an extension of the notion of social class (Bourdieu 1987) has helped feminist researchers to theorize the experiences of women in a variety of contexts and situations in a more sophisticated way. This type of theorization has enabled us to address what Aitchison refers to as the 'socio-cultural nexus of leisure relations' (Aitchison, 2000: 133). However, while recognizing the impact of difference and diversity, we also need to scrutinize the everyday contexts of most women's leisure.

Analysing leisure as an everyday practice which occurs in and around the home and exploring how leisure practices have been affected by an accelerated entry of ICTs into the majority of contemporary western households allows us to do a number of things. First, it enables an exploration of the complex social relations which constitute contemporary 'family life', asking questions about relationships between household members and the place and meaning of leisure practices. Second, it poses questions about the nature of leisure. Is it sensible to talk of 'family leisure'? And if so, as argued by feminist leisure theorists (Wearing 1998), is family leisure still facilitated mainly by the emotional labour of women? Or might the expansion of ICTs into the domestic space, especially artefacts such as game boys, etc., which are identified with masculinity, facilitate a sharing of the emotional labour (Hothschild 1989) which accomplishes family harmony, between men and women? If such emotional labour includes the use of increasingly technical ICTs to accomplish family entertainment, will male partners and fathers incorporate it into their domestic responsibilities? Such considerations require us to re-examine the technology as masculine culture debate, asking questions about the gendering of particular artefacts as they enter and find a place in the home. In the next section I shine the spotlight on the leisure context, exploring the potential of ICTs to enhance or interrupt women's opportunities and spaces for leisure.

Consuming virtual leisure

As suggested at the beginning of the chapter, the contemporary scramble for the latest ICTs in the workplace and the home carries with it an assumption that the newest forms of technology are highly desirable. It is implied that the emphasis upon individuality, self-expression and, above all, electronic speed of access to where and whatever we so desire will improve the quality of our lives in general and the quality of our leisure experiences in particular. Recent statistics seem to confirm some of this picture, while at the same time revealing inequalities of access and a consistent relationship between patterns of ICT ownership, household income and class position.

Access to affordable technology is the key to understanding such inequalities and the divide between the information rich and the information poor. Ownership of consumer durables such as television, CDs and VCRs continues to rise in the UK; over 80 per cent of households had a VCR in 1998 (ONS 1998), and by 1996, 99 per cent of households had a television but the class dimension remains stable. Professional households are more than twice as likely to own both VCRs and CD players than those headed by unskilled manual workers (ONS 1997). Ownership of home computers has risen much more slowly and, although an estimated one in four families now own a computer, only about 20 per cent of these have Internet access. Levels of Internet access are hard to establish but Mintel Leisure Intelligence suggests that by the year 2000 the UK will have 4–5 million households online (Ody 1998). Although women users are reportedly catching up, young, male professionals still vastly outnumber any other groups on the Internet which may be related to work-related access and the prioritizing of time for such activities. Lack of time, followed by financial resources, appears to be the biggest barrier for women. This lack of resources also restricts their leisure opportunities.

Arguably more interesting, are the ways in which individuals and household groups use the above commodities. As Silverstone and Haddon (1996) argue it is the domestication process which reveals the crucial interface between design and use and, perhaps more importantly, sustainability. To comprehend fully what is going on here, we need to know what meanings and processes are involved in 'taking technologies and objects home or into other private cultural spaces, and in making, or not making, them acceptable and familiar' (1996: 45).

This acceptance and familiarization process is governed by what Silverstone et al. (1992) refer to as the 'moral economy' of households – a set of shared meanings and value systems which are grounded within and expressed through the home. Such values and meanings are expressed in the symbolic and material boundaries that emerge both around and within the household. Silverstone et al. (1992) suggest that such moral economies are gendered, with men and women accepting responsibility for maintaining different spheres, but imply the existence of a *household* moral economy, rather than the co-existence of a multiplicity of different and at times conflicting moral economies. Decisions about the purchasing of new ICTs and their regulation within particular households will be influenced by such moral economies which are continually evolving and expressed at an everyday level through articulated decisions which include the consumption of specific artefacts: who watches and uses what, in which spaces and places.

There now exists a substantial body of work on television preferences and ownership patterns but similar studies of the placing and use of home PCs are surprisingly few, despite the rapid expansion in ownership over the last five years. Will the stand-alone PC be replaced by sophisticated versions of interactive digital televisions that incorporate its function and purpose? Or will the PC inhabit a different space and meaning in the household, moving from the relative privacy of the bedroom or study, to kitchens or living rooms? In communal living space, PCs could be used for games, emails or work purposes by a variety of family members, especially by women engaged in regulating and interpreting the emotional 'flow' of the household while on call to the needs of others. But such use by women could hardly be labelled 'women's leisure'.

Maintaining and enhancing family relationships is a key part of the emotional labour which women routinely perform (Hochschild 1989) and includes framing the spaces for family intimacy. Silva's work on the politics of consumption at home is important here and provides a fascinating glimpse of the 'active role of users/consumers in shaping technological artefacts and their meaning' (2000: 9). Her detailed ethnography of family life suggests evidence of the operation of not one moral economy at work in particular families and households, but several. Such moral economies will influence both the purchase of ICTs and their placing and use. Adopting ICTs creatively, for example, and placing PCs in central living spaces where they become part of the familiar everyday can transform them and other technological artefacts into comfortable 'virtual spaces' which can themselves be inhabited. In such situations, technophobia can be transformed into technofamiliarity. The key is the process of familiarity itself. PCs on kitchen tables lack the mystique of PCs in private spaces like the study. Moreover, extending the familiar to encompass the new,[3] is a crucial element in the sustainability of new ICTs.

Space, place and time

Turning to insights from cultural geography theorists, if we constitute space (including virtual space) as not only an arena in which social life occurs but also as a medium through which social life is reproduced (Rose 1993), then the adoption and level of use of new ICTs is closely related to the everyday contexts into which they are introduced. Thinking about leisure and the spaces in which it occurs, I have argued in this chapter that leisure is highly gendered and that women's opportunities for leisure are constrained by geographies of space and time. Taking that a step further, and picking up the strand of leisure theory which cites women's leisure as defined by relational activities such as community-based friendships and talk as leisure (Green 1998), the suggestion emerges that the social process of gender may alter our understanding of the meanings of particular places and spaces, not just the activities which take place in them. The construction of identities like motherhood through everyday negotiation of meanings in specific spaces may affect conceptions of space and therefore the appropriateness of what is allowed to occur. If an area of the home has been designated as space for relaxation and leisure and invested with emotional meanings attached to family space or 'adult' space, introducing ICTs which clash with or disrupt those meanings may result in them being resisted or subverted from their original design. ICTs appropriated for children's leisure, for example, electronic games, may dominate family leisure space in such a way as to encourage parents to re-assign space for personal leisure to technology-free spaces where they can relax secure in the knowledge that their children are both entertained and safe within the home. Equally, adults importing laptop computers for work purposes into communal bedroom space may disrupt seriously the intimacy and meaning of such places as an escape from the pressures of everyday work. Approved activities and the artefacts which enhance or support them will depend upon the meanings assigned to such spaces, which individuals are allowed to inhabit them and the moral economies which prevail.

Television as leisure

Studies of television use continue to demonstrate its popularity as a major source of relaxation and leisure (Gauntlett and Hill 1999). The most common home-based leisure activity for both men and women in the UK is watching television (ONS 1998). This kind of survey data is unable to shed light on the extent to which television viewing is combined with other activities but it is well documented by feminist leisure theorists that women routinely combine television with housework and childcare, or 'being on call' for the family (Deem 1986; Green et al. 1990). Morley's classic study of television conducted in the 1980s concluded that because home was the site of leisure for men, they could watch television uninterrupted whereas women, engaged in unpaid work in the home, viewed distractedly and often guiltily (1986). More interestingly for our purposes, Morley found evidence of a gendered use of remote controls with men 'flicking channels' while others attempted to watch programmes (1986). Building upon our previous discussion of contemporary family and household practices, we can speculate that despite continuing inequalities of access to free time between men and women (Bittman and Wajcman 1999), millennium households are characterized by more fluid gender relations. Gauntlett and Hill (1999) confirm this, citing recent survey research which found that both sexes used the remote controls frequently, although men were more likely to 'channel hop' and express pleasure at using the remote control. A finding reinforced by the 1997 Audience Tracking Study (cited in Gauntlett and Hill 1999) suggests that, when they do get to sit down, women have greater television power than the original studies by Morley (1986) and Gray (1992) imply. Data from the 244 households studied shows that although men continued to dominate the *use* of the television remote control in the 1990s, in four out of five homes the decision about what to watch was made jointly by household members.

Leisure as 'personal space'

A major finding from international feminist research conducted on the meaning of leisure for women over the last two decades (Deem 1986; Green et al. 1990; Wearing 1998; Wimbush and Talbot 1988) suggests that the concept of leisure as uncommitted time or personal space remains closely identified with women. Wearing (1998), adopting a Foucauldian model of space as a site of power and resistance, argues that leisure as personal space affords women a chance to resist 'inferiorized subjectivities'. No longer constructed in contrast to work (paid or unpaid), personal space, i.e., that which one chooses and has some control of, allows the exploration of self and identity which may not be possible within lives characterized by the family and the caring responsibilities traditionally associated with women. Of course women may choose to fill such personal spaces with ICTs designed for leisure and pleasure but as yet there is little empirical material which sheds any light on women's use of ICTs to gain either personal space or autonomous leisure.

Conclusion

This chapter has explored the complexity of the relationship between new technologies or ICTs and leisure patterns and practices within the household which constitute 'everyday practices'. Asking questions about the potential impact of ICTs on the use of space and time, and in particular women's space and time for leisure, it argues for the need for more qualitative research that examines the everyday. More understanding of the social practices associated with the appropriation of 'ordinary' ICTs in the home would tell us, first, about the continued maintenance of, or challenge to gendered leisure practices and, second, about the factors which are critical to the sustainability of specific technologies designed for household consumption.

Silva's (2000) thesis – that women develop a 'habitus' or disposition which encourages them to become major facilitators of the emotional well-being of others within a household or family context, complements data from studies of women's leisure conducted over the last two decades (Deem 1986; Green et al. 1990; Wearing 1998) which reports women's experiences of a blurring between work and leisure-time activities with very little uncommitted time for themselves. What recent studies of ICT use in the home reveal is data on the complexity of negotiations entered into by household members around particular artefacts and the prioritization by mothers of children's access at the expense of their own (Livingstone and Bovill 1999). As with leisure, central to any analysis of the gendered meaning and use of ICTs in the household or home is an awareness of the complex politics of the household, the relationships between adults, adults and children and groups of children, and the persistence of gendered social relations of the household. More research on the micro-processes involved here would be invaluable in furthering our understanding of the complex ways in which everyday life is both transformed and reproduced with technology assuming an integrated dimension of such transformation and reproduction processes.

Notes

1 By 'the habitus' Bourdieu means ways of doing things and being which individuals acquire during the process of socialisation. Habitus is therefore

acquired through what he terms 'lived practice'. See Bourdieu (1990) *The Logic of Practice*, Cambridge, Polity, for a full discussion of these ideas.

2 See Henwood (1993) and Grint and Gill (1995) for an overview.

3 I am indebted to Zoë Sofoulis for clarifying my thinking on this point as I listened to her unpublished paper delivered at the seminar on Cyberfeminism on 16 May 2000 at the University of Surrey. Third in the ESRC-funded research seminar series 'Equal opportunities on-line' (1999–2000) and co-organized by the editors, this seminar has provided a valuable space in which to explore cutting-edge debates on feminism and technology.

References

Adam, B. (1995) *Timewatch: The Social Analysis of Time*, Cambridge, Polity Press.

Aitchison, C. (2000) 'Poststructural feminist theories of representing others: a response to the "crisis" in leisure studies', discourse, *Leisure Studies* 19 (3): 127–44.

Balsamo, A. (1996) *Technologies and the Gendered Body: Reading Cyborg Women*, Durham, NC: Duke University Press.

Bittman, M. and Wajcman, J. (1999) *The Rush Hour: The Quality of Leisure Time and Gender Equity*, Sydney: Social Policy Research Centre (SPRC), University of New South Wales.

BT (2000) *Future Talk: A Special Millennium Initiative*, London: Forward Publishing.

Bourdieu, P. (1987) *Distinction*, London: Routledge.

Bourdieu, P. (1990) *The Logic of Practice*, Cambridge: Polity Press.

Braverman, H. (1974) *Labor and Monopoly Capital*, New York: Monthly Review Press.

Carvel, J. (2000) 'More women delay starting their families', The *Guardian*, 21 June.

Cockburn, C. (1983) *Brothers, Male Dominance and Technological Change*, London: Pluto Press.

Cockburn, C. (1985) *Machinery of Dominance, Women, Men and Technical Know-how*, London: Pluto Press.

Cockburn, C. (1992) 'The circuit of technology, gender, identity and power' in R. Silverstone and E. Hirsch (eds) *Consuming Technologies: Media and Information in Domestic Spaces*, London: Routledge.

Cockburn, C. and Ormrod, S. (1993) *Gender and Technology in the Making*, London: Sage.

Cockburn, C. and Furst-Dilic, R. (1994) *Bringing Technology Home: Gender and Technology in a Changing Europe*, Buckingham: Open University Press.

Cowan, R. S. (1983) *More Work for Mother: The Ironies of Household Technology – From the Open Hearth to the Microwave*, New York: Basic Books.

Deem, R. (1986) *All Work and No Play? The Sociology of Women and Leisure*, Milton Keynes: Open University Press.

Deem, R. (1996) 'No time for a rest? An exploration of women's work, engendered leisure and holidays', *Time and Society* 5 (1): 5–25.

Faulkner, W. and Arnold, E. (1985) (eds) *Smothered By Invention: Technology in Women's Lives*, London: Pluto.

Game, A. and Pringle, R. (1983) *Gender at Work*, North Sydney: George Allen and Unwin.

Gauntlett, D. and Hill, A. (1999) *TV Living: Television, Culture and Everyday Life*, London: Routledge.

Giddens, A. (1991) *Modernity and Self-Identity, Self and Society in the Late Modern Age*, Cambridge: Polity Press.

Gray, A. (1992) *Video Playtime: The Gendering of a Leisure Technology*, London: Routledge.

Green, E. (1998) 'Women doing friendship: an analysis of women's leisure as a site of identity construction, empowerment and resistance', *Leisure Studies*, 17 (3): 171–83.

Green, E. and Adam, A. (1998) 'Online leisure: gender and ICTs in the home', *Information, Communication and Society*, 1 (3): 291–312.

Green, E., Hebron, S. and Woodward, D. (1990) *Women's Leisure, What Leisure?* London: Macmillan.

Green, E., Owen, J. and Pain, D. (eds) (1993) *Gendered by Design? Information Technology and Office Systems*, London: Taylor and Francis.

Green, N. (2000) *Gendering Virtual Selves: Technologies, Social Practices and Identity Transformation*, http://www.surrey.ac.uk (24 June 2000).

Grint, K. and Gill, R. (1995) *The Gender–Technology Relation, Contemporary Theory and Research*, London: Taylor and Francis.

Hamill, L. (2000) *The Introduction of New Technology into the Household*, http://www.surrey.ac.uk (24 June 2000).

Henwood, F. (1993) 'Establishing gender perspectives on information technology: problems, issues and opportunities' in E. Green, J. Owen and D. Pain (eds) *Gendered by Design? Information Technology and Office Systems*, London: Taylor and Francis.

Hochschild, A. (1989) *The Second Shift*, Berkeley: University of California Press.

Le Feuvre, N. (1994) 'Leisure, work and gender: a sociological study of women's time in France', *Time and Society*, 3 (2): 151–78.

Livingstone, S. and Bovill, M. (1999) *Young People, New Media, Research Report*, London: London School of Economics.

Mackenzie, D. and Wajcman, J. (eds) (1985) *The Social Shaping of Technology*, Buckingham: Open University Press.

Morgan, D. (1996) *Family Connections: An Introduction to Family Studies*, Cambridge: Polity Press.

Morgan, D. (1999) 'Risk and family practices: accounting for change and fluidity in family life' in E. B. Silva and C. Smart (eds) *The 'New' Family?* London: Sage.

Morley, D. (1986) *Family Television: Cultural Power and Domestic Leisure*, London: Comedia.

Ody, P. (1998) 'Non-store retailing: exploiting interactive media and electronic commerce', *Financial Times* Retail and Consumer Publishing.

Office for National Statistics (ONS) (1997) *Social Trends 27*, London: The Stationary Office.

Office for National Statistics (ONS) (1998) *Social Trends 28*, London: The Stationary Office.

Office for National Statistics (ONS) (1999) *Social Trends 29*, London: The Stationary Office.

Rose, G. (1993) *Feminism and Geography: The Limits of Geographical Knowledge*, Cambridge: Polity Press.

Schor, J. B. (1991) *The Overworked American*, New York: Basic Books.

Silva, E. B. (1999) 'Transforming housewifery: dispositions, practices and technologies' in E. B. Silva and C. Smart (eds) *The 'New' Family?* London: Sage.

Silva, E. B. and Smart, C. (1999) 'The "new" practices and politics of family life' in E. B. Silva and C. Smart (eds) *The 'New' Family?* London: Sage.

Silva, E. B. (2000) 'The politics of domestic consumption @ home: practices and dispositions in the uses of technologies', Pavis Papers No. 1, Faculty of Social Sciences: The Open University.

Silverstone, R. and Haddon, L. (1996) 'Design and the domestication of information and communication technologies: technical change and everyday life' in R. Mansell and R. Silverstone (1996) *Communication by Design: The Politics of ICTs*, Oxford: Oxford University Press.

Silverstone, R., Hirsch, E. and Morley, D. (1992) 'Economy of the household' in R. Silverstone and E. Hirsch *Consuming Technologies: Media and Information in Domestic Spaces*, London: Routledge.

Smart, C. and Neale, B. (1999) *Family Fragments*, Cambridge: Polity Press.

Stepulevage, L. (1999) 'Becoming a technologist: days in a girl's life', *Information, Communication and Society*, 2 (4): 399–418.

Vehviläinen, M. (1991) 'Social construction of information systems, an office workers' standpoint', a licentiate thesis, University of Tampere, Finland, Department of Computer Science (unpublished).

Wajcman, J. (1991) *Feminism Confronts Technology*, Cambridge: Polity Press.

Wearing, B. (1992) 'Leisure and women's identity in late adolescence', *Loisir et Société*, 15 (1): 323–42.

Wearing, B. (1998) *Leisure and Feminist Theory*, London: Sage.

Wimbush, E. and Talbot, M. (eds) (1988) *Relative Freedoms: Women and Leisure*, Milton Keynes: Open University Press.

Woolgar, S. (2000) 'Where is the paperless office?' *The Times Higher Educational Supplement*, 23 June 2000.

Chapter 10

Men, masculinities and 'mundane' technologies

The domestic telephone

Maria Lohan

Introduction

Technology is a significant site of gender negotiations where both masculine and feminine identities are constructed and deconstructed. Technologies are incorporated into our gender identities in the way we negotiate them as part of our own – 'mine' or 'not-mine' – feminine or masculine identity. By interpreting their usage in our lives, they become part of the gendered division of labour and, through social relations, technologies are assigned gendered symbolic values. Most notably, feminist researchers of technology (for example, Wajcman 1991; Sørensen 1992; Cockburn and Ormrod 1993; Berg and Lie 1995; Lie 1995; Faulkner 2000) have noted that men and technology are so often placed together that some of the defining characteristics of masculine culture are welded to technology in terms of male technological competence and interest/fetish. Images of men and heavy technologies, such as bulldozers, men and sophisticated technologies, such as high-spec computers, or men and military technologies, such as fighter planes, prevail in everyday life.

Yet with notable exceptions (Hacker 1989; Gray 1992; Cockburn and Ormrod 1993; Murray 1993; Lie 1995; Faulkner 2000; Oldenziel 2000), feminist scholarship on the gendering of technologies has mainly concentrated on researching and theorizing women's experience of technologies and exclusion from technological labour markets and training. This is because, as McNeil has suggested, 'women are seen (including frequently in social science research) as the "exclusive carriers" of gender relations – the bearers of the meaning of sex and gender. In contrast, men are easily positioned outside of the realm of gender relations as the agents of versions of "human history" in which gender is not significant' (McNeil 1992: 111–12).

This chapter is premised on the argument that in order to understand gender and information communication technologies, we need also to turn the camera angles on this implicit relationship between men and technology. In studies of masculinity, a mirror is placed before the male gaze. The reflection reveals not the lives of generic human beings or a singular masculinity but, as others have now come to argue, a complex of masculinities (Connell 1987; Brittan 1989; Brod and Kaufman 1994; Hearn and Collinson 1994; Kimmel 1994; Segal 1997). In particular, too, ICTs that have been domesticated into our everyday lives can be seen to disrupt implicit relationships of masculinities and technologies. This chapter observes the symbolic associations and men's everyday use of one such ICT: the domestic telephone.

The domestic telephone is a technology that no longer quite fits the stereotypical relationship between masculinities and technologies. Women's domestication of the telephone into family and friendship networks is said to have subverted the designer's interpretation of the telephone as an instrument of telegraphic business information (Fischer 1991, 1992; Martin 1991; Frissen 1995; Lohan 1998). In-depth studies using qualitative methods also focussed on how women have incorporated the domestic telephone for the sustenance of family relationships (Moyal 1989, 1992; Martin 1991; Rakow 1992; Lohan 1997; Maddox 1977). In these studies, and other surveys of men and women's usage of the telephone (Schabedoth et al. 1989; Dordick and La Rose 1992; Lange 1993; Fortunati 1995; see Haddon 1997 for review) the domestic telephone has emerged as an object of both (female) love and (female) labour. As a domesticated and feminized technology, it has also become a 'mundane' technology.

This is potentially a technology, then, which highlights the tensions between stereotypical associations of gender and technology, as outlined above. Technical apparatuses that do not fit descriptions of being 'heavy', 'advanced'/'high-tech' or 'dangerous' and are, instead, 'familiar', 'easy to use' and predominantly used by women can find it difficult to retain their definition as technologies. Conversely, men who use and identify with such technologies may have some difficulty of meeting definitions of 'hegemonic masculinity' (Connell 1987). The apparently contradictory stance of looking at men in relation to a feminized and mundane technology, such as the domestic telephone, is a useful research perspective in that it opens up spaces for examining the processes of variation and change both within genders and in gender–technology relations. In addition, if the stereotypes of masculinity and femininity can be broken down around this technology, they will be more difficult to sustain around some of the newer communication technologies.

This chapter seeks out this diversity of experience and change in both gender relations and gender–technology relations by focusing on how *men* describe their incorporation of the telephone into their *everyday* family lives. The methodology used in this research has also been designed to capture some of the *diversity* in the possibilities of masculinities and technological identities. The primary source of analysis for this research is male narrators' descriptions of the integration/non-integration of the telephone in their lives. From November 1995 to June 1996, I interviewed 21 men living in Ireland (the exception being one narrator who was living in London). I sought to include diversity not only in traditional 'background variables' such as age, class and, to a limited extent, ethnicity, but also in the narrators' adoption of masculinities. Thus I interviewed one priest, one transvestite, 'new men', as well as elderly bachelor farmers, 'family patriarchs' and so on. The interviews are based on a non-random snowball sample of men, such that whatever variability I may have found represents at least the minimum variability of masculinities and the technology found in Ireland at the time.[1] The empirical material presents two contexts of familial relations. The first context is concerned with looking at telephone communication in the relationships between fathers and their adult children and between sons and their parents. The second context is concerned with how the domestic telephone is negotiated within the domestic environment of (mostly heterosexual) couples.

The importance of the telephone in fathers' everyday lives: 'I was terribly chuffed that she rang'

Martin is a father in his late 50s. At the time of the interview he had a temporary job working as a plasterer on new houses being built in the area but had been unemployed for a long period previous to this. His successful construction business had declined in the recession of the late 1970s and early 1980s and his current re-employment reflects a resurgent economy and the associated building boom. When asked about his domestic phone usage he said he used the phone very rarely now. He explained that it was very important to him at one time when his construction business was at its height, in order to cope with architects who kept changing their minds and to move men accordingly.

Nowadays, he said, the main usage of the phone for him was to *receive* calls from his sons and daughters living abroad. He told me the following story of his daughter who had been working as a nurse in Manchester but who had recently gone to live in Auckland, New Zealand, for a year. On the evening that she left for New Zealand, Martin stayed in and waited for a telephone call:

> I had an intention of going out earlier but I had this kind of pre-monition, knowing Una [that she might call]. The rest of them were all gone out and I just hung on from half-hour to half-hour until quarter to twelve, she rang. You see, there is 12 hours difference. She was only after getting there. I had misjudged that. Then the phone rang. The first thing she said was: 'You know Dad I'm reversing the charges.' And I said: 'Well let that not worry you, Una' I said, 'because even if it takes a day's or a week's wages now, it is that good to hear from you.'
>
> [He confirmed to me that this was indeed how he felt.] And it wouldn't bother me. That's a type of phone call now that I consider worth its money. Let it cost 35 or 40 pounds or even more than that. It is the first call we ever had from New Zealand or that far out in 32 years, so I just put her at ease there. That kind of thing you couldn't do other wise. You would still be sitting there wondering if she got there. To get going to the international date line, I mean if she kept going, wouldn't she be coming back? Little things like that.

What was apparent in Martin's description of the call was the joy. That, which he had dared to expect as a father had happened. He had very little real concept of what the call had cost, nor how much he would have to earn to provide for it. The call was instead about being a father. 'Things like that now. I was terribly – what do they say in England, "chuffed" that she rang to tell me how she got there.' Indeed, for all of the fathers who had adult children living outside their home, it was fatherhood which defined the importance of the telephone. The telephone was thus integrated into the lives of men in ways which approximated studies of female telephony in which it has been suggested that the telephone could be seen as a metaphorical umbilical chord (Moyal 1989; Claisse 1989) helping to retain contact with next of kin and enhancing women's sense of participation and well-being (Moyal 1992; Rakow 1992).

Conflicting readings of family calls: 'I always come off stressed out after talking to my parents'

At the same time, however, the young male interviewees described phoning their parents, and particularly their fathers, as an effort (if not a struggle). The following narratives present stories of how divergent value systems between parents and siblings made communication somewhat stifled, as did the telephone not being completely socialized into the family home (especially, though not exclusively, by older male parents). Most striking of all was the greater difficulty of talking to fathers on the telephone despite the stated value, as we saw above, of their *receiving* calls. This suggests that changing relationships of masculinities and domestic technologies can be a slow process since the process is related to the division of labour in households. Gullestad, for example, has argued that ideological changes might have limited effects since certain tasks (and, I would argue, certain technologies) themselves 'have accumulated symbolic value, which makes changing the division more than a practical and organisational matter' (Gullestad 1992: 109).

Diverging value systems

For example, Damien, a young accountant, reported ringing home as a bit of an ordeal. He said he rings his parents once every two weeks but would prefer to ring a lot less: 'I always come off the telephone stressed out after talking to my parents.' Contrary to convention, however, he says it is his parents, in his view, whose values need to be controlled: 'When we were at home, we could keep them in check. As soon as you go away there is nothing, so any kind of bizarre idea can run free.'

Brendan's narrative is another example of troubled calls home. Brendan lived in England until two years ago and described how he found it especially difficult to ring his parents since having lived in England. His reasoning suggests that the discomfort has arisen on the telephone owing to a mixture of geographic and social mobility but also that the telephone accentuates these distances.

> I never really rang my parents much. I don't know what it is with England but I think you grow apart. Well that's me anyway. I find I can't speak to them as easily now. A lot of people get like that. I was very close to me Mother and Father, but like, the way we think is totally different now since I bought a house, have a good

job and a couple of bob behind me. When you get on the phone
you'd ask them how is this and how is that and, as soon as you've
asked them all that, the conversation ends. That's it. But when you
see them, it's completely different. Like I'm very close to them that
way.

This social mobility might be overlooked in orthodox class analysis since
he remains working class, similar to his parents, but through *his own*
descriptions of his economic status, including his great pride in house
and car ownership, we learn that he probably fits closer to middle-class
consumption patterns. Differing value systems also permeated more than
social mobility.

Difference over appropriate sexual relations was also a hurdle. Jim,
a student in his late 20s for example, described this to me in hypo-
thetical terms:

Like, say I had been on holidays with my girlfriend. Well there would
just be so many gaps in what I'd be telling the folks about it. It
would be like as if we (his girlfriend and he) didn't have to sleep
at all, sort of to make out we walked through the night too. 'There
were seven days and no nights.' If I started to talk about the hotel,
my Mother would start to get uneasy and start to talk about the
weather again.

In this we see the use of contrived silence from both sides on certain
aspects of their lives, particularly sexual morals. The constructed silence
is used as a means of negotiating new and traditional moral standards
while avoiding conflict and a breakdown of communication altogether.

Socializing the phone into the family network

What was also evident in the narratives, was that the telephone itself
also was an extra barrier in this communication. It has been noted by
others (Aronson 1971; Lange 1993) that the very ubiquity of the telephone in our homes has made it disappear from view, or that it has
been fully domesticated (Frissen 1995). Yet in these narratives in
everyday calls between men and their families, the telephone seems, at
times, not fully socialized into men's familial communication. This was
apparent above in Brendan's problems of communication with his
parents on the phone: 'When you see them it is completely different.'
In Father Finian's narrative (a priest who lived with a religious com-

munity) this is more pronounced. The telephone for him is simply not an instrument of family communication but is used to appease his mother. He will, so to speak, turn the phone on and let it run for a while.

> Yeah, I'm the world's worst because I don't ring every week. When I have to ring my Mother she goes into some kind of 'thing'. You just have to agree occasionally and let her go. Just follow the tone of her voice. But if I was sitting in front of her, I'd talk to her. I drop out a lot without arranging. My Dad is the same as me anyway. He doesn't like the phone.

In Jim's parents' home, the telephone seems very much part of the front hall of their home. It has, as in many homes, its own seat. However, his father's encounters with it suggests it's more of a stranger in the home.

> But you *know* he is uncomfortable on the phone, even by his body language. We have this silly thing, a table with a chair attached. Most people sit on the chair right? Well he sort of crouches down looking at the phone. He wouldn't lounge on the chair and go 'ba da ba da'. He's not in 'someone's going to attack me mode' but he is not fully relaxed.

He shared with me a further quirk of his father's habit of combing his hair in front of the hall mirror before he made a call. The phone was formal for Jim's Dad. It is a moment of the presentation of self (Goffman 1971) which is why, as I outline below, the presentations of self are also gendered presentations.

'I'll get your mother'

Already implicit in some of the above conversations is the greater propensity to talk to mothers on the telephone than to fathers. The above examples were of young heterosexual men. With the group of gay men whom I interviewed there was a similar consensus on it being easier to talk to one's mother than it is to one's father: 'I've a great relationship with my mother but not with my Father. I don't think it is just a gay thing. Most fathers and sons are like that' (Jack). According to Damien, it was the British Telecom advertisement in which the father passes the phone straight away to the mother, saying 'I'll get your mother' that he found most perceptive.[2] It has its corollary in the infamous family phrase: 'Wait until I tell your father' in which the father is projected as the primary agent of discipline in the family. In the phrase 'I'll get your mother' we see gender being done in that it is *she* who is being delegated the responsibility of family communication.

The most notable exception to this mode of delegation among the interviewees was in my case of a single father. He explained that on reprimanding his children, they often rang their mother for consolation but also probably as a means of retrieving power in the father–child relationship again. His children's telephone calls to their mother, and calls from her, were viewed by the single father as a nuisance and an incursion into his attempts for both caring and authority in the household. We get a further view of this division of labour in Adrian's description of his parents. He described there being no difference in his communication with his parents only that: 'My mother is much more long-winded on the phone than my father. My father would be more to the point and would be more conscious of the length of time than she would be.' Their communication is otherwise equal, he maintains, except too that his father would mainly be 'out during the day and in the evenings too as he is involved in all kinds of committees'.

It is in the diversity of these stories then that I find an answer to the question I posed about why is there a discrepancy between a father's pleasure of receiving calls, a son's pain in making them or in a son's reported minimal communication with his father? It is precisely because the domestic phone is part of the ordinary everyday life of the family. If men's voices are not part of that everyday life, it is harder to be part of the domestic phone. Many (though not all) of the older fathers in this collection were less participative in the labour of day-to-day communicating and distanced themselves from the ideology of small talk. Yet, at the same time, fathers in the study reported wanting to be included, wanting to be participative fathers and loved fathers. It was this disconnection here which makes telephone connections more uncomfortable. The fathers openly acknowledged the love brought to them by telephone calls from their sons and daughters living away from home. Yet, they were much less willing to, or less sure about, actively taking on the labour of communication. For this group of middle-aged fathers, they were not quite sure how to *undo* traditional masculinity in this way. Nor, it must be said, were they quite sure they wanted to.

I spoke of Martin's call from his daughter earlier. In his home, though, the division of labour went largely unchallenged despite (or perhaps because of) his period of unemployment. This division was also explicit in the labour of communication. According to Martin: 'I haven't written a letter, since I was married. I'd be only telling the same story' (as his wife). This included letters to his sisters living in England which his wife took over on marriage. This trend in the division of communication labour was not universal of course, even among my narrators. Hugh, for example, regularly wrote and called his son who had been living in Mexico. Yet the masculine protest to such a traditional order came most strongly from the younger men and I will explore the tensions of this within the homes of heterosexual couples in the next section.

Domestic telephony and the division of communication within couples

For the older men among my narrators, the division of labour in their homes was a natural order reflecting – as it were – men and women's natural differences. Complementarity rather than equality in the division of communication tasks was also consequently emphasized. For example, Senan (an elderly man from the Cayman Islands who lived most of his adult life in London and is now living with his partner in the West of Ireland) described a strong division of labour in his household in terms of telephone communication – she does it and he doesn't. This included calls made to his children from his previous marriage: 'One I don't like it and two she loves it so why interfere?' In the course of our interview, Senan himself repeats over and over again his belief that men and women are '*completely* different' and what is more he regards this difference as being 'instinctive' that 'maybe society reinforces it but they are born with this difference'. Nevertheless, he does not regard telephone communication as being at all affected by gender: 'Some people like to talk. Period.' His staccato sentences performed onomatopoeically his non-party to this category 'some people'. As far as he is concerned, rather than communication being a gender issue, *he* is extremely introverted and Paula, his partner, extroverted. However, he does acknowledge that though men and women are no more 'fanatical about the phone', as he puts it, 'the conversation *might* be different'.

> In that, women talk about the more subtle part of emotions in situations. Whereas, men talk about material things like cars. You know, and what's happening on the farm and this type of thing. But they are more emotional, the women, and whether that constitutes, emm, stupid talking is a matter of opinion.

Yet people's biographies are pluralized and, during our life, changing circumstances might also call us to question values and knowledge. What we regard as natural and right can take unexpected turns, creating contradictions in our lives. This was also the case for Senan. Paula, Senan's partner, developed an illness and now has limited mobility. Consequently, Senan actually does most of the housework. Our interview, in fact, was finally drawn to a close when he had to prepare dinner. Disrupting the traditional or stereotypical division of labour between the sexes – which Senan still sees as a product of the natural differences between men and women – was a source of reflexivity and discomfort for him. His necessity to renegotiate this labour makes him worried about his natural difference to his partner: 'You know, I look at myself doing all this women's work and I wonder which side of the fence I'm on.' When I asked him if he was sure there was such a fence, he said: 'Of course there is. Men and women are completely different. But I don't know, I've got to do it anyhow.' I shall return to analyse his story further in the light of some of the younger men's narratives.

In the younger couples' homes, the traditional division of labour was not an option. In Giddens' terms these relationships represented a transformation of intimacies to the 'pure relationship' defined by emotional and sexual equality (Giddens 1992). Among the younger men whom I interviewed, there was a strong rhetoric of full equality and sharing in daily life. Their home life was undoubtedly radically different to that which I described in their fathers' generation above. To illustrate the point I will compare Senan to Noel. Noel is a telesales operator in a large manufacturing plant in Dublin. Geraldine, his wife, works as a personal assistant in a publisher's office. At the time of the interview, they had been married three years and were in their early 30s, late 20s respectively. In Noel and Geraldine's home, household tasks appeared to be evenly distributed. Take, for example, his description of his use of the answering machine as a means of planning when to 'throw the dinner in the oven', and consider how this might have been different 20 years ago, in Ireland at least:

> I work to Continental times, so if I have just left work and Geraldine was just told that she had to stay on or knew that she was going to be late, she just leaves a little message on the answering machine for me, so I come in take a message. Or, if she has to go to her Mother, or go down town, then there is no problem. Like, I'm not out there cooking the dinner expecting her home or wondering where she is.

Nor was there a question of Geraldine taking on his communication with his family. Noel rings his mother twice a week or more, depending on whether his Dad is commuting to Brussels that week or not.

Interviewer	And would they be fairly long conversations?
Noel	Emm, not really, maybe just five, ten minutes. It's more just seeing how she is getting on and everything else. I mean if she needs anything, even though it is a journey across town, of course I will go over and get whatever she wants.

Thus, equality and similarity seem to be the order of the day. It might have appeared, then, that gender was not so pertinent in such family homes: for example, that masculinity was not being confirmed or contested around the telephone. That gender was not so relevant to younger couples' telephony might, in fact, have been my conclusion, were it not for the curious repetition of the phrase by more than one of the narrators of: 'Her family is very different to mine.' Its appearance was not arbitrary but rather tightly associated with those households where wives/partners no longer were, or had never become, the 'family communicator'.[3] In such households, distinguishing masculine and feminine usage of the telephone, were it to be achieved, had to be done so in more subtle ways. Noel, for example, not only describes his calls as being short and task oriented as in the above quotes – fetching things – but also, in the following illustrations, he describes his calls as being very different to calls which his wife makes to her family. Indeed, communication in her family is not only different to his. Through his descriptions, her usage of the phone is made to sound silly and unnecessary.

> Her family life is totally different to mine. I mean she comes from a very, very close-knit family, am, sometimes a little too close-knit. I mean, my Mother-in-law is always ringing my wife asking her opinion on what is happening with my sister-in-law or my mother-in-law's sister, that's my wife's aunt. The whole family and extended family on her side are very, very involved with each other in a certain respect. They are always involved in practically every situation.

Interviewer	Is that a good or a bad thing?
Noel laughs and says	It's not a good thing at all. It's just ahh, they are too involved. Am, you know and they are all kind of putting their two pence ha'peny worth in or whatever and every one is involved.

In this we see the gender difference is not located between him and his wife (the relationship of equality and sameness) but rather just outside, between *his* family and *hers*. Performing gender in this way might also be a way of performing class. Noel's wife comes from a lower-middle-class family, while we are left in no two minds of the professional status of his parents. According to Delphy and Leonard, 'continuing to rely on your mother or sister (for emotional support) is not fully approved of. It may be regarded as a symptom of emotional immaturity or downgraded as being "traditional working class" behaviour' (Delphy and Leonard 1994: 163).

In the narrative of Senan, the chronic illness of his wife had forced him to take on much of what he regarded as 'feminine work' thereby leading to a reflexive questioning of his gender identity and gendered dichotomies. Or, as he described it, the feeling of not knowing 'which side of the fence' he was on. This co-existence of gender stability and gender transgression was also relevant in the younger men's narratives. In Noel's narrative, he presented himself and his wife as doing and sharing the same things in the household. Yet, he presented their domestic telephony as being different. He described himself and his wife as having different types of families to explain how they had different types of conversations on the telephone. The use of this phrase, 'her family is very different to mine', was a more subtle way of creating a gender difference. The difference was not located between him and his wife (the relationship of equality and sameness) but rather just outside, between his family and hers.

Noel's construction of gender may also be contrasted to a different type of masculinity expressed by a young gay man (Jack). Jack's report of his calls suggests that it is not simply a difference between 'types' of families, but it is about *making* a difference; about taking on the responsibility to call and share regularly: 'I'd ring my Mother every weekend. I offer her support and she offers me support. We always have had a very honest relationship. What I notice about him (father) is that he will never sit down, even if there is a seat or not.' We also heard how Noel's mother makes valiant efforts to act as a lynchpin in her disparate family 'She will ring my brothers and she would ring me just to let me know if something happened to a relation or something. My mother would be the one to, emm, to pass on the news.' However, unlike in Geraldine's family and the gay man above (Jack), this form of communication is not reciprocated by her sons.

Concluding discussion

Technologies gain gender identities when they enter into our everyday structural relations and our cultural meaning systems and, as such, technologies can become actors or agents in the material and symbolic practices of our everyday lives. Technologies and masculinities are typically written about as being symbolically aligned in our culture to the extent that some of the qualities of masculinity and technology are regarded as co-terminus – for example, 'advanced', 'skilled', 'remote' and 'dangerous'. However, this chapter has looked instead at how meanings of masculinities and technologies are both deconstructed and reconstructed around a *mundane and domestic* technology which is familiar, easy-to-use and which previous research has suggested is predominantly used by, and associated with, women – that is, it is a feminized technology (Moyal 1989; Schabedoth et al. 1989; Dordick and La Rose 1992; Rakow 1992; Lange 1993; Fortunati 1995; see Haddon 1997 for review). This chapter investigated how a group of men living in Ireland described their domestication of such a mundane and feminized technology: the domestic telephone as part of their family relationships. Clearly this also requires an understanding of men's positions and responsibilities in family life more generally, whether as sons, fathers, grandfathers, spouses/partners or brothers.

In one exploration of the material, I discussed an intergenerational paradox in the experience of familial telephony. This was the apparent discrepancy between the joy and pleasure fathers reported from receiving calls from their sons and daughters (especially those abroad) on the one hand and, on the other hand, the perceived awkwardness expressed by sons of such calls to their fathers. A reason for this discrepancy could also be ascertained from within the narratives. I concluded that this could be partly attributed to the very contradiction of love and labour. While fathers loved these calls, they were frequently (though not always) less participative than their wives and partners in the labour of communication, in the everyday life of the household and in the ideology of small talk. This participation was, therefore, difficult to reconstruct on a moment's notice in a phone call and fathers were often reported as running for their wives. Where there were exceptions to this, where fathers were involved in the day-to-day running of the home, such as a single father and a teacher who was the main communicator with his son in Latin America, the telephone was entirely a much more sociable technology.

What was also evident was that the telephone itself was an additional actor in the negotiation of satisfactory/dissatisfactory telephone relationships for the narrators. In particular, the part social/part technical aspects of the telephone as an artefact were being negotiated in each call. For example, for some of the fathers (usually middle-aged men, many of whom had not grown up with a phone in their home) the telephone was not fully socialized into their homes or relationships, despite having its own seat in their households.

The second exploration of the empirical material focused on the negotiation of the telephone by men as husbands and partners, again in the context of the changing involvement of men in families, households and domestic telephony. What I found was that in the different narratives of men's lives which make up this study, there is a co-existence of the more traditional ideology of gender with a modern vision of equality and sharing of formerly dichotomous life-spaces – or modernity and reflexive modernity (Beck 1992). This I have illustrated by comparing Senan and Paula, an elderly couple whose narrative suggested the ideology of gender dichotomies, to the younger couple, Noel and Geraldine, whose narrative highlighted an egalitarian ideology of gender. However, I have also suggested that the transition into reflexive modernity or the breakdown of gender dichotomies between the generations is not complete. Not only was there a co-existence of 'traditional' and 'modern' gender ideology between the narratives but also one that exists *within* the narratives.

Overall, the narratives do present a multiplicity of genders within masculinity and a multiplicity of men's interpretations of the domestic telephone in their family relations. The material also presents significant challenges to traditional masculinity between and within the generations of men. However, on a number of occasions in the narratives of men's use of the domestic telephone, I have paused to remark on the sense of *gender vertigo* (Segal 1997) or a hesitancy in the breaking down of gender dichotomies or, conversely, in the opening up of life spaces for masculinities and femininities. In ways that are sometimes hard to follow, younger men in heterosexual couples re-embroidered the 'his' and 'her' back into their telephony and relationships so as to distinguish a masculinity (and hierarchy!). Though summarized by the phrase 'her family is very different to mine', there were new names and new words for gendering difference in almost all the narratives.

Notes

1 This research was conducted as part of my PhD thesis entitled 'The transvestite telephone: a male technology dressed up in women's clothes' (Trinity College, Dublin 1998). I'd like to thank Professor Ann R. Sætnan of Norwegian University of Science and Technology (NTNU), Trondheim, and Dr Brian Torode, Trinity College, Dublin, for their comments on earlier drafts of this chapter.

2 British Telecom ran a domestic telephone advertising campaign in the early 1990s entitled 'It's Good to talk'. The campaign was primarily aimed at men. It sought to challenge the feminine image of the domestic telephone, to encourage men to talk more and longer on the phone and to provide cultural legitimacy for women talking on the phone. The campaign was also viewed in Ireland.

3 In Claisse's study of French households he concluded that married women, especially housewives, most often took on the role as 'family communicator' (Claisse 1989, author's translation). This means that such women often took on responsibility for communications, not only with their own family but also with their in-laws, as Martin described.

References

Aronson, S. (1971) 'The sociology of the telephone', *International Journal of Comparative Sociology*, 12 (9): 153–67.

Beck, U. (1992) *Risk Society: Towards a New Modernity* (translated by Mark Ritter), London, Thousand Oaks, New Delhi: Sage.

Berg, A.-J. and Lie, M. (1995) 'Feminism and constructivism: do artefacts have gender?' *Science, Technology and Human Values* 20 (3): 332–51.

Berg, A.-J. (1996) 'Digital feminism', unpublished PhD thesis, Centre for Technology and Society, Norwegian University of Science and Technology, Trondheim.

Brittan, A. (1989) *Masculinity and Power*, Oxford, UK: Blackwell.

Brod, H. and Kaufmann, M. (eds) (1994) *Theorizing Masculinities*, Thousand Oaks, London, New Dehli: Sage.

Claisse, G. (1989) 'Telefon, Kommunication und Gesellschaft: Daten Gegen Mythen' in U. Lange, K. Beck and A. Zerdick (eds) *Telefon und Gesellschaft: Beitrage zu einer Soziologie der Telefonkommunikation*, 1, Berlin: Volker Speiss.

Cockburn, C. and Ormrod, S. (1993) *Gender and Technology in the Making*, London: Sage.

Connell, R. W. (1987) *Gender and Power*, Cambridge, UK: Polity Press.

Connell, R. W. (1995) *Masculinities*, UK: Polity Press in association with Blackwell Publishers.

Delphy, C. and Leonard, D. (1994) 'The variety of work done by wives' in *The Polity Reader of Gender Studies*, Cambridge: Polity Press.

Dordick, H. and La Rose, R. (1992) *The Telephone in Daily Life: A Study of Personal Telephone Use*, Philadelphia: Temple University.

Faulkner, W. (2000) 'The power *and* the pleasure? A research agenda for "making gender stick" to engineers', *Science Technology and Human Values*, 25 (1), 87–119.

Fortunati, L. (1995) *Gli Italiani al Telefono*, Milano: FrancoAngeli.

Fischer, C. S. (1991) 'Touch someone: the telephone industry discovers sociability' in M. C. La Foilette and J. Stine, *Technology and Choice: A Technology and Culture Reader*, Chicago: University of Chicago Press.

Fischer, C. S. (1992) *America Calling: A Social History of the Telephone to 1940*, Berkeley and Oxford: University of California Press.

Frissen, V. (1995) 'Gender is calling: some reflections on past, present and future uses of the telephone' in K. Grint and R. Gill (eds) *The Gender–technology Relation: Contemporary Theory and Research*, London: Taylor and Francis.

Giddens, A. (1992) *The Transformation of Intimacy*, Cambridge: Polity Press.

Goffman, E. (1971) *The Presentation of Self*, London and New York: Penguin Books.

Gray, A. (1992) *Video Playtime: The Gendering of a Leisure Technology*, London: Routledge.

Gullestad, M. (1992) *The Art of Social Relations: Essays on Culture, Social Action and Everyday Life in Norway*, Oslo: Scandinavian University Press.

Hacker, S. (1989) *Pleasure, Power and Technology: Some Tales of Gender, Engineering, and the Co-operative Workplace*, Boston: Unwin Hyman.

Haddon, L. (1997) *Empirical Research on the Domestic Phone: A Literature Review*, CulCom Working Paper, No. 2, Falmer, Brighton: University of Sussex.

Hearn, J. and Collinson, D. (1994) 'Theorizing unities and differences between men and between masculinities' in M. Kaufmann and H. Brod (eds) *Theorizing Masculinities*. Newbury Park, CA, London, New Delhi: Sage.

Lange, U. (1993) 'Telefonkommunikation im Privaten Alltag und die Grenzen der Interpretation' in S. Meyer and E. Schulze (eds) *Technisiertes Familienleben: Blick Zurück und Nach Vorn*, Berlin: Sigma.

Lie, M. (1995) 'Technology and masculinity: the case of the computer', *The European Journal of Women's Studies*, 2: 379–94.

Lohan, M. (1997) 'The feminisation of the domestic phone space: women and the domestic telephone in Ireland' in A. Byrne and M. Leonard (eds) *Women in Ireland: A Sociological Profile*, Belfast: Beyond the Pale Press.

Lohan, M. (1998) 'The transvestite telephone: a male technology dressed up in women's clothes', unpublished PhD thesis, Department of Sociology, Trinity College, Dublin.

Kimmel, M. (1994) 'Masculinity as homophobia: fear, shame and silence in the construction of gender identity' in M. Kaufmann and H. Brod (eds) *Theorizing Masculinities*, Newbury Park, CA, London, New Dehli: Sage.

Maddox, B. (1977) 'Women and the switchboard' in Ithiel de Sola Pool (ed.) *The Social Impact of the Telephone*, Cambridge, MA: MIT Press.

Martin, M. (1991) *'Hello Central' Gender Technology and Culture in the Formation of Telephone Systems*, Montreal and London: McGill Queen's University Press.

McNeil, M. (1992) 'New information technologies, English heroes and English lifestyles' in V. Frissen (ed.) *NICTS and the Changing Nature of the Domestic*, Amsterdam: GRANITE, Siswo.

Moyal, A. (1989) 'The feminine culture of the telephone' in *Prometheus*, 7 (1): 5–31.

Moyal, A. (1992) 'The gendered use of the telephone: an Australian case study', *Media Culture and Society*, 14: 51–72.

Murray, F. (1993) 'A separate reality: science, technology and masculinity' in E. Green, J. Owen and D. Pain (eds) *Gendered By Design*, London: Taylor and Francis.

Oldenziel, R. (2000): *Making Technology Masculine: Men, Women and Modern Machines in America, 1870–1945*, Amsterdam: Amsterdam University Press.

Rakow, L. F. (1992) *Gender on the Line, Women, the Telephone and Community Life*, Urbana and Chicago: University of Illinois Press.

Segal, L. (1997) *Slow Motion, Changing Masculinities, Changing Men*, revised edition, London: Virago Press.

Schabedoth, E., Storrl, D., Beck, K. and Lange, U. (1989) 'Der Kleine Unterschied, Erste Ergebnisse einer repräsentiven Befragung von Berliner Haushalten zur Nutzung des Telefons im Privaten Alltag' in U. Lange, K. Beck and A. Zerdick (eds), Berlin: Volker Speiss.

Sørensen, K. H. (1992) 'Towards a feminized technology? Gendered values in the construction of technology', *Social Studies of Science*, 22 (1): 5–31.

Wajcman, J. (1991) *Feminism Confronts Technology*, Cambridge: Polity Press in association with Blackwell Publishers.

Part III

Citizens at work and in the community

Chapter 11

Cyberstalking
Gender and computer ethics

Alison Adam

Introduction

The task of this chapter is twofold. First, I argue that the newly emerging discipline of computer ethics could benefit from insights into feminist theory, particularly in areas where there may be substantial differences in men's and women's experiences online. Second, I illustrate how feminist theory can be used to make a more extended analysis than is usually available in discussions of computer ethics through examples of 'cyberstalking', an extreme form of Internet-based harassment.

As a discipline, computer ethics has arisen in response to the apparently new social and ethical dilemmas that have resulted from the widespread adoption of information and communications technologies. These include issues such as hacking and viruses, copying software and electronic invasions of privacy. Opinions differ as to whether computer ethics problems really are novel or are best characterized as new variations of older problems. One of the most influential writers in the field, Deborah Johnson (1994), emphasizes the latter approach. Reading computer ethics problems in the light of existing and older ethical dilemmas has the advantage of connecting information technologies to their history. Such a view is less likely to be determinist in trajectory as it looks at the ways that other technologies may have developed in the past and may have been seen as completely novel and unlike anything else. In other words, it offers a more grounded view of technological innovation rather than seeing it as determined and inevitable. This more historically rooted approach may avoid the problems of determinism yet, at the same time, it may compound errors and inequalities committed in the name of more traditional ethical theories. This is especially problematic if the traditional ethical approaches are individualist and rationalist views of ethics that render invisible, and hence level out, inequalities of power.

Considering more radical approaches to ethics brings to the fore the question of power structures. Gender and technology studies have proved successful in exposing power relations in the development and use of technologies in relation to men's and women's experiences of information and communications technologies which represent one of the most substantial areas of potential inequality (for example, Adam et al. 1994). At the same time, major developments in feminist ethics over the last two decades make this an area at least as important as computer ethics and probably more important on the theoretical front in terms of overall contribution to philosophical ethics (Tong 1998). Feminist ethics, coupled with other relevant aspects of feminist theory, applied to computer ethics promises a novel and fruitful alternative to current directions in computer ethics in three major ways. The first offers the possibility of countering the technological determinism inherent in views of computer ethics that see the trajectory of computer ethics as substantially different from other technologies and at the same time threatening and out of control. The second reveals continuing inequalities in power and how these are often 'gendered', i.e., the experiences of men and women are often substantially different and are different in relation to their respective genders. The third aspect of this process involves offering an alternative, collective approach to the individualism of the traditional ethical theories encapsulated in computer ethics.

In this chapter I concentrate on the second aspect outlined above, namely thinking through how feminist ethics can be used as an explanatory tool in relation to computer ethics problems, taking the topic of cyberstalking, an extreme form of harassment on the Internet, as an example. Three case studies are discussed. I argue that, given that the majority of victims are women and the majority of perpetrators men, the kind of liberal measures advocated in current policy documents are unlikely to be effective in stemming the problem, unless a better understanding of the gendered nature of the phenomenon can be obtained. We need to look to feminist ethics and related theory to achieve such an understanding.

Gender and information and communications technologies

One of the clearest power imbalances that exists in the use of information and communications technologies is the difference between men's and women's access and usage of computers which continues to be one of the major inequalities running throughout the whole of computing. There now exists a fairly substantial literature on gender and computing which spells out that relationship in the context of home, work and virtual communities.[1] Much of this literature looks to feminist theory for its inspiration and therefore offers the possibility of alternative ethical approaches which have the potential to open up and expose latent power relations.

Despite the increasing theoretical sophistication of research on gender and information and communications technologies few authors have yet chosen to take on the domain of computer ethics to examine its potential gender implications. Such studies as currently exist tend to focus on statistical measures of men's and women's ethical decision-making in order to say whether women are more ethical than men or vice versa (Khazanchi 1995; Kreie and Cronan 1998; Bissett and Shipton 1999). This focus on the minutiae of statistics tends to detract from the need to theorize the reasons for any underlying differences in men's and women's behaviour, meaning that the whole area remains undertheorized especially in relation to the substantial body of literature in feminist ethics.

Some of these studies mention Carol Gilligan's (1982) well known study of men's and women's moral reasoning, *In a Different Voice* (for example, Bissett and Shipton 1999). This is such a well known work that we can refer to it as a base level of theorizing from feminist ethics and we expect it to be cited in any piece of research which purports to deal with some aspect of gender and ethics. Yet none of these studies uses substantially more than Gilligan and several of them are without reference to feminist or gender ethics theory at all (for example, Kreie and Cronan 1998). If these authors had located their work against the debate surrounding Gilligan's work, which also centred round an empirical study, they would have been able not only to apply her results, where appropriate, but also to counter the criticisms of her work which also potentially apply to their studies. For instance, Larrabee (1993) notes that one of the criticisms of Gilligan's research was that she asked her respondents to work through a number of artificial case studies rather than observing them making real, live ethical decisions. This remains an important consideration for any such work and it seems that we are still far from understanding how ethical reasoning in response to an artificial scenario maps on to ethical reasoning in a more realistic setting. However a more appropriate approach towards the use of scenarios or 'vignettes' for exploring moral reasoning can be found in Silva's research (2000) where the emphasis is less on the use of turbo-charged statistical techniques and more on understanding morality as grounded experience, changing with life course and personal circumstances.

While potential gender differences in computer ethics decisions remain important, given the caveats above, current studies appear to be taking the subject of gender and computer ethics down something of a cul-de-sac, especially on the theoretical front. Importantly the focus of current studies offers no challenge to the determinism and tacit power relations vector prevalent in computer ethics which I have emphasized. Indeed the statistical studies can be seen as reinforcing rather than challenging such issues. They do not challenge the apparent inevitability of the introduction of new information technologies, nor do they question the organizational structures within which their ethical scenarios are set, nor indeed do they challenge the tacit power relationship that exists between researcher and researched.

The approach taken in this chapter involves starting off from the theoretical to consider (albeit briefly) what feminist ethics and related feminist theory might offer the study of gender and computer ethics. Then, rather than homing in on the minutiae of statistical results from a questionnaire survey, I offer a new analysis of examples, deriving from the arena of cyberstalking, to argue that the traditional liberal ethical response does not get to the heart of the problem and that feminist theory may offer a more promising alternative.

Feminist ethics and feminist theory

Feminist ethics embrace attempts to rethink and revise the facets of traditional ethics which devalue the moral experience of women (Tong 1998). Arguing that traditional ethics fails women in that it regards their experiences as uninteresting, at the same time it overemphasizes traditional masculine ways of ethical reasoning which look to individual, rationalistic, rule-based ethical models. In developing various women-centered approaches to ethics the overall aim of feminist ethics is 'to create a gender-equal ethics, a moral theory that generates non-sexist moral principles, policies and practices' (Tong 1998).

Importantly, feminist ethics can offer help in exposing the power inequalities which exist in our case studies which traditional computer ethics renders invisible in its pursuit of mainstream ethical views and its lack of critique of professional roles and structures. It is this critical bite which has proved appealing to many feminist authors and this is reflected in the critical tone of much writing on feminist theory. The challenge is then to harness this energy into a constructive critique of computer ethics.

However it would be wrong to suppose that feminist ethics sets out its theoretical stall in splendid isolation from other branches of feminist theory. The empirical examples that I discuss towards the end of this chapter relate strongly to privacy, which provides an excellent example of the way in which several aspects of feminist theory come together. Privacy is not just a matter for feminist ethics, there are also strong legal and political dimensions to the concept. There is the question of whether privacy is different for women and men and also how this difference can be captured in legislation (MacKinnon 1989; DeCew 1997).

What can feminist ethics offer computer ethics?

In this section I wish to consider whether concepts from feminist ethics may offer alternative readings of computer ethics problems. Johnson (1994) regards new responses to new computer-based behaviours as the fundamental job of computer ethics. A view from feminist ethics may offer an alternative to the responses of computer ethics. What insights can be offered on computer ethics problems which may potentially affect men and women in different ways? In looking at these issues through examples I want to return to the problem of technological determinism which was raised earlier in the chapter as being problematic in current constructions of computer ethics. Having argued, in particular, that determinism is problematic in relation to gender, i.e., these views can do little to alleviate inequalities in power and participation, I want to discuss the ways in which alternative readings from feminist ethics and feminist theory can be used to alleviate these problems through thinking about how such arguments may be applied to the phenomenon of cyberstalking.

Sexual harassment online

Before looking at the more extreme examples of cyberstalking I introduce the topic by discussing online sexual harassment, the milder form of behaviour from which cyberstalking apparently derives. A leading feminist legal theorist, Catharine MacKinnon (1979: 1) writing in the 1970s, defined sexual harassment as '. . . the unwanted imposition of sexual requirements in the context of a relationship of unequal power. Central to the concept is the use of power derived from one social sphere to lever benefits or impose deprivations in another.' Sexual harassment *can* involve unwanted explicit sexual attention and it *can* be applied by women to men, but in a world where power relationships most often put men in a superior position it has come to be used to define, more generally, behaviour by men, often in the workplace, which demeans women or otherwise makes them feel uncomfortable and which arises, at least in some part, because of the differential power relationships between the genders.

Looking at empirical studies suggests that the picture is extremely complex and ambivalent. On the one hand, there is evidence of women feeling empowered by their use of information technology and actively resisting the paternalistic protection. For instance witness the responses to the formation of a direct-action feminist group against Internet censorship at Carnegie Mellon University: 'We're big girls who don't need to be protected from horny geek fantasies' (Riley 1996: 159). Yet we must recognize that only relatively few women are in the privileged position of taking part in this empowerment.

On the other hand, there are some negative experiences and some authors take the view that, for example, the Internet reinforces and magnifies stereotypical gendered behaviours rather than smoothing them out and acting as the great leveller that some desire. Susan Herring's well-researched study of interactions on the Internet (1996) shows that computer-mediated communication does not neutralize gender. As a group she found women more likely to use supportive behaviour while men were more likely to favour adversarial interactions. These she linked to men favouring individual freedom while women prefer harmonious interpersonal interaction. Such behaviours and values can be seen as important in reinforcing male dominance and female submission.

There are a number of issues at stake here. The liberal values which have often been taken for granted in relation to Internet interactions (Winner 1997) start from a position of assuming free and equal interactions and that everyone has equal abilities on the Internet. They also contain a determinist view that the spread of Internet usage is inevitable; we have to take part or be swept aside by the technological tide. On the other side, an analysis of sexual harassment on the Internet from any traditional ethical theory, either from a utilitarian or deontological position, would surely condemn it. From a utilitarian point of view, making some women very unhappy does not seem to add to the greatest good for the greatest number; on the other hand, we have the paradox that this behaviour could make a few women very unhappy but many men happy, thus increasing overall happiness. However few people would be comfortable with such arguments.

A more reasonable position is offered by a Kantian analysis that would condemn cyberstalking as treating women as a means to an end rather than as individual moral agents with rights. However both these traditional approaches to ethics seem to offer little scope for offering measures to stop it, other than, perhaps, legislation with no guarantee as to whether or not that legislation can prove effective. However, as the cyberstalking examples described below demonstrate, the victims clearly felt unhappy about the level of protection that the law currently affords them. As I shall argue, this reflects a typical liberal position that does not get to the heart of the problem of why threatening behaviour occurs in the first place. Only when we have a better understanding of why the behaviour occurs can we then begin to think about policy measures which may be effective.

Cyberstalking

Online sexual harassment may be something of a problem but, as Herring (1996) argues, it tends to mirror the levels of harassment that women often find in real life. Latterly, a more extreme version of online sexual harassment in the shape of cyberstalking has reached the attention of the media, the government and law enforcement agencies. In this section I describe briefly three cyberstalking cases where women were victims and compare some aspects of these cases against an example, with some similarities and differences, where a man won redress after being defamed on the Internet. I analyse the reactions to cyberstalking in the media and at government level in the USA and describe how the lack of analysis of why cyberstalking has become such a menace, encapsulated in the traditional liberal and deterministic view of ethics, threatens to dilute the measures being taken to combat the problem. I conclude the discussion by arguing that a contrasting view of this issue from a feminist ethics position could offer a better understanding of the causes of the problem and thereby offer more hope for future solutions.

Online sexual harassment raises the question of individual privacy but cyberstalking really hammers home what is involved in violations of individual privacy. Stalking has become a familiar term but more recently the term 'cyberstalking' has been coined to describe stalking behaviour perpetrated through some aspect of information and communications technology and even then it is probably not useful to draw too distinct a line between 'cyber' and traditional versions as, for instance, the telephone has traditionally been a tool of the stalker (Case 2000). However cyberstalking more usually involves the use of the Internet to perpetrate stalking behaviour and this has prompted a flurry of legislation and other interest culminating in US Vice President Al Gore's commissioning of a report on the subject by the Attorney General in the summer of 1999 (Reno 1999).

Cyberstalking examples

Jayne Hitchcock's experience of cyberstalking is typical of the phenomenon (Mingo 2000). She is an author of children's books who, when she first became connected to the Internet, contacted Woodside Literary Agency which advertised its services over a number of Usenet groups. Woodside accepted her as a client and then immediately asked for up-front fees. She realized that she had been rather naïve in contacting them and that the organization was probably of dubious legitimacy. She began warning fellow Internet writers on Usenet groups. A number of her contacts were already peppering the Woodside agency with queries to which it never responded, angered by its insistent 'spamming' of advertisements. Although Hitchcock was not its only critic, Woodside began posting attacks on her over the 'misc.writing' Usenet group and posted claims that she was a pornographer over various newsgroups. After this someone began to post counterfeit messages in her name all over the Internet. These messages of an explicit sexual nature invited people to contact her or come to her house. The phone rang constantly. Eventually a friend of Hitchcock's was able to gather enough evidence from the headers of the counterfeit messages that had allegedly been sent by Woodside and a case was brought to the legal courts.

A second case, which is in some ways similar to the Hitchcock case, involved a man from California who was jailed for six years for offences resulting from cyberstalking (*Guardian* 1999). Angry that a woman had spurned him, he assumed her identity and posted personal information about her, including her address, in Internet sex chat rooms where he claimed sado-masochistic fantasies in her name. As a result of this a number of men tried to break into her house. The man thought that his anonymity was preserved on the Internet. He was eventually caught after the victim's father spent hours on the Internet posting messages that he hoped would attract the stalker. When the stalker eventually made contact, the woman's father turned the case over to the FBI resulting in the prosecution.

A third, somewhat older example, involves Stephanie Brail's experience of harassment bordering on stalking which dates from 1993 (Brail 1996). She rationalizes this as resulting, not just because she was a women online, but because 'I dared to speak out in the common space of the Internet, Usenet' (Brail 1996: 144). Brail found herself drawn into a 'flame war' on a news group about underground magazines, defending another woman who had been verbally attacked by a number of men for views on an alternative women's publication. She started to become the victim of anonymous obscene postings. The perpetrator posted her name and details on sex chat rooms and so other people began contacting her. Finally the anonymous stalker threatened to visit her house. She began to feel fearful of her personal safety. But he had left a loophole in the header of his anonymous email and she was able (after having felt forced to learn both self-defence and UNIX) to trace him and email him back whereupon the threats stopped.

Analysis of cyberstalking examples using feminist ethics

In this section I draw together an analysis of the cyberstalking phenomenon through an examination of the above examples in relation to feminist ethics and related theory. In all three cases the victim is a woman. In one case the perpetrator is definitely male; in the Woodside case it is a small group of men and women and in the Brail case the perpetrator styled himself 'Mike' and is assumed to be male by the victim although, as the case was never brought to the law, we cannot be sure. In all the cases the victims and/or friends and associates used some aspect of the Internet to help track down the perpetrator. Indeed both Mingo's article (2000) on the Woodside case and Brail's own description of her experiences (1996) explicitly use the rhetoric of 'frontier justice' and so they are both indicating that the normal channels of law and justice are either not available or are not sufficient. This opinion would seem to be justified given the efforts of the victims' friends and families in these cases. Hitchcock enlisted the help of a 'volunteer cyberposse' reinforcing the rhetoric of the Internet as frontier territory. Only in the California case is there the traditional 'spurned lover.' The other two cases are unusual in comparison to traditional stalking in that the women became victims not as ex-lovers or distant objects of desire but use they chose to speak up publicly on the Internet about ɪjustices. They then became the victims of those they were

Both men and women can be the victims of conventional stalking and cyberstalking. In the typology of stalking behaviour (*Stalking Behavior* 2000) one substantial category involves the obsessive personality who fixates on a figure of authority whom the stalker regards as above them in status, for example, a medical doctor or a media figure. In this case the stalker can be a man but is often a woman fixating on a man.

In all three cyberstalking examples given, the perpetrators impersonate the victim in anonymous Internet postings. This has the effect of defaming the victim and, because the postings contain some kind of pornographic invitation, they caused others to display threatening behaviour towards the victim. This threatening behaviour was not confined to the Internet, as the victim's telephone number and address are given and unwanted visits and telephone calls were made. So the cyberstalker can hide behind the anonymity of the Internet and, at the same time, can trigger real life stalking behaviour in others, thereby creating a whole new sinister turn to the phenomenon of stalking.

Clearly men can also be the victims of anonymous, defamatory Internet postings posted in their name. But the features of a case involving a man, although it has some similarities, demonstrate aspects which are interestingly different from the women's cases I describe above. In this example, a physicist, Laurence Godfrey, successfully obtained a small amount of damages, but a large amount of legal expenses, in a libel case against the Internet service provider, Demon in the UK (Yahoo 2000). The Godfrey case is quite complex and long running; he was involved in a number of actions for defamation. However the action that he eventually won involved the Internet service provider, Demon. Godfrey was a contributor to a newsgroup about the politics of Thailand. Anonymous postings containing 'squalid, obscene and defamatory' material were posted in his name. He asked Demon to remove the forged material on several occasions but it did not. He is reported to have taken the action in a bid to force Internet service providers to behave more responsibly. It is not clear, however, how this will affect Internet law in the UK, which is different from US law, as many see it as unrealistic for service providers to police their newsgroups rigorously. At the moment US laws treat Internet service providers analogously to telecommunications providers, i.e., not responsible for content. Current UK law treats Internet service providers more akin to publishers where there is a level of liability for content. In the shorter term, however, UK service providers appear to be very nervous of anything contentious and already there is evidence of their removing controversial material at the slightest suggestion that it is problematic (*Guardian* 2000).

There are distinctions to be made between the Godfrey case and the three examples I use above. The Godfrey example does not appear to have been construed as an instance of cyberstalking and there is no mention of Godfrey feeling under threat in that way in media reports (although that is not to say he did not feel a similar threat). The media portrayal of his case, rather, revolved round the idea of the consumer winning out against the Internet service provider who has now been given a sharp reminder of its duties to its customers. This is set against the freedom of speech that individuals may expect to have on the Internet as elsewhere in life. It is a measure of Godfrey's confidence in winning the case that he was able to run up legal bills of some £200,000 in the expectation that he would win his case. Of course Godfrey's case was against the service provider and not the anonymous individual or individuals who defamed him and it is clear that Godfrey would have struggled to bring his case against the service provider in a different legislative framework whose laws were substantially different to those in the UK.

Despite the fact that both women and men can be victims of stalking and cyberstalking, the majority of reported cyberstalking cases involve women as victims and men as perpetrators. The US Attorney General's report (Reno 1999) which represents the major public policy document on the subject to date, other than recording this fact makes virtually nothing more of this, seemingly treating it as an accidental rather than fundamental aspect of such behaviour. The report suggests the following:

> The first line of defense will involve industry efforts that educate and empower individuals to protect themselves against cyberstalking and other online threats, along with prompt reporting to law enforcement agencies trained and equipped to respond to cyberstalking incidents.
>
> (Reno 1999: 2)

The strong, clear message of the Reno report is that cyberstalking is to be tackled by an industry–law enforcement agencies partnership. Online providers must educate their customers in avoiding unwanted and threatening messages and must respond promptly and effectively when threatening behaviour is reported to them. 'Self-protection' is the term used (Reno 1999: 11). Similarly the Reno report argues that policy-makers and law enforcement agencies have a duty to ensure appropriate legislation is in place, to enable their own training, to share information across states and, internationally, to build up expertise, to work with victims' groups and to co-operate effectively with industry.

> Both industry and law enforcement benefit when crime over the Internet is reduced. In particular, the Internet industry benefits significantly whenever citizen and consumer confidence and trust in the Internet is increased.
>
> (Reno 1999: 12)

The Attorney General's report offers a number of traditional, liberal ethical measures to counteract the problem of cyberstalking. In looking to industry for a large part of the solution to the problem it borders on advocating a free-market economics which, when coupled with the last quote, purveys a strongly utilitarian argument. Framing the argument starkly, it is as if we appeal to industry to help with the problem as it makes good business sense for it to do so, not because we expect it to care about its customers as individuals.

Now no one would advocate that industry does nothing; the Godfrey case indicates that the Internet service provider was too slow in responding to his requests to remove offensive messages. Similarly no one would advocate that we should *not* try to protect ourselves against cyberstalking and other threatening behaviour. Finally we would all hope for protection from the law, although my three examples above suggest that one cannot rely solely on the standard sources of justice. The official version firmly advocates a mixture of trust in free-market utilitarian arguments in relation to industry with a strong measure of self-protection and trust in the law, in other words the traditional forces of capitalism and state. This must also be balanced with that most liberal of concepts, free speech. Hence the balance between industry and legislative bodies in the education and empowerment of the individual is meant to take care of the problem. But why should it if we do not properly understand why the phenomenon occurs in the first place? Such arguments are not radical enough.

Important though these measures may be in looking towards the protection of the individual, they do not get to the root cause or causes of cyberstalking. The official argument of the Reno report barely mentions the important fact that cyberstalking behaviour is strongly gendered. An argument from feminist ethics and related theory could, at least, help us to understand why the behaviour takes place in the first place and can begin to suggest policy measures to tackle the problem.

The liberal tradition maintains a firm separation between the public and private spheres. Only after a long fight, well into the nineteenth century, did married women have legal rights regarding property, person and children. But as MacKinnon points out (1989), in the private sphere, traditionally the domain of women and the family, women may have limited rights as the state is reluctant to interfere. As women have traditionally had few rights to privacy (DeCew 1997) it is not always easy to see when their rights are being violated. This may partly explain the reluctance of official bodies to see cyberstalking as a problem that affects women to the extent that they may need special measures to counteract it.

Feminist ethics emphasizes the web of responsibilities we have towards one another in an 'ethic of care' rather than seeing us as individual moral agents as implied by traditional liberal ethics. This too suggests that rather than individual 'self-protection' we need to understand the interconnectedness of the effects of the problem. The Reno report was balanced towards counteracting cyberstalking behaviour when it happens but said little of how we may stop the behaviour in the first place. If it is a crime mainly perpetrated by men against women, we need to understand how men become perpetrators and women victims. Current measures against the problem are couched in terms of relying on a mixture of free-market economics, self-help and the actions of legislative bodies. This, then combines right-of-centre liberalism in terms of reliance on the free market to sort out social ills coupled with exhortations for us to trust in the state to look after us. This is a position of which feminists and others have rightly been wary. The self-help actions that the three women and their allies took in the case studies above, rather than purely being measures to protect themselves, represented rather much more active pursuits of justice against those perpetrating the crimes. Once more a more active agency is implied by the empowerment involved in feminist ethics measures rather than the weaker more passive version of empowerment offered by the liberal state/industry/self-protect version in the Reno report.

Only when the causes of cyberstalking are better understood can we offer policy measures that have any hope of being effective in counteracting the problem. The feminist analysis involves trying to understand the nature of relationships between men and women by examining the fundamental structures of the way we organize ourselves in society. These structures, of course, involve government, industry, law enforcement bodies, etc. Suggesting that all bodies in public and private life require dissection for gendered power relations is understandably too radical a message for powerful authorities to swallow. To require that all institutions be examined need not, however, imply that all require radical overhaul.

The 'ethic of care' espoused in Gilligan's (1982) and related work offers an alternative to many of the current possibilities on offer. The individual need not see him/herself as an isolated moral agent protecting him/herself in between the moral rationalism of state and free market implied by the Reno report. For both the Brail (1996) and Woodside (Mingo 2000) cases there are extended accounts either written by the victim or a close associate. In both cases an extended network of friends helped the victim reach a solution. The power and importance of these informal networks that are present in some walks of life are perhaps the nearest thing we get to an ethic of care in society. Yet in the official response to the problem of cyberstalking the importance of these informal yet vital networks is not acknowledged.

Conclusion

In this chapter I have taken a step backwards to view a wider picture in understanding the development of computer ethics and its individualist, rationalist stance towards ethical issues. I have taken up one of the major inequalities in the use of ICTs, namely the position of women. In beginning to explore these alternatives, my key example is sexual harassment and, more specifically, cyberstalking on the Internet. I contrast a view from feminist ethics with the liberal arguments found in computer ethics and which are already being enshrined in important policy documents to argue that the way forward arises from an understanding of these problems which is only achievable through a better analysis of the gendered nature of the causes of the phenomena currently found under the banner of computer ethics. Cyberstalking displays clearly gendered aspects. In that case it may well be that new understandings of other problems may be desirable. For instance, it has often been noted that hacking is largely a masculine phenomenon (Taylor 1999) suggesting that it too would benefit from a more thorough-going analysis in terms of feminist ethics. This is just a beginning. I argue that feminist ethics holds much promise both in forming alternative analyses of computer ethics problems and in offering a more collectivist vector for computer ethics theory.

Note

1 A fairly comprehensive bibliography of gender and ICTs can be found at the following website: http://www.library.wisc.edu/libraries/WomensStudies

References

Adam, A., Emms, J., Green, E. and Owen, J. (eds) (1994) *Women, Work and Computerization: Breaking Old Boundaries – Building New Forms*, IFIP Transactions A-57, Amsterdam: Elsevier/North-Holland.

Bissett, A. and Shipton, G. (1999) 'An investigation into gender differences in the ethical attitudes of IT professionals', ETHICOMP99, October, Rome.

Brail, S. (1996) 'The price of admission: harassment and free speech in the wild, wild west' in L. Cherny and E. R. Wise (eds) *Wired_Women: Gender and New Realities in Cyberspace*, Seattle, WA: Seal Press.

Case, D. O. (2000) 'Stalking, monitoring and profiling: a typology and case studies of harmful uses of caller ID', *New Media and Society* 2 (1): 67–84.

DeCew, J. W. (1997) *In Pursuit of Privacy: Law, Ethics, and the Rise of Technology*, Ithaca and London: Cornell University Press.

Gilligan, C. (1982) *In a Different Voice: Psychological Theory and Women's Development*, Cambridge, MA: Harvard University Press.

The *Guardian* (1999) 'Cyber-stalkers make computer new tool of terror', 29 November, broadsheet section: 13.

The *Guardian* (2000) 'Freedom fear on website closure', 3 April, broadsheet section: 8.

Herring, S. (1996) 'Posting in a different voice: gender and ethics in CMC' in C. Ess (ed.) *Philosophical Perspectives on Computer-Mediated Communication*, Albany: State University of New York Press.

Johnson, D. (1994) *Computer Ethics*, second edition, Englewood Cliffs, NJ: Prentice-Hall.

Khazanchi, D. (1995) 'Unethical behavior in information systems: the gender factor', *Journal of Business Ethics*, 14, 741–9.

Kreie, J. and Cronan, T. P. (1998) 'How men and women view ethics', *Communications of the ACM*, 41 (9): 70–6.

Larrabee, M. J. (ed.) (1993) *An Ethic of Care*, New York and London: Routledge.

MacKinnon, C. A. (1979) *The Sexual Harassment of Working Women*, New Haven, CT: Yale University Press.

MacKinnon, C. A. (1989) *Toward a Feminist Theory of the State*, Cambridge, MA: Harvard University Press.

Mingo, J. (2000) 'Caught in the net: an online posse tracks down an Internet stalker.' Available online: http://www.houston-press.com/extra/cyber-stalk.html (24 March 2000).

Reno, J. (1999) 'Cyberstalking: a new challenge for law enforcement and industry. A report from the Attorney General to the Vice President.' Available online: http://www.usdoj.gov/ag/cyberstalkingreport.html (30 November 1999).

Riley, D. M. (1996) 'Sex, fear and condescension on campus: cybercensorship at Carnegie Mellon' in L. Cherny and E. R. Wise (eds) Wired_Women: Gender and New Realities in Cyberspace, Seattle, WA: Seal Press.

Silva, E. (2000) 'Domestic dilemmas: ethics of everyday living', paper presented at Gendering Ethics/The Ethics of Gender Conference, Centre for Interdisciplinary Gender Studies, University of Leeds, 23–5 June 2000.

Stalking Behavior (2000) 'Stalking behaviors, definitions and links'. Available online: http://onour.com/stalking (28 March 2000).

Taylor, P. A. (1999) Hackers: Crime in the Digital Sublime, London and New York: Routledge.

Tong, R. (1998) 'Feminist ethics' in Edward N. Zalta (ed.) The Stanford Encyclopedia of Philosophy (Fall 1999 edition). Available online: http://plato.stanford.edu/archives/fall1999/entries/feminism-ethics/ (23 September 1998).

Winner, L. (1997) 'Cyberlibertarian myths and the prospect for community', ACM Computers and Society, 27 (3): 14–19.

Yahoo (2000) 'Service provider Demon settles Internet libel case'. Available online: http://uk.news.yahoo.com/000330/91/a2nba.html (31 March 2000).

Chapter 12

Gender and citizenship in the information society
Women's information technology groups in North Karelia

Marja Vehviläinen

Introduction

> 'NiceNet is the Marjala women's own information technology circle, in which information technology is harnessed for everyday life, work and leisure. One studies, experiments, practices, networks, makes development happen to oneself and others.'
>
> (NiceNet 1998)

The NiceNet group was formed in North Karelia, Finland, and has supported its members in the creation of opportunity for action, home and active citizenship related to information and communication technologies and networks. In this chapter I examine the practices of citizenship in the information society from the perspective of women and gender. The NiceNet group and its home pages form the beginning of my analysis.

It is common policy for western governments, including the Finnish government, to aim for the provision of equal access to information technology for all citizens. To attain this goal governments provide computers, network connections and sometimes training and support for schools, libraries and other public institutions. These policies commonly define citizenship in the information society narrowly, in terms of machines and technical user skills. They hardly notice that women and men relate differently to networks and computing, that information technology and electronic networks are mainly worlds for young men, both statistically and culturally (for example, Spender 1995; Herring 1996; Wakeford 2000) or that it is generally only western cultures whose inhabitants can realistically expect to use electronic network connections (for example, Holderness 1998). The social setting of technology is not included in their analysis and policies implicitly carry a western, male and middle-class bias, without reflecting upon or questioning it. In this context the NiceNet women's information technology group, located in a particular setting of a neighbourhood centre, allows me to acknowledge broadly the practices of citizenship which have room for situated social differences and, at the same time, to explore how these practices can be made to work locally for women.

I present the NiceNet group and the home pages produced in the group as well as the practices that have made the group and its activities possible. I explore social and textual relations (Smith 1990) that organize the women's group's activities and practices, and look for the material construction of active citizenship in the information society. The local women's information technology group needs support from various institutions and from local and (trans)national sources. I challenge the stereotypical 'equal access' view of citizenship that claims to make space for women's active agency in a technically mediated society. I discuss the possibility for making a home within the networks; firstly, through the possibility of changing the dominant network practices; secondly, by means of the cultural space that a local women's group can provide for the development of alternatives. I initiate this analysis by elaborating the problem of gender and citizenship.

On gendered citizenship in the information society

The goal of equal access to information technology connects with the liberal tradition of citizenship. It contains the idea of citizens as individuals. Individuals are interested in using information technologies and individuals have a universal desire for using them as soon as public sites are furnished with computers. The liberal understanding of citizenship bypasses the structural displacement of various groups, notably women (Lister 1997). It relates to the idea of a coherent information technology culture that sees technology as neutral, with no regard for people's gender, age, race or local situation. It assumes that the technical terms of dominant computing companies suit the activities of all humans regardless of their different situations and positions. It does not make room for counter discourses or resistance, for local (for example, women's) development work or for the formation of one's own perspective. Although the argument for equal access is important as a citizen's right, it also remains very limited.

Ruth Lister (1997) conceptualizes citizenship both as a status carrying a wide range of rights (for example, access to technology) and as a practice including political participation. The two sides of citizenship are woven together within human agency: 'Citizenship as participation represents an expression of human agency in the political arena, broadly defined; citizenship as rights enables people to act as agents' (Lister 1997: 36). Human agency as a core element of citizenship may generally refer to any human activity or more strictly to conscious political activity but in both cases it makes space for women's – as individuals and as groups – own definitions of technology. Women need equal access as their self-evident right but as they live in a society of gendered social orders they also need to develop particular practices for their participation in the societal life.

Human agency sets the question of subjectivity in the centre of citizenship. Electronic networks 'are changing the way we think, the nature of our sexuality, the form of our communities, our very identities'. We learn to step 'through the looking glass', like Alice steps into Wonderland, 'we learn to live in virtual worlds . . . Other people are there as well' (Turkle 1995: 9). One's subjectivity, human agency and citizenship get their shape when people connect to networks and meet other people there. Moreover, the subjectivities of people who use computers and enter networks have bodies and life histories in local, historical and socially constructed practices. Although they want to go into virtual worlds, they are still ordinary men and women. Networks and computers are meaningless until people, or actants, interpret them or produce new meanings through them.

If people are to be active and creative in and through networks they need to be able to connect the networks and technology to their local situations and use their local situations, bodily beings and the differences embedded in them as point of departures (Escobar 1999; Wakeford 2000). As Lister (1997) points out, the practices of citizenship should have room for situated and local differences (Wise 1997), wide societal orders and people's activities of connecting these in their everyday settings. Mere Internet surfing and the practices of citizenship based on individual interests do not acknowledge the agency of women thoroughly enough and it is now time to have a look at the citizenship and human agency in locally based groups which are part of wider social worlds.

My analysis has been inspired by Donna Haraway's (1991) and Kathy Ferguson's (1993) notions of subjectivity embedded in social relations taken to be simultaneously local and bodily, global and textual, even technical. The self is an acting subject who defines her/himself and her or his activity in society. This subject has links with the multi-tier construction of citizenship introduced by Nira Yuval-Davis (1997): people are members in more than one community, in local, ethnic, state and often trans-state communities, and citizenship includes domains of the state, civil society and the family. In communities people feel accepted, they become one of 'us', but communities also reject and define the 'other' (Griffiths 1995). In particular, I trace the communities that have been referred to in the women's group's home pages.

I look for a citizenship that has room for women's active definitions of information technology. I am interested in the possibilities for action and the tension between local situations and global technology.

The Finnish and North Karelian setting

The Finnish economy benefits extensively from the Nokia mobile phone industry and there has been little criticism of the seeming necessity of information society development. To a large extent the governmental goal of the equal access to information and communication technologies has been reached. Since the 1980s both women and men, and in fact women slightly more than men, make frequent use of computers in their workplaces (Lehto and Sutela 1999). In the 1990s libraries as well as various citizen and neighbourhood centres have supplied opportunities for computer use. Schools in most parts of Finland have good computing facilities. People do use mobile phones, computers and networks more than almost anywhere in the whole world. Yet although 'equal access to computers', as defined by governmental policies, generally takes place, not everyone uses them equally nor even desires to use them. The global divisions of gender, class and region are present in Finland, too (Nurmela 1997).

In this chapter, I adopt the perspective of the women's information technology group, NiceNet, in North Karelia province on the eastern border of Finland and the European Union. North Karelia is a region of high unemployment (20 per cent and in parts even 25–30 per cent) and long distances. These have prompted the regional authorities to develop information technology in order to transform this peripheral position into an advantage – to have a good life in a beautiful environment – which is how the information strategy of the North Karelian Council described it in 1996. Furthermore, as a region of a Nordic welfare state, North Karelia aims to take care of its inhabitants and to include them all in societal development. There are a number of ongoing development projects focusing specifically on citizenship and the information society in the area.

I have undertaken interviews and observations in the neighbourhoods and citizens' centres in Joensuu (the capital of the province with 50,000 inhabitants). The subjects were residents, social workers, city planners and a neighbourhood centre computer support person. The data also includes reference to information society texts that are specifically related to the area and especially to the NiceNet group, for example, the home pages and meeting notes of the group. The research took place between autumn 1996 and spring 1998.

NiceNet – information technology in a women's group

The NiceNet women's group (the pronunciation of 'Nice' closely resembles the pronunciation of the Finnish word 'nais', which roughly means 'women's'; hence NiceNet can be thought of as both a women's electronic network and as a nice setting) has met since the summer of 1997 in the neighbourhood centre in the Joensuu suburb, Marjala. The women have various backgrounds, from busy working women to students and mothers doing part-time work. They have in common living in the locality of the Marjala suburb. They have approached information technology beginning with their everyday lives, work and leisure with conscious attempts to develop their own understanding and that of others. During the summer they make labels for canning bottles; in December they produce Christmas cards. They have used the Internet to search for information on, for example, child care and cooking as well as their work activities.

Thirty-six-year-old Sari, a mother of three young children, says in an interview: 'I want to be at home as long as the children are small. I work (sell cosmetics, study for a new occupation) while the children sleep . . . in the NiceNet I have learnt how to do letters, registers and time schedules for my work with the computer. We have a computer at home, bought by my husband, for example for games for the girls. I did not, however, first see how I could use it myself but it was first in the NiceNet that I learnt to see my needs.'

NiceNet started when Ritva, a female resident of Marjala, participated in a computer study group arranged by the neighbourhood centre. She was the only female participant which had surprised her. This prompted her to develop the idea of an information technology group for women only. She called Sari who lived nearby and together the women sat down at the centre's computer. Ritva was using computers in her work and she was able to show things to Sari. Sari realized that a computer was helpful in her everyday tasks, for example in letter writing. With the help of the computer support person they were able to continue for hours. After a couple of months they announced the new women's group in the neighbourhood news bulletin and, in July 1997, they formed a group of five to seven women interested in computing. Sari says: 'I was asked: what are you doing there? Have you used computers? I had not been using, and then other women also felt that they could join us although they had no experience . . . first we made canning labels. Each woman was able to say what they wanted to be done. The group first met every fortnight. In NiceNet we speak about other things, too.'

Information technology studies in the group create a sense of community which might otherwise be absent in the neighbourhood where most people are newcomers. Information technology studies provide a legitimate excuse for the residents to keep coming back to the centre. By doing this they get to know other people in the neighbourhood and get an opportunity to speak about their shared living conditions and lives. People move back and forth but it would be difficult to get acquainted with other people without particular projects.

In NiceNet everybody can make proposals for study topics. Although Ritva took the initiative in forming the group, the group did not nominate any supervisor or co-ordinator. If the group had problems with technical matters it consulted the computer support person or other 'nice men in the neighbourhood' (minutes of the group). The support person answered and helped but did not act as a teacher or a mediator for the group. The NiceNet group has all the appearance of sisterly groups in the women's movement (Bono and Kemp 1991). Some of the 'sisters' have been more knowledgeable than others; two of the members have used computers in their work and studies but their knowledge has not given them hierarchical authority over others. The group members have discussed the study programme together as well as taking care that nobody feels rejected (Griffiths 1995). They write summaries of the meetings in order to allow the members who have been unable to attend to follow their activities. The summaries often include the names of those who were absent.

Both Sari and the computer support worker say that studies in the women's group have differed from the 'general' information technology sessions in the centre still attended only by men. In the men's group they are interested primarily in the technology while, in NiceNet, Sari and the other women are more interested in 'how things can be done'. The NiceNet programme has included concrete tasks: making canning labels and Christmas cards with the help of a computer, making one's own home pages, including a section for advertising second-hand items and making access easy to recipes (which includes Internet searching and making new titles). The women have also made detailed algorithms (40 steps) for scanning operations, web surfing and label production. Sari has noticed that the computer support worker, who tries hard to make himself understood, speaks differently on different kinds of topics and uses different terms when speaking to her and to her husband.

Global technology is a foreign language to all but a small group of white middle-class men in western societies. Similarly, a particularly serious divide in citizenship in the information society takes place along gender lines. Boys seem to acquire information technology through their fingertips and learn the ability to shape it accordingly. Girls seem to learn it as a foreign language, although maybe as a well spoken foreign language (Kristeva 1992; Nurmela 1997). In a women's group in a neighbourhood centre information technology can be defined from one's own position: from the point of view of both the local culture and one's bodily situation. The NiceNet group tries to make an alternative information technology to that of the 'general' men's group. At the same time, the NiceNet group is taking part in the process of identity formation. The group produces a new kind of communal life. It is a group of 'our own' where the women do not need to feel themselves as strangers or 'others' as they do in the men's information technology group. The NiceNet women challenge the masculine culture of information technology by creating new kinds of information technology practices for themselves.

The gender difference in the information technology groups relates to concrete life situations. Women choose topics that arise from their particular lives. While doing this they create, at least to some extent, an alternative way of learning and using information technology. They bring gender difference into the otherwise singular (male) gender dominated world of information technology and networks. However, they themselves never questioned their reliance on the ultimate expertise of the 'nice men of the neighbourhood'.

Home pages – the domain of publicly defined agency

Home pages are texts which give information about their authors ('self portraits') and how citizenship is represented. The main page of

NiceNet (1998) shows a group of smiling women in a photograph and lists what is available on this site: shopping, banks, work, the Marjala neighbourhood, the Internet chat channels, a regional information society development project, a non-governmental service system and 'goodies'. Furthermore, the page includes links to local, national and European Community decision-makers, especially to women's organizations and equal opportunity officers, and also to leisure and pleasure: to arts, travelling, delicacies, the library and to the home pages of *The bold and the beautiful* soap opera.

On the second page the group presents its agenda (see 'Introduction' at the beginning of the chapter) and the names of the group members. The page is the home for the group advertisement board and for selling second-hand items. The individual home pages present the women's hobbies (crafts, outdoor activities, sports, baking, films and music), competencies ('I am familiar with the beauty business and have worked in the field for five years, if you need guidance or care for your skin . . .'), family (if they have one), pets and their relationship to information technology ('At the moment I am interested in these gifts and possibilities provided by the ICT field, because these skills are currently needed in almost every professional field. I have been a user for almost ten years but it was a quite narrow activity.'). The pages also lead to various services that can be transmitted in the networks, especially to sharing recipes.

The NiceNet women introduced themselves by locating themselves in their concrete surroundings. They wrote about their situations, family members, friends, their favourite hobbies and the competencies they have for local activities, work and leisure. They gave a special emphasis to baking and cooking which represents a very concrete and bodily expression of care of their families, friends and themselves. They entered the networks as concrete, living humans who strongly acknowledged their local positions.

The NiceNet home pages indicate a subjectivity where the local and situational has a dialogue with global networks along the lines which Haraway (1991) suggests. The group home page illustrates this dialogue most clearly. On the one hand, it gives a rich picture of the locality: the neighbourhood, work places, shopping and banking. On the other hand, it can be used as an opening to regional, national and international decision-makers, including members of the European Parliament and it allows one to reserve tickets for travel to the other parts of the world. In the group page, the global paths originate from the women's concrete lives.

Of the three tiers of Nira Yuval-Davis' model of citizenship (1997) – familial relations, civil society and the state – the group's home pages can be seen to cover civil society and some aspects of the democratic decision-making of the state and to connect to leisure and family as well. In individual home pages it is especially the individual's and the family's activity in civil society that tend to be described. Finnish women participate in working life, education and other civil society activities similarly to Finnish men and all these activities are visible in the NiceNet home pages. The group is therefore significant for women citizens making and defining their connection to the state. The group acts as a link between private and public space. It makes possible a simultaneous view of familial communities as well as those of civil society and the state. It enables the broadening of activity and one's subjectivity to include, for example, the political.

A room of NiceNet's own – supportive practices

A woman cannot write unless she has a room and money of her own, as Virginia Woolf pointed out, and the same is true of a women's group. The women's information technology group is based on various textual and social practices. An important condition for the women's information technology group has been the availability of the neighbourhood centre, primarily meant for the use of residents. During the day, the doors are open and during the evenings the key can be obtained freely from a small corner shop. The centre has cosy furniture and computers with access to the Internet available for residents. However, the availability of computers and the use of the centre were far from enough.

The activities became possible only when the city of Joensuu started to provide social work services in the centre. While the social worker struggled with the problems of her often unemployed customers and considered their individual rights to social benefits she, at the same time, was able to observe the whole variety of life situations of the residents, even of those in the most disadvantaged situations: 'We made coffee and talked; I heard what was needed.' She encouraged residents to start activities independently and invited people to join the already established activities. She says that, in practice, she 'co-ordinated so that the inhabitants became actors'. In an area where people move often (38 per cent had moved within a few years) 'there is a need for information for new people'. Soon there were activities in the neighbourhood centre every evening: for example information technology groups for men (the 'general' ones, open for all), women, the young and children.

The social worker was supported by a network that took care of the running of Marjala suburb. The network was partly funded through a European Commission development project, 'Socio-technology in North Karelia 1995–1999', and partly through the city's welfare funds. The network included various professionals (for example, youth work, health care, land use planning, day care, church social work and city social work) and residents: 'in the group we practised doing things together with the residents . . . using the system side by side with the residents: not as authorities as before' (interview of a group member). The special goals of the town planning in the area have been 'a city for all' and 'a barrier free environment' in terms of physical movement, services and social interaction, including electronic networks (Savela 1998).

The network was able to arrange for a computer support worker to be hired in the neighbourhood centre to support both individual people and group activities in the evenings. He found himself among the unemployed residents in the area. The network was able to get machines and electronic networks as well as programs and computer-based services installed for the free use of the inhabitants: 'The information networks may open Marjala to the world and this may prevent it from becoming a slum' (interview with a network member).

The North Karelian Council's information strategy puts emphasis on the activity of citizens. The executive director of the provincial council, Tarja Cronberg, a former researcher of technology in daily life, supports the principles of the social shaping of technology: information technology is made by people in the interaction between people and technology and most importantly it should not be discussed only in technical terms. The NiceNet group has become visible in local and national newspapers, magazines and radio. Although there may be other opinions and people who resist or ignore these ideas, there certainly is also a discursive space for various experiments and the space is close enough to the economic decision-makers in order to guarantee at least some funding.

The formation of the group did not happen by chance. Instead, it is rooted on welfare networks, an information strategy that puts emphasis on the activity of citizens as well as on the facilities of the neighbour-hood centre – place, machines and personal guidance. The neighbourhood centre seems to be a place for a new kind of a space in between, a new kind of activity and perhaps a new kind of citizenship (Karjalainen and Virtanen 1997). In information technology groups residents get to know each other and they can develop aspects of their local communities. Women in the NiceNet group exchanged news and discussed the coping strategies needed for their everyday problems.

The Nordic Welfare State exists as a provider of resources and as a guarantor of the basic necessities and in some measure it also channels (preprogrammed) EU funding which represents another major resource. Furthermore, it has an important role in starting and supporting the residents in their initiatives and activities. The women's group was born through an initiative of an active resident but the group would only have been able to form in the context of the neighbourhood centre. The neighbourhood centre and the welfare networks, the initiative of local social workers, are creating a space for the projects of defining one's self and citizenship based on local culture.

Home in the nets – towards located and communal citizenship

Susan Leigh Star (1996: 31) argues that thinking about Greek and Roman domestic goddesses and gods

suggest(s) three modes of approaching the idea of home:

1. That which is omnipresent, taken-for-granted and which enlivens the rest of life in a background fashion.
2. That which rests comfortably in particular locales (such as jars and cupboards), embodying a place to be secure and fed.
3. That which must be defended and tended, often in a very public fashion, under the rule of the state and church.

Home is a location that includes all the rights and activities of citizenship.

What is women's (for example in the eastern province of Finland, North Karelia) home in the information society? Networks and information technologies intertwine with women's citizenship in both their being and their active participation in society (Lister 1997: 41). Networks and information technologies as an equal right can enable women as agents if (and only if) women can inhabit them as they do their own homes. Do NiceNet or other local women's information technology groups provide a space for women to meet electronic networks as in the 'jars and cupboards' of security and nourishment in a taken-for-granted but supportive manner?

When the world of information technology is structurally dominated by men any women's agency in information technology necessarily requires resistance: women need to build rooms of their own within the networks. Ruth Lister (1997) writes about creative acts of resistance and the self-esteem that is needed in this endeavour. Manuel Castells' argument (1997: 8) points to the resistance 'generated by those actors that are in positions/conditions devalued and/or stigmatized by the logic of domination, thus building trenches of resistance and survival on the basis of principles different from, or opposed to, those permeating the institutions of society'. By resisting projects, Castells argues that women are building 'a new identity that redefines their position in society and, by so doing, seek the transformation of overall social structure' (Castells 1997: 8). The secure agency in electronic networks is related to the practices of groups and communities as well as to the deep processes of subjectivity and identity.

In NiceNet women acted differently from the 'general' men's group and simultaneously they built definitions of themselves in their home pages and in shared talks. There was a new kind of communal setting and new information technology practised which challenged the masculine culture of information technology. The projects of resistance, transformation and identity met in the very same practices.

In NiceNet, women's identities also become intertwined with technology built from men's outlooks based on men's lives and on men's terms. This cannot entirely happen in a taken-for-granted, background manner which showed up as an ambivalence in the NiceNet group. For serious technical problems, the women readily came to rely on the neighbourhood centre men – like strangers far away from home.

Agency means involvement in local citizenship. This citizenship is based on identity processes rather than on the interests of individuals. The identity processes may organize themselves through the welfare state but primarily, in people's subjective experience, they are organized through the communities and networks of people who live in particular times and places (Ferguson 1993; Lister 1997). Women's citizenship in the information society is created in neighbourhoods, women's projects and rural women's organizations. Citizenship originates out of everyday practices (Turner 1993; Gherardi 1995).

The neighbourhood centre is an extension of the home for many residents, a space in which one can build a home between one's own familiar one and the strangeness of electronic networks. In NiceNet women have started from their daily practices and made the first steps in order to move safely in the home of networks with the support of their local community. They have found words to define home in relation to machines and they have concretely made it a place of nourishment with their recipes. Yet, in the public defence of their homes the support of the welfare network has been important. There may not have been such good facilities and certainly no computer support person would have been hired without the welfare network. The articulation and practices of locality have much to gain from supporting processes. In the Finnish society the support processes seem to be connected to state and government but in other societies they relate to other institutional practices such as non-governmental groups, for example.

The new citizenship is related to the 'spaces-in-between' as well as to various communities: local sisterly groups as well as broad networking (Escobar 1999). These also make the public defence of the home possible. NiceNet as a group had more connections to the state and the various public bodies than the individual members. Without the spaces-in-between and the communities embedded in them most women in the NiceNet group would have been excluded from information technology groups within a male-dominated culture of information technology which defines women as 'others'. Having a right to equal access to computers would not have been enough to start the group and Turkle's charming vision of the step behind the looking glass would have remained totally beyond the women's reach.

The local and situational NiceNet meetings and home pages are a part of building an alternative information technology culture. Technology includes social practices, and the entering and writing positions of network users are of crucial importance. Women's and women's groups' home pages, with their practices of location, challenge the dominant approach to technology (technology beyond social: objective and deterministic) and participate in a culture which recognizes the social formation of technology. They make room for various differences and local knowledge, different homes in the networks and active citizenship.

Conclusion

In the chapter, I have followed the women's information technology group, NiceNet, which meets together in a neighbourhood centre in North Karelia on the eastern border of Finland. The group provides the women participants with a place for active citizenship, a place in which they can define the practices of their own and create a home of their own, related to their local existence and knowledge, within the world of information and communication technologies. It is difficult to acknowledge the local community when one faces the network world as an individual, separated from the others sharing the same locality and it is especially difficult to articulate the relationship between the local and the global. The group served as a link between the public and private necessary for the practices of local agency and resistance, and of the situated, local and communal citizenship, distinct from the individual 'equal access' citizenship present in most governmental policies of information society. The group practices, however, required particular institutional support to develop. In the Finnish context, this support was organized through the welfare state but in other societies the non-governmental groups may provide the support needed in local communities.

The NiceNet group is an example of rooted and place-based women's politics and of a women's local agency which Arturo Escobar (1999) has also advocated. In addition Escobar points out that women could use the cyberworld to transform local places away from patriarchal practices. To do this even more thoroughly, the NiceNet women could have tried to develop technical expertise for themselves, instead of requesting help from the neighbourhood centre men which left the nexus between men and technical expertise (Wajcman 1991) partially untouched. This may have required help from an outside facilitator who would have helped women to build critical development and evaluation (instead of only user) skills of information technology. In the NiceNet neighbourhood context such a facilitator was not available. Furthermore, Escobar suggests that networks could be used to build alliances between local struggles. In NiceNet the Finnish language limited the number of alliances that could be made but the group home page linked NiceNet to women's activities both nationally and internationally. Critical citizenship means both making the 'otherness' related to information technology more visible and also means struggling to deconstruct it simultaneously through local agency and global connections via information technology and networks.

Acknowledgements

I would like to thank Laura Tohka and Alison Adam who have made my English more readable.

References

Bono, P. and Kemp, S. (eds) (1991) *Italian Feminist Thought*, Oxford: Basil Blackwell.

Castells, M. (1997) *The Power of Identity*, Oxford: Blackwell.

Escobar, A. (1999) 'Gender, place and networks: a political ecology of cyberculture' in W. Harcourt (ed.) *Women @ Internet: Creating New Cultures in Cyberspace*, London: Zed Books.

Ferguson, K. E. (1993) *The Man Question: Visions of Subjectivity in Feminist Theory*, Berkeley and Los Angeles: University of California Press.

Gherardi, S. (1995) *Gender, Symbolism and Organizational Cultures*, London: Sage.

Griffiths, M. (1995) *Feminism and the Self: The Web of Identity*, London: Routledge.

Haraway, D. (1991) *Simians, Cyborgs, and Women: The Reinvention of Nature*, London: Free Association Books.

Herring, S. (1996) 'Gender and democracy in computer-mediated communication' in R. Kling (ed.) *Computerization and Controversy: Value Conflicts and Social Choices*, second edition, London: Academic Press.

Holderness, M. (1998) 'Who are the world's information poor?' in B. D. Loader (ed.) *Cyberspace Divide: Equality, Agency and Policy in the Information Society*, London: Routledge.

Karjalainen, P. and Virtanen, P. (1997) 'Työttömyys ja urbaani toiseus: pohjoiskarjalainen näkökulma' ('Unemployment and urban otherness: a North Karelian view' in Finnish), *Sosiologia* 4/1997: 281–94.

Kristeva, J. (1992) *Muukalaisia Itsellemme* (*Strangers to Ourselves*), a Finnish translation, Helsinki: Gaudeamus.

Lehto, A.-M. and Sutela, H. (1999) *Gender Equality in Working Life, Labour Market*, 1999: 22, Statistics Finland, Helsinki: Hakapaino.

Lister, R. (1997) *Citizenship: Feminist Perspectives*, London: Macmillan.

NiceNet (1998) Available online: http://www.jns.fi/palvelut/marjala/nicenet (September 1998).

Nurmela, J. (1997) *Suomalaiset ja Uusi Tietotekniikka* (*Finns and the New Information Technology*) Katsauksia 1997, Helsinki: Tilastokeskus.

Savela, A. (1998) 'Barrier free city and technology applications, Marjala, Joensuu, Finland', a paper given at United Nations Headquarters, New York City, 29–30 April 1998.

Smith, D. E. (1990) *The Conceptual Practices of Power: A Feminist Sociology of Knowledge*, Toronto: University of Toronto Press.

Spender, D. (1995) *Nattering on the Net: Women, Power and Cyberspace*, North Melbourne: Spinifex.

Star, S. L. (1996) 'From Hestia to home page: feminism and the concept of home in cyberspace' in N. Lykke and R. Braidotti (eds) *Between Monsters, Goddesses and Cyborgs*, London: Zed Books.

Turkle, S. (1995) *Life on the Screen: Identity in the Age of the Internet*, New York: Simon and Schuster.

Turner, B. S. (1993) 'Contemporary problems in the theory of citizenship' in B. S. Turner (ed.) *Citizenship and Social Theory*, London: Sage.

Wajcman, J. (1991) *Feminism Confronts Technology*, Cambridge: Polity Press.

Wakeford, N. (2000) 'Gender and the landscapes of computing in an Internet café' in G. Kirkup, L. Janes, K. Woodward, F. Hovenden (eds) *The Gendered Cyborg: A Reader*, London: Routledge.

Wise, J. M. (1997) *Exploring Technology and Social Space*, London: Sage.

Yuval-Davis, N. (1997) *Gender and Nation*, London: Sage.

Chapter 13

Gender in the design of the digital city of Amsterdam

Els Rommes, Ellen van Oost and Nelly Oudshoorn

Abstract

This chapter analyses the social shaping of the Digital City of Amsterdam – 'De Digitale Stad' (DDS) – from a gender perspective. It aims to contribute to an understanding of the overwhelming dominance (more than 90 per cent) of male DDS users, a fact which is more than surprising given that the designers had high ideals about making the Internet accessible to a wider public. The analysis is rooted in the social constructivist tradition in technology studies. As such, it analyses technology as a product of social, political and cultural negotiations among designers, policy-makers and other social groups. The concept of 'genderscript' is used to examine the gender relations embedded in the design of DDS. In our analysis we show that the design process was gendered at three levels: the structural, the symbolical and the identity level. As the design-process was highly informal and no conscious attempt was made to focus on specific user-groups, the designers unconsciously projected their own masculine-biased interests on the future user. Thus they affected the choices concerning the goals, content and interface of DDS, providing it with a masculine genderscript.

Introduction

On 15 January 1994, Amsterdam's alderman De Grave officially opened the virtual city gates of DDS by sending an email to Al Gore, who was Vice President of the USA at the time. Although DDS was to be an experiment of ten weeks, the publicity it generated and the interest it aroused was overwhelming. Within one week this new city comprised more than 3,500 residents and drew more than 2,000 visitors a day (NN 1994). In Amsterdam, modems were sold out within a few days, and the initial 20 modem lines providing access to DDS had to be doubled in order to cope with the queue outside the virtual city gates.

DDS was built in order to stimulate political discussion in Amsterdam and to make the relatively new Internet technology available to a wider public. To make DDS easier to use, it was built as a virtual analogue to an actual city. Thus, for example, after passing the city gates, you had to go to the post office to send or receive electronic mail, in a kiosk you could read electronic newspapers, from the central station you could start your worldwide Internet trip and the town hall provided citizens with information on local politics. Beyond making information available, DDS provided discussion platforms on various political issues. To improve the accessibility of DDS, free email accounts and Internet access were offered. Moreover, several public terminals were installed in publically accessible locations in Amsterdam. One was even located in an old people's home, thus emphasizing the initiators' ideal of 'access for all'.

Despite the policy of accessibility, the residents of DDS were by no means representative of the population of Amsterdam. A survey of DDS users carried out in April 1994 (Schalken and Tops 1994) revealed that the city was primarily 'inhabited' by young, highly educated people of whom only 9 per cent were female.[1] Thus, although DDS was successful in attracting participants with no prior experience of using computer networks (33 per cent had little or no experience), it failed to attract a population which is more diverse than the traditional group of Internet users. This phenomenon of the lopsided resident group was known to the organizers of DDS. It was, however – especially with regard to gender – not defined as an urgent problem.

DDS was the first community network in The Netherlands and one of the first in Europe (Bastelaer 1998). It set an example for many other digital cities and organizations of which there are now hundreds in The Netherlands.

A gender analysis of this pioneering project may reveal some of the roots of the gendered character that is still reflected in many of these kinds of Internet applications. Moreover, many (Rheingold 1993; Castells 1996) expect the Internet, or its successor, to become one of the most – if not the most – important technologies for future communication and information retrieval. Given this, means of avoiding the exclusion of specific social groups becomes a crucial social issue. In discussing these inequalities, the gender dimension is often considered to be less important than factors such as age, ethnicity or social status (Brouns 1998). In this chapter gender is placed in the limelight again.

Research and policy concerning the under-representation of women as designers and users of new information technologies often focus particularly on the so-called deficiencies of women (Henwood 1993). Policies for change are thus restricted to educating women to fit the requirements of the technology, rather than designing the technology in such a way as to encourage a diversity of users. We want to reformulate the problem by exploring the extent to which the under-representation of women users can be understood in terms of technological choices made in the design of this technology. We aim to deconstruct the 'black box'[2] of DDS and analyse how gender has influenced both the design process as well as the actual design that emerged. To do this we draw on studies of technological development introduced by scholars in social and feminist studies of science and technology.

In the theoretical section, Akrich's concept of a script and the multi-level theory of gender is conceptualized and explained. These form the theoretical basis of this chapter. Following the multi-level theory, the empirical section starts by describing gender at the structural level of the organization of DDS and in terms of the identity of its founders and developers. In the next part of the empirical section, gender is examined at a symbolic level within a context of the goals and content of DDS. Following on from this, we focus on the interface of DDS. Although the designers tried to develop a system for everybody, many of their design choices were gender biased because they used themselves as exemplary of the users. We finish the chapter with some concluding remarks.

Theoretical perspectives on gender and technology

The British sociologist Flis Henwood distinguishes between two ways of looking at the problem of gender and information technology (Henwood 1993). First, there is a liberal perspective that focuses on women's exclusion from technology and seeks solutions in equal opportunity policies. Second, Henwood analyses the gendered constructions of skills and power in relation to technology, here the nature of technological work is analysed. A third position is then distinguished, one involving the social construction of the technology itself.

Social constructivist theories of technology reject the positivistic notion that technological objects have intrinsic properties. In this view, technology is seen not as autonomous from society but as the product of social, political and cultural negotiations among innovators, policy-makers, and social groups (Pinch and Bijker 1987; Bijker 1995). Although most attention has been focused on the role of innovators in the construction of technological objects, recent social studies of technology also include analyses of the role of users in technological development (Green et al. 1993).

Traditionally, users have been regarded as important actors in the diffusion and acceptance of new technologies (Von Hippel 1976, 1988). More recently within the sociology of science and technology, attention has shifted away from the analysis of users in the sociological sense (i.e., as identifiable individuals involved in the diffusion of technologies) towards users in the semiotic sense (as imagined by the designers of a technology). As Madeleine Akrich has suggested, 'innovators are from the very start constantly interested in their future users. They construct many different representations of these users, and objectify these representations in technological choices' (Akrich 1995: 168). As a result, technologies contain scripts: they attribute and delegate specific competences, actions and responsibilities to their envisioned users. When these scripts reveal a gendered pattern, we can call them gender scripts (Oost 1995; Oudshoorn 1996).

The concept of 'script' is an important tool in analysing the politics of technological objects. A script analysis enables us to understand how technologies play a role either in normalizing behaviour or in (re)allocating responsibilities and dependencies among people and between people and things. Scripts may also contribute to the exclusion of specific users if, for example, the designers' image of users represents only a selective set of competences, interests, attitudes and values. Given the heterogeneity of users, designers will, consciously or unconsciously, favour certain representations of users and use over others. Studies of the development of information technologies, for example, indicate that design practices are dominated by the so-called 'I-methodology' in which innovators consider their own preferences and skills to be representative of those of the future user (Akrich 1995; Oudshoorn 1996). Technological objects become attuned to the interests and skills of young middle-class men rather than women or other groups under-represented in the world of technology. The concepts of 'user representation' and 'gender script' thus appear to be useful tools for analysing the extent to which the problem of under-representation of women as Internet users can be understood as a mismatch between the designers' image of users and the actual users.

Gender analysis

To understand whether and how technologies embody gender scripts, a gender analysis of the design process of DDS will be undertaken. Adopting Sandra Harding's multi-level theory of gender, we will take into account gender processes at the structural, the symbolic and the identity level (Harding 1986). The gender structure of DDS will be analysed by mapping the gendered division of tasks and the delegation of responsibilities among designers and policy-makers. Unlike many other design communities in the world of the Internet, DDS involved designers of both sexes. This enables us to explore the extent to which women designers are committed to a different design style than their male colleagues and particularly whether they are more likely to acknowledge the diversity in the interests and needs of female and male users.

Feminist studies of technology have emphasized that, in addition to gender structures, gender symbolism is important in making technologies a male domain. Technologies have a masculine image, not only because they are dominated by men, but also because they incorporate symbols, metaphors and values which have masculine connotations (Wajcman 1991). As Pacey suggests, technologies often represent a specific set of values. Thus some may prioritize the values of virtuosity and others may emphasize user or need values. Whereas the latter are linked to hegemonic feminine values, the former express hegemonic masculine values (Pacey 1983). High-tech areas such as space technologies emphasize the power of mankind to control the universe, thus creating and reinforcing the image of technology as a world of virtuosity. In contrast, technologies that are developed to improve the living conditions of the elderly may stress care and user-friendliness as their main values. Adopting Pacey's framework of gender symbolism will help us to determine which values are dominant in both the designers' documents as well as in some media reports about DDS.

Finally, we try to map the gender dimensions of the technology's design by analysing the gender identities of the designers and users of DDS. We examine the designers' attitudes, interests and learning styles regarding technology. Using Cockburn and Ormrod's distinction between projected identities ('potential, actual, or desired gender identities as others perceive or portray them') and subjective identities ('the gendered sense of self, the identity, created and experienced by the individual'), we also focus on the projected identities of users by analysing the designers' representations of them (Cockburn and Ormrod 1993).

The social shaping of DDS

> It is not a linear process – like there is money, there is a plan, consequently there is a project plan, a project manager, and that person decides how it should work functionally and goes to another person and that person builds it. It was not like that. We got drunk every night in the Winston, so to speak, and then the plan got adjusted.
>
> (Interview, Flint 1998b: 1)

This quotation by one of the founders of DDS is characteristic of the way in which the project got started. The organization of DDS was very informal and the enthusiasm, idealism and personal initiative of the contributors were indispensable for its survival. The organizational structure can be characterized as a network organization (Krogt and van der Vroom 1989: 122, 123). Diverse organizations and private individuals connect with parts of the project on the basis of their own private goals, knowledge and interests, thus helping to shape the project. However, the 'ordinary citizens' for whom DDS was designed were not a part of the network.

In the following paragraphs we describe in greater detail the mutual development of the organization and the design of DDS. We analyse how the interests and goals of the participating social groups were reflected both in the design process and in the actual design of DDS. This process resulted in a script that implicitly attracted users whose socio-cultural attitudes were similar to those of the initiators. DDS is a project reflecting very high ideals, such as the realization of a 'non-hierarchical space for everybody' (van Meerten 1993: 2). Nevertheless, we are left with an image of an organization in which personal goals and style unconsciously result in design choices that run counter to these idealistic goals.

The birth of the concept of DDS

In the spring of 1993, Marleen Stikker helped to organize a series of debates about the cultural boycott of Yugoslavia in 'De Balie', an important political and cultural centre in Amsterdam.[3] During this project Stikker, who has vast experience in the field of new media, art and politics, became aware of the importance of email as a means of communication for people in war-zones.[4] As a consequence she became involved in the Internet and especially in Free Nets where she did not, however, feel at home, meeting 'boys, mostly science students': 'They were not my kind of people, so to speak, and they weren't discussing my issues' (interview, Stikker 1998a: 4). Stikker became convinced that the Internet could be made more attractive to 'her kind of people' and that the arts and politics could play a bigger role so, in April 1993, she started a new De Balie project.

Inspired by the metaphor of the 'digital town hall' that was being promoted at that time by the American presidential candidate Ross Perot, Stikker started formulating a plan. The metaphor was appealing because it combined computer networks with politics. This perspective was not only of interest to De Balie but also to the city council of Amsterdam which she had approached with her ideas. Local elections had been scheduled to take place in March 1994 and the city council was extremely interested in new ideas to stimulate the involvement of citizens in local politics as the number of voters had reached rock bottom during the previous elections. The city council thus subsidized De Balie for the DDS project which was then defined as a ten-week project organized around the elections of 2 March 1994 (van Meerten 1993: 1).

As a 'political tool' aimed at stimulating democracy, DDS had to be for everybody. In the project proposal the initiators promised that 'access will be extremely public-friendly, so that computer illiterates can participate too' (van Meerten 1993: 2). Indeed, as we shall see, the initiators put a great deal of effort into achieving this goal. They had, however, underestimated the fact that the computer was already a strongly gender-biased machine in our society (van Oost 1994; Brosnan 1998). Moreover, in the process of developing DDS, choices were made that resulted in a masculine-oriented gender script.

Organizing DDS: who did it?

Stikker gathered a group of about 30 volunteers to help shape her ideas. She used her own network consisting of artists, graphic designers and people working on media projects of whom very few had experience with the Internet. Some were asked to moderate discussion groups or to provide information or art for the content of DDS. Most of them were involved in the so-called 'city-plan group' comprising four women and about 15 men. In brainstorming sessions, this group helped to develop metaphors and a new language to replace traditional technical computer terms. By providing them with a space for their ideas, initiatives and ideals, their enthusiastic contribution was ensured.

As such, the individual backgrounds, personal goals and motivations of the workers were important factors in shaping the project.

This was particularly true for the core-group of three people who decided whether the ideas of the city plan group could be programmed. This group included Stikker, who remained the project leader, Joost Flint, who wrote most of the policy documents and a user's manual, and Félipe Rodriguez, who together with Stikker did most of the programming work. Although Stikker herself was fascinated by the potential of the new technology, she lacked the skills to implement the technological part of the project on her own. This core-group spent days and nights discussing and creating DDS.

Rodriguez was a member of a group of four male hackers who worked together under the name of HackTic-Network. Based on their ideal of free access to information for everyone, the hackers were the first group in The Netherlands to create an Internet connection for private individuals, naming their computer 'XS4ALL' (pronounced 'access for all'). As passionate idealists, the founders of the HackTic-Network were easily convinced to take part in DDS. They were responsible for the hardware and for system management. Their contribution to the project was so vital that DDS was called a joint project of De Balie and Hack.

HackTic-Network

Rodriguez, who was the main participating hacker, described his motives for joining DDS as follows:

> DDS was a way to prove what is possible with the Internet, with that technology. And also an attempt to make it accessible . . . XS4ALL was terribly complicated. A prompt was given, and from then on, the users had to do it themselves . . . I was at that time striving to introduce the Internet, to make it bigger, to show all those people who did not understand me what it really was about.
> (Interview, Rodriguez 1998: 6)

Thus Rodriguez's personal goals in joining DDS were twofold: a fascination with what is technologically possible and a desire to make the Internet more accessible. In addition he was interested in the political potential of the Internet.[5]

Joost Flint was the third person to join the core-group. Flint, who at the time of writing is the present director of DDS, had been a volunteer with HackTic for a few weeks when he heard about the project.

He had been active as a journalist and writer so he joined in order to write the user's manual.

An informal organization

Strikingly, none of the core-group's members had any form of computer-related education. Stikker studied philosophy, Flint had taken courses in political science, and Rodriguez, DDS's main programmer, had managed a restaurant. Although he calls himself a computer-nerd who has played with computers since childhood, he explicitly stated: 'I am not a programmer, just someone who understands computers.' This lack of a computer-related education may have contributed to the informal way in which the interface was built, as well as to the lack of a systematic user's profile. However, the informal style also facilitated the inspired, enthusiastic, creative and often chaotic process which was characteristic of this phase of the project. Time pressures intensified this specific character:

> It was such a huge chaos ... The week before DDS was opened, we moved to a new office ... there was no light, no doors, the ceiling was just installed, no heating. We had to sleep alongside the computers, with a gas-heater, and we had to borrow power from the neighbours.
>
> (Interview, Rodriguez 1998: 15)

The recruitment of journalists, graphic designers and people from non-profit organizations by Stikker seems to have been one of the more successful ways of gathering together a diverse group of designers. This personal networking did attract women to the project, most of whom are very active in computer networks. Nevertheless, looking at the gendered division of labour within DDS, women were mostly found in creative, assisting and policy-making positions, whereas male hackers dominated the programming tasks. Moreover, Stikker's network was biased towards people who were already interested in computers and their new possibilities – these were mostly men – and because she was not personally interested in women's issues, she did not specifically recruit women to correct this imbalance. In this respect, DDS became gendered at the structural level.

As an informal network organization, DDS had many faces. As various groups – including the city of Amsterdam, the HackTic-Network and individuals with diverse backgrounds – were drawn into the project, the identity and goals of DDS came to reflect this diversity. Organizations and private individuals could find their own points of interest in the project, thus making it worthwhile for them to help build or subsidize it. In this way the project remained viable. Notwithstanding this diversity, all the people involved in the design process shared a fascination with new information technology. This fascination was reflected in the design of DDS because of the informal and chaotic character of the organization (Francissen and Brants 1998: 35).

Goals and content of DDS

It is commonly believed that for women to adopt a new technology, its usefulness must be of particular relevance to them (for example, van den Boomen 1996: 10). Despite this, the founders did not give much thought to the question of why users would want to use DDS. Owing to the network and voluntary character of the organization, they designed DDS mainly according to their own preferred goals. As described in the previous sections, the designers shared a fascination with new technologies and an interest in politics. These interests were reflected in the two main goals of DDS presented to the public in policy documents, the user's manual and the press.[6] They can be labelled as technological goals, reflecting virtuosity values and political ideals. We will argue that neither the goals nor the content reflecting them are gender-neutral.

With regard to the first goal, DDS was seen as a way of introducing people to the Internet with all its potential for communication and information. The designers of DDS wanted to introduce the possibilities of data communication to users; they wanted them to use the technology for the sake of technology itself. What the users themselves would want was not a consideration:

> What users themselves want? [Laughing] Well . . . the system of course was not built because people wanted it so badly; the system is built because we thought that a social function was connected with it, because we thought the Internet was important, that it needed to be introduced, and to show all that is possible with technology . . . These people had to get free e-mail to discover the rest [of the Internet].
>
> (Interview, Rodriguez 1998: 30)

In the user's manual and newspaper articles, this technological goal was linked to travelling around the world, to excitement and adventure. With regard to technology, these kinds of values have been described as 'virtuosity' values. Like designing technology for its own sake, virtuosity values are connected with hegemonic masculinity in our society (Pacey 1983; Connell 1987; Wajczman 1991).

The second dominant goal of DDS was to stimulate political involvement among the citizens of Amsterdam. Given that politics in The Netherlands is more often practised by men than by women,[7] this probably served to attract more men than women to DDS. The political issues discussed in DDS included urban city planning, the expansion of Schiphol Airport, ICT in society and racial discrimination. Given that these topics have either a gender-neutral or a masculine connotation in our society, they strengthened the gendered nature of DDS.[8] The latter was further strengthened by the format of political discussions. Shade (1993) and Herring (1993, 1994) argue that the discussion style on mailing lists, which are comparable with the discussion platforms in DDS, is generally more attractive to masculine users than to feminine users.[9] The presence of female moderators in DDS did not change this bias.[10] As one of the female moderators explained, 'she changed her moderating style quickly to adopt existing Internet conventions' (interview, van den Boomen 1998: 10).

In light of the main reasons presented to potential users for using DDS, it was overall more attractive to male users. Nevertheless, for both goals – introducing the Internet and creating a political platform – the accessibility of DDS 'to everyone' was of vital importance. Thus the accessibility and user-friendliness of the interface is discussed from a gender-perspective.

Designing the accessibility of the hardware

The designers of DDS paid close attention to the accessibility of the hardware and the usability of the DDS software. First, the way in which the designers tried to overcome the societal bias determining who has access to computers is discussed. Second, the design of the interface itself is considered: what kind of choices were made and in what way was the interface gendered?

One of the most important ways in which access to DDS could be obtained was by using a PC and a modem with a phone line to DDS. The instalment of a modem was described as a difficult job, even by the designers. As the founders of DDS knew that not everyone had access to a PC and modem or the money to buy one, public terminals were installed. This plan was inspired by the freenets in America, a project that had even succeeded in attracting homeless people to public terminals (Varley 1991; Rogers et al. 1994). There was, and still is, a gender-bias in the distribution of computers, in who possesses computers: the majority of computer owners are men, making it easier for them to obtain access to DDS. Thus, it seems reasonable to assume that public terminals help to compensate for this inequality. Figures in Santa Monica do not, however, support this thesis (Rogers et al. 1994: 407; Collins-Jarvis 1993: 61). No research has been done on the usage of DDS terminals by men and women.[11] Designers, however, stated that the typical public terminal user was a 20-year-old male (Diemen 1998: 6).

Designing the interface

The DDS designers tried to build an interface that would be easy to use. To do this, several decisions were made. First, they chose to use FreePort software, which was developed for Free Nets in the US. It is a user-friendly menu-based program that allows users to navigate by selecting options from a menu (see Table 13.1). By choosing options, the user finally ends up with the required information or software, for example, the email program. To enhance easy usage of DDS further, the city metaphor, which can also be found in the original FreePort software (Stallings 1996), consequently was used far more. In this way, much technical language was avoided. Moreover, the decision was taken to translate most of the software into Dutch. However, owing to a shortage of time, the command keys were not changed. As can be seen in Table 13.1, which shows a later version of the interface, the following options were offered at the bottom of the screen: 'x = Exit; h = Main menu; v = Previous Menu, Choice?' In DDS's original interface, which is no longer available online, the main menu contained the following (Flint 1994: iii–2): '1 Help; 2 The Post Office; 3 Public Forum; 4 The Library; 5 Building for Art and Culture; 6 Town Hall; 7 Office District; 8 Plaza; 9 Central Station; 10 Configuration Centre'.

Apart from user-friendliness, there were other reasons for choosing the FreePort software. The sourcecode[12] of this software was available which made it easier for the designers to make changes to the original program. This was exactly what the founders wanted to do: partly because of what they themselves called the 'not invented here syndrome', they

Table 13.1 De Digitale Stad

1	Belangrijk: De Digitale Stad 2.0
2	Helpdesk
3	Het Postkantoor
4	Openbaar Forum
5	De Bibliotheek
6	Gebouw voor Kunst en Cultuur
7	Het Stadhuis
8	Kantoorwijk
9	Verkiezingscentrum
10	De Kiosk
11	Een Plein
12	Universiteit van Amsterdam
13	Centraal Station
14	Configuratie-centrum

Note
x = Exit, h = Hoofdmenu, v = Vorig Menu, w = wie zijn er? Keuze?

wanted to leave their own mark on the program. They also wanted to offer users more functionalities than the original FreePort software allowed for. There was almost no discussion of this decision. The founders of DDS wanted to offer users all the functionalities of the Internet, not just an 'amputated' version (interview, Stikker 1998b: 7). This meant that Rodriguez integrated about six different software packages into the FreePort software. This made the interface far more complicated to use since the functions of the keys varied as the user shifted between programs.

At the same time, the program did not start with the possibility of consulting a help menu, so users were expected to know how menus and tree structures work. This indicates that DDS was actually meant for more experienced computer users but it also means that one particular learning-style was supported by DDS, one which all the designers of DDS shared:

> You have to keep things exciting; discovering is important. This has to do with the way in which I discovered the Internet and all its possibilities, you discover more and more, and that is fascinating. So you will have to let people discover things; that is fun.
>
> (Interview, Rodriguez 1998: 27, 28)

Thus, users were expected to find their way around DDS by trial and error. For this style of learning, one has to feel at ease with computers and be self-confident enough to try out things. As Turkle has shown, in our society this particular style of learning how to use technology and computers is more often found among boys than girls (Turkle 1991: 48, 49).

Designing for everybody?

To assist with the use of the software, DDS opened a telephone help desk and a user's manual was written (however it was distributed only in Amsterdam). It was an apparent success with its author, Joost Flint, estimating that about 2,000 copies were sold. People came from all over The Netherlands to buy one. Flint wrote it using the I-methodology: 'it is very much written from my own experience. So I learned it myself and then wrote it down' (interview, Flint 1998a: 13).

When reading the manual, one thing stands out. During the design process, the designers must have realized that, in spite of their attempts to make DDS more user-friendly, it was still too complicated for 'computer-illiterates'. In other words, DDS and the manual were made for people 'who have little experience with data communication' but who do have some experience with computers:

> Both XS4ALL as well as DDS are advanced systems. They offer very much and are therefore, at first sight, maybe not so simple as you would want them to be. You will, however, discover that all the basic actions are fairly easy to learn for anyone who has worked with a computer before.
>
> (Flint 1994: 2–3)

Of course there is an important difference between offering DDS to 'everybody' and offering it only to 'everybody who has worked with a computer'. Given that, in Dutch society the percentage of men with computer experience exceeds that of women,[13] the gender consequences of this perception of the intended user has been negative for women.

Somehow, during the design of the interface itself, the diversity of the users and the user-friendliness of the design were no longer the main focuses of attention. Moreover, no conscious choices were made about the user-groups for which DDS was intended. The problem of 'designing for everybody' is that the designers did not consider what kinds of skills, knowledge or cognitive capabilities they expected the user to have (van Lieshout 1998: 35). Again, it is understandable that the designers saw themselves as being typical users and hence that the design practice of DDS was dominated by the I-methodology. The question of the user-friendliness of the system became less relevant as the designers developed a system according to their own preferences, technical capabilities and learning style. Although not all designers were male, they were masculine in their use of, experience with and attitude towards technology, making the design of DDS more suited to masculine users.

Conclusions

In summary, we can conclude that DDS clearly embodies a gender-script. Our analysis shows the gendered nature of this technology at the structural, the symbolic and the identity level. This is all the more remarkable given that the designers of DDS were very idealistic and wanted to design a system that was accessible to everyone.

At a structural level, DDS represents a gendered division of tasks. We have shown how the founders of DDS personally approached non-profit organizations and private individuals to help them design the project. This resulted in a more diverse group of collaborators than is usually seen in this type of organization. At the time of writing, some of the women who were asked to join are still actively working with computers and the Internet. However, the founders of DDS could not totally overcome the already gendered character of society's interest in the new technology and computer networks. Most of the people whom they successfully approached had already got an interest in computers and consequently were mostly male, young and highly educated. Moreover, the design process shows a traditional gendered division of tasks where most of the programming activities were done by male hackers. Although the main founder of DDS is a woman, and the brainstorming group included several women, this mixed membership did not result in extra attention being devoted to the position of female users.

On the whole, the designers had a masculine attitude towards technology. As they did a lot of work voluntarily and were encouraged to bring their own ideals into DDS, the prevalent user-representation technique came to be the 'I-methodology'. Designers made choices on the basis of what they themselves found attractive in the new technology. Thus, at the symbolic level, the design practices of DDS reflect a world in which using technology for excitement and adventure, and designing it for its own sake, emerged as dominant technological choices, reflecting the masculine attitude of the designers towards technology.

At the identity level, the designers were personally interested in politics, fascinated with all the new technical possibilities of computer networks, and were endowed with a masculine learning style. This masculine identity was reflected in their representation of users and thus in the technology they designed. This is remarkable given that, at a conscious level, the designers of DDS were very idealistic and took great pains to make their design user-friendly for everybody. They made the hardware more accessible by choosing user-friendly software which was translated into Dutch, by integrating the metaphor of a city and by installing a help desk and writing a manual to support users. On the other hand, they prioritized a masculine learning style and made the software more complicated by adding other software packages with more functions. As a result, the initial DDS policy of making the digital city maximally accessible to everybody was transformed into one of making a technology for 'everybody who has worked with a computer', a user representation that more readily accommodates male rather than female users. We thus may conclude that the DDS can be portrayed as a technology that incorporates a clear gender-script.

The fact that the DDS embodies a gender-script is not the result of conscious choices. On the contrary, our analysis of the organization of DDS shows that the ideal of making Internet technology accessible to everyone was at the heart of the project. The gender-script of DDS could, however, emerge in a design practice in which the designers took their own skills and interests as guides in making technological choices.

Acknowledgements

We would like to thank Marleen Stikker, Joost Flint, Félipe Rodriguez, Reineke van Meerten, Michaël van Eeden, Marianne van den Boomen, Rob Gonggrijp and Nina Meiloff for their kind help and the opportunity they gave us to interview them. Moreover, we would like to thank the two anonymous referees of this journal for their useful comments on a previous version of this chapter.

Notes

1 North American FreeNet Communities did slightly better with, for example, 18 per cent female users in the Canadian National Capital FreeNet and 17 per cent female users in Cleveland FreeNet, as opposed to the World Wide Web's 10 per cent of female users (Patrick 1997). Santa Monica's Public

Electronic Networking system (PEN) had 30 per cent women registered as users after it was initiated (Collins-Jarvis 1993).

2 The notion of 'opening the black box' of technology is rooted in the field of sociology of technology. During the last two decades a new social constructivist perspective on technology has been developed (Bijker et al. 1987). Scholars in this tradition analyse technology as the result of a social process in which different involved actor groups interact and give meaning to the technology.

3 De Balie is a centre for politics and society, arts and technology. Its 'programme makers', such as Marleen Stikker, are encouraged to develop experiments on the tangent planes between theatre and discussion, technology and art, politics and society.

4 Earlier, Stikker had generally been interested in the potential of new information technology but had no interest in the Internet because – as she put it – there was no one with whom she would want to communicate on the Internet (interview, Stikker 1998a: 3).

5 These two goals are part of the hackers' ideology (Håpnes and Sørensen 1993).

6 Press-reviews show that four major newspapers in The Netherlands devoted five articles to the opening of DDS. About 100 lines were written about using DDS for political purposes, 80 lines related virtuosity values to DDS (such as excitement and travel around the world) and about 50 lines were written about using DDS for information and communication in general (Bosman 1994; Limburg 1994; van der Nederlanden 1994; van Jole 1994).

7 In 1994, only 34 per cent of the members of the national parliament were female. The political participation of women was considerably lower than the participation by men, specifically as far as contacting politicians and dealing with societal issues are concerned. These kinds of participation by women did not increase between 1974 and 1979 (Elsinga 1985: 154–5).

8 A few weeks after the opening of DDS, a female user took the initiative to ask for a discussion platform for women: DDS.femail. After DDS was opened, female users became active in creating spaces for women. This phenomenon was also noted in Santa Monica's PEN System (Collins-Jarvis 1993) and was discussed in a paper presented in Autumn 1999.

9 Shade and Herring argue that 'flame wars', heated arguments which tend to appear on such discussion lists, are particularly unattractive to women. Moreover, a more masculine style of discussion generally seems to be facilitated by the mailing list's software which makes it easy to 'cut and paste' in messages from other contributors. An extensive discussion about masculine and feminine styles of discussion on mailing lists, and how these are encouraged or discouraged, is beyond the scope of this chapter.

10 Research conducted in 1995 indeed showed that less than 2 per cent of the contributions to a political Internet discussion organized by DDS were made by women (Ministerie van Binnenlandse Zaken 1995).

11 Moreover, because these terminals kept breaking down and were consequently very expensive to maintain, they were removed in the course of the first year and a half of DDS's existence.

12 The sourcecode of software is the original programming in the programming language in which it was written. Having access to the sourcecode means that the programmer is able to rewrite the original program.
13 The percentage of women studying and working in the field of computer science, for example, in The Netherlands is, compared to other western countries, one of the lowest. In the 1990s the enrolment of women in engineering studies of computer science did not exceed 5 per cent. Business-oriented IT studies attracted only 15–20 per cent of female students (van Oost 1994).

References

Akrich, M. (1995) 'User representations: practices, methods and sociology' in A. Rip, T. J. Misa and J. Schot (eds) *Managing Technology in Society: The Approach of Constructive Technology Asssessment*, London and New York: Pinter Publishers: 167–84.
Bastelaer, B. van (1998) 'Digital cities and transferability of results', 4th EDC Conference on digital cities, Salzburg, 29–30 October. Available online: http://www.ed.ac.uk/~rcss/SLIM/SLIMhome.html (11 June 1999).
Bijker, W. E. (1995) *Of Bicycles, Bakelites, and Bulbs: Toward a Theory of Sociotechnical Change*, Cambridge, MA: MIT Press.
Bijker, W. E., Hughes, T. P. and Pinch, T. J. (1987) *The Social Construction of Technological Systems: New Directions in the Sociology and History of Technology*, Cambridge, MA, and London: MIT Press.
Boomen, M. van den (1996) *Internet ABC voor vrouwen, een inleiding voor D@t@d@mes en modemmeiden*, Amsterdam: Instituut voor Publiek en Politiek.
Bosman, F. (1994) 'Discussie in Digitale Stad', *Het Parool*, 12 January.
Brosnan, M. (1998) *Technophobia: The Psychological Impact of Information Technology*, London and New York: Routledge.
Brouns, M. (1998) 'Leeftijd en sekse in een digitale wereld', *Facta*, 6 (1): 6–8.
Castells, M. (1996) *The Rise of the Network Society*, Malden, MA, and Oxford: Basil Blackwell.
Cockburn, C. and Ormrod, S. (1993) *Gender and Technology in the Making*, London, Thousand Oaks and New Delhi: Sage Publications.
Collins-Jarvis, L. A. (1993) 'Gender representation in an electronic city hall: Female adoption of Santa Monica's PEN system', *Journal of Broadcasting and Electronic Media*, 4: 49–65.
Connell, R. W. (1987) *Gender and Power: Society, the Person and Sexual Politics*, Stanford, California: Stanford University Press.
Diemen, D. van (1998) *The Public Internet Terminal in Amsterdam: Embodying the Ideal of Citizenship in Technological Design*. Available online: http://www.sussex.ac.uk/EMTEL/dani.htm (14 January 1998).
Elsinga, E. (1985) 'Politieke participatie in Nederland, een onderzoek naar ontwikkelingen in politieke participatie in Nederland gedurende de jaren zeventig', Proefschrift Technische Hogeschool Twente, 18 October 1985.
Flint, J. (1994) *Handleiding XS4ALL/Digitale Stad*, Archive DDS, January.

Francissen, L. and Brants, K. (1998) 'Virtually going places, square-hopping in Amsterdam's digital city' in R. Tsagarousianou, D. Tambini and C. Bryan (eds) *Cyberdemocracy, Technology, Cities and Civic Networks*, London and New York: Routledge.

Green, E., Owen, J. and Pain, D. (eds) (1993) *Gendered by Design? Information Technology and Office Systems*, London and Washington: Taylor and Francis.

Håpnes, T. and Sørensen, K. H. (1993) 'Competition and collaboration in male shaping of computing: a study of a Norwegian hacker culture', STS Working Paper 4/93, Senter for teknology og samfun.

Harding, S. (1986) *The Science Question in Feminism*, Ithaca/London: Cornell University Press.

Henwood, F. (1993) 'Establishing gender perspectives in information technology: problems, issues and opportunities' in E. Green, J. Owen and D. Pain (eds) *Gendered by Design? Information Technology and Office Systems*, London and Washington: Taylor and Francis: 31–49.

Herring, S. C. (1993) 'Gender and democracy in computer-mediated communication', *Electronic Journal of Communication*, 3 (2).

Herring, S. C. (1994) 'Gender differences in computer-mediated communication: bringing familiar baggage to the new frontier', Keynote talk panel 'Making the Net*Work*: is there a z39.50 in gender communication?', American Library Association annual convention, Miami, 27 June. Available online: gopher://gopher.cpsr.org:70/00/cpsr/gender/herring.txt (27 February 1997).

Jole, F. van (1994) 'De Digitale Stad van start', *de Volkskrant*, 15 January. Available online: http://www.xs4all.nl/~fvjole/archief/artikelen/Volkskrant/1994/dds.html (18 January 1999).

Krogt, T. P. W. M. and van der Vroom, C. W. (1989) *Organisatie is Beweging*, Culemborg: Lemma.

Lieshout, M. van (1998) *The Digital City of Amsterdam: Between Public Domain and Private Enterprise*.

Limburg, D. (1994) 'Amsterdam heeft er een kleine stad bij', *NRC*, 17 January.

Meerten, R. van (1993) 'Projectvoorstel De Digitale Stad', Archive Municipality of Amsterdam, BBI/93/103/1, 27 September.

Ministerie van Binnenlandse Zaken (1995) 'Eén maand Binnenlandse Zaken Discussie @ Internet, Verslag van een door De Digitale Stad georganiseerde discussie op het Internet over Beleidnota Informatiebeleid Openbare Sector 3 "Terug naar de Toekomst"', Den Haag, Ministerie van Binnenlandse Zaken, 26 April 1995.

Nederlanden, F. van der (1994) 'De Balie als elektronische navel van de wereld', *Het Parool*, 15 January.

NN (1994) 'Digitale stad trekt duizenden bezoekers', *NRC*, 22 January.

Oost, E. van (1994) 'Nieuwe functies, nieuwe verschillen: Genderprocessen in de constructie van de nieuwe automatiseringsfuncties 1955–1970', *Eburon*, Delft.

Oost, E. van (1995) 'Over "vrouwelijke" en "mannelijke" dingen' in M. Brouns and M. Grunell (eds) *Vrouwenstudies in de Jaren Negentig: Een*

Kennismaking Vanuit Verschillende Disciplines, Bussum: Coutinho: 289–313.

Oudshoorn, N. (1996) 'Noodlot of uitdaging' ('Genderscripts in technologie'), inaugural speech, University of Twente.

Pacey, A. (1983) *The Culture of Technology*, Cambridge, MA: MIT Press.

Patrick, A. S. (1997) 'Media lessons from the national capital FreeNet', *Communications of the ACM*, 40 (7): 74–80.

Pinch, T. J. and Bijker, W. E. (1987) 'The social construction of facts and artefacts or how the sociology of science and the sociology of technology might benefit each other' in W. E. Bijker, T. P. Hughes and T. J. Pinch (eds) *The Social Construction of Technological Systems: New Directions in the Sociology and History of Technology*, Cambridge, MA: MIT Press.

Rheingold, H. (1993) *The Virtual Community: Homesteading at the Electronic Frontier*, Addison-Wesley, 1993.

Rogers, E. M., Collins-Jarvis, L. and Schmitz, J. (1994) 'The PEN project in Santa Monica: Interactive communication, equality and political action', *Journal of the American Society of Information Science*, 45: 401–10.

Schalken, K. and Tops, P. (1994) 'The digital city: a study into the backgrounds and opinions of its residents', paper presented at the Canadian Community Networks Conference, Carleton University, Ottawa, Canada, 15–17 August. Available online: http://cwis.kub.nl/%7Efrw/people/schalken/dceng/html (20 January 1999).

Shade, L. R. (1993) 'Gender issues in computer networking', talk given at Community Networking, the International Free-Net Conference, Carleton University, Ottawa, Canada, 17–19 August.

Stallings, B. (1996) *A Critical Study of Three Free-Net Community Networks.* Available online: http://www.ofcn.org/whois/ben/Free-Nets (7 October 1997).

Turkle, S. (1991) 'Computational reticence: why women fear the intimate machine' in C. Kramarae (ed.) *Technology and Women's Voices*, New York: Routledge and Kegan Paul: 41–61.

Varley, P. (1991) 'What's really happening in Santa Monica?' *Technology Review*, 6: 43–51.

Von Hippel, E. (1976) 'The dominant role of users in the scientific instrument innovation process', *Research Policy*, 5: 212–39.

Von Hippel, E. (1988) *The Sources of Innovation*, Oxford: Oxford University Press.

Wajcman, J. (1991) *Feminism Confronts Technology*, Cambridge: Polity Press.

Wajcman, J. (1994) 'Een Digitale Stad mèt onderwereld', Trouw, 15 January.

Interview list

Marianne van den Boomen (moderator), 13 November 1998.

Joost Flint (author user's manual), 27 January 1998a and 12 March 1998b.

Reineke van Meerten (Civil Servant Municipality Amsterdam), 27 January 1998.

Félipe Rodriguez (programmer), 2 September 1998.

Marleen Stikker (co-ordinator), 22 June 1998a and 12 August 1998b.

Archives

Archive DDS.
Archive Municipality of Amsterdam.
Marleen Stikker, personal archive, Centrum voor Oude en Nieuwe Media De
   Waag.

Part IV

Identity and self
Gendered play, virtual reality and cyborgization

Chapter 14

The social geography of gender-switching in virtual environments on the Internet

Lynne D. Roberts and Malcolm R. Parks

Abstract

The virtual social worlds of the Internet give people unparalleled control over the construction and presentation of their identities. Gender-switching is perhaps the most dramatic example of how people exercise this control. It occurs when people present a gender that is different from their biological sex. While gender-switching figures prominently in academic commentaries and popular writings about online social life, there is little systematic research on the phenomenon. Online surveys of two stratified random samples (Ns = 233 and 202) of MOO users were conducted. The majority of participants (60 per cent) in social MOOs (popular text-based Internet social venues) had never engaged in gender-switching, while the majority in role-playing MOOs were either gender-switching currently (40 per cent) or had done so in the past (16.7 per cent). More than half of those who currently gender-switched did so for less than 10 per cent of their time online. In spite of the freedom to use indeterminate or even plural gender identities, most participants who switched genders (78.7 per cent) did so within traditional binary conventions (male to female, female to male). The primary reason for gender-switching was the desire to play roles of people different from one's self. The primary barrier to gender-switching was the belief that it is dishonest and manipulative. Attitudes towards gender-switching and online participation were better predictors of gender-switching than personal background demographics or personality measures. The images of gender-switching that emerge from this first systematic study of the phenomenon are considerably more benign than that usually portrayed in the literature. Gender-switching appears to be practised by a minority of MOO users for a small percentage of their time online. Gender-switching within MOOs of all kinds might best be understood as an experimental behaviour rather than as an enduring expression of sexuality, personality or gender politics.

Introduction

People possess extraordinary freedom to construct their identities in the electronic environments of the Internet. In face-to-face interaction one cannot easily escape being categorized according to age, race, biological sex, and a host of other social factors. Many of these can also be readily identified in telephone conversations. In the virtual text-based social worlds of the Internet, however, people possess unparalleled control over the construction and presentation of their identities (Parks 1998). Perhaps the most dramatic example of how people exercise this control is the case of online gender-switching. Thus, men may present themselves as women, women as men, and either sex may use plural, indeterminate or non-gendered identities.

The fluidity of gender presentation online, coupled with the intense popular and academic interest in gender, has made the Internet a prime site for gender studies. The topic has yielded an increasing number of academic commentaries (including those of Bruckman 1993; Savicki et al. 1996; O'Brien 1997; Senft 1997) and has figured prominently in popular writings about the social aspects of online life. The phenomenon of gender-switching has been discussed extensively in books like Rheingold's *Virtual Community: Homesteading on the Electronic Frontier* (1993), Turkle's *Life on the Screen: Identity in the Age of the Internet* (1995), Stone's *The War of Desire and Technology at the Close of the Mechanical Age* (1995) and a variety of edited volumes (for example, Benedikt 1994; Jones 1995; Cherny and Weise 1996). In short, gender has been 'problematized' by the freedom afforded by the Internet and gender-switching has become a standard topic in discussions of the Internet.

It is surprising, therefore, that so little is actually known about gender-switching in an empirical sense. Most discussions focus on controversial cases, on anecdotal data or on critical commentaries about limited data sets. Basic information about how often gender-switching occurs, who is doing it and why they are doing it is lacking. The purpose of this study is to begin to fill these gaps in the empirical record. We begin by situating the process of identity construction in general and gender presentation in particular within the social environment of the Internet. We then advance several basic research questions and address them by drawing on two data sets gathered in a variety of MOOs, popular online social venues.

The nature of online identities

The Internet is best understood not as a single medium but rather as a digital metamedium that carries several different types of distinctive media including email, hyperlinked webpages, file transfer protocols and a variety of virtual social environments. The virtual social environments range from the descriptively spare textual worlds of chat rooms and discussion groups to the more contextualized worlds of graphical and textual MUDs (multi-user dimensions, domains or dungeons). MUDs provide a virtual environment, usually described in text, in which participants create and describe characters, virtual places and objects. They allow synchronous discussion among geographically dispersed participants. While MUDs tend to be oriented around social role-playing games, MOOs (a type of MUD that uses object-oriented programming) are frequently purely social (Parks and Roberts 1998). We focus on these virtual social venues because they have figured so prominently in the academic and popular discussions of gender in computer-mediated communication (including Bruckman 1993; Rheingold 1993; Turkle 1995, 1998).

To illustrate the diversity of MOO environments, we will briefly describe two MOOs and the types of activities undertaken in each setting. LambdaMOO is the original and largest social MOO. Currently there are more than 5,000 people from more than 50 countries with characters on LambdaMOO. More than half of these users reside in the USA. Each person is assigned a character that they can name, gender and describe in text. In addition to their primary character, individuals can create any number of 'morphs', alternate characters with their own names, genders and descriptions, that can be switched between instantaneously. At any one point in time there are usually in excess of 100 people logged in to the MOO. LambdaMOO's virtual setting is a large house and grounds. Users socialize in groups in popular areas of the house (the living room, the hot-tub and sensual respites) or interact in smaller groups in private rooms. The social dynamics of LambdaMOO have been described by a number of observers in the popular literature (including Dibbell 1998).

Ghostwheel is a smaller role-play MOO that provides a game world set in a post-apocalypse wasteland 600 years in the future. Creatures on the wasteland include 'rous' (rats the size of small dogs), 'executioner birds' and 'cougarites'. Each individual is assigned one main character and one alternative character that are developed for role-play purposes. There are different classes of characters including 'soulmech', 'dragonrider', 'mage', 'crystal hunter', 'submariner', 'recomb' and 'bionic' (see Ghostwheel MOO's homepage: http://www.nexus.net/~bholmes/). Characters, their body parts and clothing are described and character points are used to buy advantages and skills. The predominant activity on Ghostwheel is role-playing and the combat rules are based on offline role-play gaming. Players must differentiate between in character (when role-playing) and out of character (social and casual) communication.

Several features of these environments combine to make them places where people can exercise maximal control over their own self-presentations. Non-verbal cues regarding vocal qualities, bodily movement, facial expressions and physical appearance are simply missing in these textual worlds. Cues regarding social position or social status may also be missing. Several theorists have suggested that this reduction in cues might account for the relative nonconformity of online behaviour relative to face-to-face behaviour (for example, Culnan and Markus 1987; Sproull and Kiesler 1991). Although these previous investigators have focused on the anti-social aspects of this nonconformity, it is important to appreciate that reduced cues also create freedom for people to explore alternative aspects of their identities or even entirely alternative identities. Two other features of virtual environments contribute to this freedom (Parks 1998). In many instances it is impossible to cross-check personal descriptions given online. There is usually no reliable way to verify that the person who claims to be a 22-year-old female really is either 22 years old or female.

Finally, online presentations generally do not create automatic offline consequences. In most cases online identities remain separate from offline 'real' lives. This is partly the result of the relative anonymity of online activity but it is also partly the result of simple physical separation. One may type seductive and sexually-inviting text, for example, without having to worry about actually being physically touched in return. All of these factors combine to turn MOOs, MUDs and their online relatives into 'identity workshops' (Bruckman 1992) where people are free to explore new aspects of self, including the freedom to experiment with gender.

Gender-switching in virtual social environments

Few aspects of self have been explored as extensively or with as much controversy online as gender. Cases of gender-switching have been reported since MUDs were first developed (see Rheingold 1993: 164) and some, like Van Gelder's 'strange case of the electronic lover' (1996), have become Net legends. Given this, the first and most basic research need is to determine just how often gender-switching occurs. Considering the amount of discussion devoted to the topic, we might hypothesize that gender-switching is indeed a frequent online event. Rheingold (1993) claimed that the prevalence of deceptive gender play in online social environments like MUDs and MOOs was a major reason that many administrators of college computer systems banned their use. Others (including Turkle 1995) suggest that gender-switching is a natural and comfortable extension of the desire to explore one's online identity and thereby imply that gender-switching should be a rather common phenomenon. To evaluate these claims, we asked two questions: what proportion of respondents report having switched gender (research question 1 – RQ1) and, for those who switch, what proportion of their online time do they spend in a switched state of some kind (RQ2)?

Assuming that gender-switching occurs with sufficient frequency to permit further analysis, we will next turn our attention to the nature of 'the switch' itself. In its simplest form one merely adopts an identity opposite of one's biological sex. This has been called 'on-line transvestism' by one commentator (Tamosaitis 1995). But one may also 'gender' themselves in any of a variety of other ways. LambdaMOO, for example, the largest and oldest of the MOOs, offers a choice of eight additional designations beyond male and female – Spivak, neuter, either, splat, egotistical, plural, second and royal. Or, one may simply choose to say nothing about gender. The ability to go beyond a 'binary' approach to gender has been touted by some feminist commentators as an important political feature of virtual environments (including Rodino 1997).

It is therefore useful to determine what proportion of the time people switch to a gender opposite their biological sex and what proportion of the time they switch to some neutral, plural or otherwise 'non-binary' gender (RQ3).

In addition we wished to determine if there were demographic differences between those who had never switched, those who were currently switching and those who had switched in the past but had not done so recently (RQ4). Some observers (for example, Rheingold 1993; Turkle 1995) imply that gender-switching should be more common among younger players, usually single college students. Some cases highlight gender switching by males (for example, Van Gelder 1996), while others have commented on gender switching by both males and females (for example, Bruckman 1992, 1993). To date, however, researchers have not described the demographics of those that do and do not switch in any systematic fashion.

It is possible that the deliberate misrepresentation of one's gender in an online setting reflects something about one's personality. We were particularly interested in determining if those who switched differed from those who did not in terms of how shy they were, how extroverted they were and how neurotic they were (RQ5). It has been suggested that shy (Roberts et al. 1997) and introverted (Carduccio and Zimbardo 1995) individuals are less inhibited online than they are in real life. As far as we know, there is no research on the personality correlates of gender-switching. There is, however, no shortage of speculation in popular commentaries. Slouka (1995), for instance, suggests that developing an online identity of any kind, particularly one that is different from one's 'real' identity, is a sign of dysfunction. Given the potential impact of influential commentaries like Slouka's, it is vital that we begin to explore the personality correlates of gender-switching.

It is equally important to understand the reasons people give for switching or not switching and their more general attitudes about gender-switching. Gender-switching appears to be a multi-functional social act with a diversity of attitudes surrounding it. A wide range of attitudes was revealed in exploratory interviews (Roberts 1999) and in existing literature (see Bruckman 1993; Rheingold 1993; Turkle 1995). Some focus on the social function of gender-switching (for example, to avoid harassment), while others emphasize more personal motives (for example, to explore the masculine and feminine sides of oneself). Some view gender-switching as a deliberate political act in defiance of gender stereotypes. One person advocating this view referred to the phenomenon as 'gender fucking' (Senft 1997). Some motivations are decidedly more pro-social than others (for example, to increase empathy with the opposite sex versus to control others). Our research thus focused on two final questions: What reasons do people give for engaging in or avoiding gender-switching (RQ6)? What attitudes distinguish those who have never switched, those who are currently switching and those who have switched in the past but have not done so recently (RQ7)?

It is conceivable that gender-switching online may have offline ana-
logues in transgendered behaviours such as cross-dressing, transvestism
and trans-sexualism. Do models of transgenderism in 'real life' shed light
on gender-switching online? King (1993) outlined four models used
to explain transgendered behaviour based on their ontology (essentialist versus constructionist) and tenability (theorists' views on the accept-
ability of the behaviours). Essentialist models view transgenderism as
persistent phenomena across cultures and history. The tenable essentialist model views transgenderism as an innate orientation or sexual preference that should be celebrated. The untenable essentialist model views
transgenderism as a condition that requires correction. The psychological
and medical literatures, for example, view transgenderism as gender
dysphoria, deviant from the 'normal' gender identity development and
gender-role behaviour. Gender Identity Disorder is classified as a
mental illness in the *Diagnostic and Statistical Manual of Mental
Disorders: DSM IV* (American Psychiatric Association 1994) and is
theorized to have its basis in a combination of biological factors and
family and situational factors during early childhood (Bradley and
Zucker 1997).

In contrast to the essentialist models, constructionist models view
transgenderism as social constructions specific to temporal and cultural
location. The tenable constructionist model views the range of transgendered behaviours as socially constructed categories that require no
treatment or censure. Butler (1990), for example, described gender
as a culturally prescribed act and identity as a 'signifying practise'.
The untenable constructionist model views transgenderism as a 'false
consciousness' or delusion on the part of the individual that requires
treatment. The findings from the seven research questions will be re-
examined in light of the four models presented here.

Method

This report is based on data collected in two separate studies. Study I
was intended to determine the basic frequency of gender-switching and
some demographics associated with gender-switchers. Study II replicated
some features of Study I, but was intended to explore the personality
correlates, attitudes, and rationales of gender-switchers, former gender-
switchers, and those who had never gender-switched. As the studies
overlap with respect to the research questions, however, they will be
discussed together.

Participants

Study I

Participants in Study I came from a stratified random sample of participants in seven popular social MOOs. The biggest social and biggest educational MOO were selected on a priori grounds. Five additional MOOs were selected randomly from a list of MOOs available on the World Wide Web and then participants were randomly sampled within each MOO.[1] Participants (N = 233) were almost equally divided between males (51.9 per cent) and females (48.1 per cent). They ranged in age from 13–74, but averaged just over 27 years. Most had never been married (63.3 per cent), although nearly a third were either married or cohabiting (29.7 per cent). The typical respondent had been using the Internet for over two and a half years and had been using MOOs for almost two years.

Study II

Participants in Study II were also drawn from a stratified random sample. The three largest social and role-playing MOOs using the standard MOO program structure were selected from lists available on the World Wide Web and two additional role-play MOOs were selected at random.[2] Responses were received from 202 individuals (53 per cent male and 47 per cent female). Of those who could be identified, about one third (34.3 per cent) were active in a role-playing MOO. Participants ranged in age from 16 to 53, but more than three-quarters were aged between 18 and 30 years of age with a mean of $25\frac{1}{2}$. Participants in Study II were similar to those in Study I in terms of marital status (67.5 per cent never married, 26.4 per cent married or cohabiting, 6.1 per cent separated, divorced or widowed). Although the duration of Internet use was not assessed in Study II, the length of time respondents had been using MOOs was. The typical respondent in Study II had been active in these venues for about a year longer than the typical respondent in Study I.

Procedures

MOO characters who had connected to the selected MOOs within the previous 14 days were randomly selected. The MOOs' internal email systems were used to send letters soliciting participation in a survey on communication patterns. The survey could be completed by research participants on a World Wide Web site or by email.

A total of 1,200 MOO characters were solicited in Study I, while 1,000 were solicited in Study II. Of these, 233 responded in Study I and 202 responded in Study II. The apparent response rates (19.5 per cent and 20.2 per cent) are likely to underestimate the actual response rates as a result of two factors. First, the surveys contained disclaimers discouraging participants under 18 years of age. An indeterminate, but possibly large, number of participants would not have met this age requirement. Second, many people have characters on more than one MOO and have more than one character on a given MOO (particularly in role-playing MOOs). We received several notes from participants suggesting that our sampling contained redundancies. Although a precise correction is not possible, we estimate that the actual responses were approximately 30 per cent when these factors were taken into account.

Measures

Study I

Study I comprises a previously unreported part of a larger survey on the development of social relationships on MOOs (see Parks and Roberts 1998). The measures relevant here include demographic items regarding the participants' age, sex, marital status and online experience, as well as two items dealing directly with gender-switching. In the first participants were asked if they had ever 'gender-switched' (used a character whose gender was different from their 'real life' gender). A second question asked people who responded affirmatively to the first question to report the percentage of time on the MOOs in the last month that had been spent using a gender-switched character.

Study II

Participants were asked to classify themselves according to whether they had ever used a MOO gender other than their biological sex and, if they had, whether they had done so in the last month. They were then presented with an open-ended question asking for one or two main reasons for their choices regarding gender-switching. Participants were also asked to respond to a series of 39 attitude statements about gender-switching. These items were developed from books and articles that examined gender-switching (Bruckman 1993; Germain 1993; Jaffe 1995;

Turkle 1995; McRae 1996; Van Gelder 1996) as well as from interviews with MOO participants by the first author as part of an unpublished grounded theory study of social interaction on MOOs. The responses were recorded on seven-point Likert scales. In addition to a series of demographic questions participants were asked to complete three personality measures: the extroversion and neuroticism scales of the Eysenck Personality Questionnaire–Revised (EPQ–R) short scale (Eysenck et al. 1985) and a shortened version of the shyness scale developed by Cheek and Buss (1981).

Results

Prevalence of gender-switching

Participants were classified into one of three categories with respect to their history of online behaviour: those who had never gender-switched, those who currently gender-switched at least some of the time, and those who had not gender-switched during the month previous to the study. Most participants were not using gender-switching as part of their online self-presentations. Indeed, the clear majority of participants in social MOOs in both Study I (62 per cent) and Study II (58.3 per cent) had never engaged in gender-switching. A minority were currently gender-switching (Study I, 22.6 per cent; Study II, 19.1 per cent) or had tried gender-switching previously (Study I, 15.4 per cent; Study II, 22.6 per cent). This was not true of those who participated in role-playing MOOs. Here the majority were either currently gender-switching (40 per cent) or had gender-switched previously (16.7 per cent), with a minority never having tried gender-switching (43.3 per cent). In Study II, people participating in role-playing MOOs were significantly more likely to gender-switch than those who participated in purely social MOOs.

We asked gender-switchers to report what percentage of their time on MOOs in the last month had been spent in a gender-switched state. In Study I (social MOOs only) 60 per cent of those who were currently switching did so for 10 per cent or less of their time online. Only 22.6 per cent of current switchers (5.5 per cent of the total Study I sample) spent more than 60 per cent of their time online in a switched state. In Study II, 40 per cent of those who were currently switching did so for 10 per cent or less of their time online. Almost a third of those who switched (31.5 per cent), however, spent 70 per cent or more of their time in a switched state and 20 per cent reported spending all their online time in a switched state. Among those who switched, there was no significant difference in the percentage of time spent gender-switched on role-playing and social MOOs.

Types of gender switches

In spite of the freedom to use indeterminate or even plural gender identities, most participants who switched genders did so within traditional binary conventions. Men presented themselves as women and women presented themselves as men. These conventional switches to the opposite sex accounted for 78.7 per cent of the cases among those who were currently or had previously switched in Study II. The remaining 21.3 per cent fell into 'non-binary' categories. The most common of these were neuter (6.4 per cent) and Spivak (4.3 per cent). Others included second, the opposite, plural, neither, shehe, royal, shemale and self-made genders. None of these, however, was represented by more than one case.

Demographic correlates of gender-switching

There were few differences in personal background demographics across the three categories of gender-switching (never, current and previous). There were no significant differences between categories on the basis of age, sex or marital status. Only two personal characteristics were associated significantly with gender-switching. Respondents in Study II were asked to report their sexual orientation (heterosexual, homosexual, bisexual or other). Heterosexuals were significantly less likely to have gender-switched than MOOers with different sexual orientations. Respondents in Study I were asked if they had some disability that affected their 'functioning or communication' when they were not on the Internet. Of those who reported a disability, 50 per cent were currently gender-switching compared to only 21 per cent of those who did not report disabilities.

The demographics of online participation were better predictors of gender-switching. It was not, however, the total length of time respondents had been using the Internet that counted. There were no significant differences in the number of months respondents had been using the Internet across the three groups in Study I. The groups did differ in terms of their experiences with MOOs. Current and former gender-switchers had been using MOOs significantly longer and spent more hours per week on MOOs than those who had never tried gender-switching. In both studies, people who were currently switching visited a greater number of MOOs in the past month than people who did not gender-switch.

Personality correlates of gender-switching

Scores on the personality measures we examined in Study II did not differ between those who had never switched gender, those who were currently gender-switching and those who had switched gender in the past. There were no overall differences on Eysenck's extroversion scale or his neuroticism scale. Nor did the three groups differ on the Cheek and Buss (1981) shyness scale.

It may be useful to set these findings in the broader context of how MOO users compare to the general populace. We compared the extroversion and neuroticism scores observed in our study to the normative data provided by Eysenck et al. (1985). Comparisons were made across three age groups (16–20, 21–30, 31–40) with separate comparisons by sex within each age group. This allowed six comparisons between observed and normative means for each of the two scales. Our tests showed that only one mean was statistically significant. Female MOO users between the ages of 16 and 20 were significantly less extroverted than females in the same age group in the general population. Levels of extroversion among females in the other age groups did not differ from those in the general population. There were no differences in extroversion among males and no differences for neuroticism among any of the age groups for either sex.

Reasons for gender-switching behaviour

Respondents in each of the three groups in Study II were asked to supply their one or two main reasons for their behaviour of gender-switching. These reasons were then grouped into more general categories by the senior author and are presented in Table 14.1.

A total of 105 respondents indicated that they had never gender-switched and together they provided 178 reasons for not gender-switching. By far the most common reason given was that respondents simply had no interest in doing so. They either had no desire (23 per cent) or saw no benefit (11.8 per cent). Other respondents either voiced a strong identification with their real gender (12.4 per cent) or expressed a desire to present themselves accurately online (12.9 per cent). A seventh (14.6 per cent) believed that gender-switching was dishonest. A tenth (11.8

Table 14.1 Reasons given for decisions regarding gender-switching and percentages of responses

Reasons for not gender-switching
No interest in or reason to gender-switch (example: 'No desire to be a member of the opposite sex in real life or on the MOO') 23%

Gender-switching is dishonest and deceitful (example: 'I feel it is dishonest and wouldn't want to think someone was doing it to me') 14.6%

Desire to present the 'real' self on line (example: 'I believe in presenting myself in as accurate a way as possible') 12.9%

Strong identification with own gender (example: 'My characters are each taken from little facets of myself and I am all female') 12.4%

Doubts about success (example: 'I wouldn't know how to act like a guy') 11.8%

There is no benefit to gender-switching (example: 'Don't really see any point in doing so') 11.8%

Reasons for gender-switching (current/former)
Role-playing (example: 'Allows for more possibilities in role-playing games') 24.0%/13.4%

Curiosity about gender (example: 'I wanted to experience what it was like to be male') 13.5%/34.3%

Fun (example: 'It's fun') 12.5%/10.4%

To avoid sexual harassment (example: 'To have a conversation without someone trying to hit on me') 7.3%/7.5%

Challenge (example: 'I thought it would be a good challenge to my acting skills') 7.3%/0

Sex (example: 'Much easier to find sexual fantasies when playing a female') 5.2%/10.4%

Reasons for no longer gender-switching
Curiosity was satisfied (example: 'I did it a couple of times and had my answers so never felt like doing it again') 18.3%

Prefer characters that match real sex (example: 'I have an established character who is female that I like to interact as') 16.7%

Spend less time MOOing in general or using the MOO containing the switched character (example: 'I haven't been on the MOO much lately') 15.0%

Easier to play a character consistent with real sex (example: 'It's too much work to remember that I'm playing male') 8.3%

Did not like the way I was treated as a gender-switched character (example: 'I realized that female acquaintances weren't joking about being frequently hit on by strangers') 6.7%

per cent) expressed doubts as to whether they would be successful if they tried to gender-switch.

A total of 97 respondents were either currently gender-switching or reported that they had gender-switched at some point in the past. The 55 individuals currently gender-switching provided 96 reasons and the 42 individuals who had previously gender-switched provided 67 reasons for gender-switching.

For those who currently gender-switch the most common reason (31.3 per cent) related to role-playing: that it was part of role-playing (24 per cent) or a challenge to their acting or interpersonal skills (7.3 per cent). The next most common reason involved a desire to satisfy curiosities about gender or to experiment with gender (13.5 per cent). In contrast, the most common reason for previous gender-switchers to begin gender-switching was curiosity or experimentation with gender (34.3 per cent), with role-playing (13.4 per cent) less important. A closer inspection of role-playing responses revealed that the majority came from people who were involved in MOOs that were structured as role-playing games. More than 10 per cent of responses from each group reported that gender-switching was a fun activity. Gender-switching was also used to engage in sexual talk and fantasies or alternatively to avoid gendered responses, usually sexual harassment. Almost all of those who said they switched genders to avoid sexual harassment were women.

The 42 respondents who fell into the category of former gender-switchers – those who had not gender-switched in the previous month – provided 60 reasons for no longer gender-switching. The most common reason (18.3 per cent) for stopping was that it was no longer interesting or that their initial curiosity about gender-switching had been satisfied. Gender-switching stopped for many respondents (15 per cent) simply because they no longer spent as much time on the MOOs. The remaining reasons given for stopping all expressed some sort of dissatisfaction with gender-switching. For some (16.7 per cent) it was expressed as a desire to be more authentic with regard to gender, while for others the reason was that gender-switching had been unpleasant (6.7 per cent) or required too much effort (8.3 per cent).

Attitudinal correlates of gender-switching

The final set of analyses explored attitudes about gender-switching gathered from the extant literature and interviews. Our goal was to determine if there were systematic attitudinal differences between those who did not gender-switch, those who did and those who did but stopped.

Participants indicated their level of agreement with 39 attitudinal items using seven-point scales. Significant differences were observed among gender-switching categories for the majority of items. Rather than detailing all the items here, we will focus on several themes that run through the results. There are comparatively few differences between current and former gender-switchers. These two groups differed significantly on only less than a third of the items. Compared to current gender-switchers, former gender-switchers viewed switching as less honest and more manipulative and deceitful. Compared to current gender-switchers, they were less comfortable and experienced less enjoyment interacting with gender-switchers, having a higher expectation that people on MOOs were the same gender in real life as their MOO character. They rated gender-switching less highly as an opportunity for identity and emotional exploration. They were also less positive about it as a form of role-play. Moreover, they were less likely than those currently switching genders to see it as a way to overcome gender stereotypes. They were more likely, however, to say that they had gender-switched just to see if they could get away with it.

Those who had never gender-switched differed from current gender-switchers on a variety of items. The largest factor separating these two groups appears to be an ethical perspective. Compared to those who were currently gender-switching, those who had never switched viewed switching as dishonest, deceitful and manipulative. They expected people to use their biological sex and were upset and uncomfortable when they did not. A second factor separating those who were currently switching from those who never did was an enjoyment of role-playing. Those who had gender-switched viewed gender-switching as a form of role-play and were more likely to endorse statements suggesting that gender-switching made life on the MOOs more interesting. Current gender-switchers also registered greater agreement with items, suggesting that gender-switching created opportunities for self-exploration and growth. They gave stronger endorsements, for instance, to statements about the potential for gender-switching to enhance one's emotional range, learn about the opposite sex and explore additional facets of their own identities.

We also sought to identify those attitudes that distinguished most powerfully between those who had never gender-switched and those who were current or former gender-switchers. Current and former gender-switchers were placed in the same group. An analysis to discriminate between items was then run to determine which items most sharply distinguished them from those who had never gender-switched. This procedure yielded five significant discriminators. Compared to those who switched genders online, those who maintained their biological sex online were more likely to believe that gender-switching was manipulative, that it was a way unwary people were lured into 'Netsex' and that it was a way to create trouble for members of the opposite sex. They expected people they met in MOOs to be the same gender online and offline. Those who switched genders, in contrast, were much more likely to hold the belief that it was fun to play a different gender online.

Discussion

The image of gender-switching that emerges from this first systematic study of the phenomenon is considerably more benign than the portrayals of both its harshest critics (including Slouka 1995) and most avid advocates (Stone 1995). First of all, gender-switching appears to be a relatively infrequent behaviour practised by a minority of MOO users. Approximately 60 per cent of social MOO and 40 per cent of role-play MOO users had never engaged in the behaviour. An additional 15–23 per cent had tried gender-switching but had stopped. Even among those who were currently gender-switching, the majority was doing so infrequently. Less than 6 per cent of the social MOO participants surveyed in Study I spent over half their time as a gender-switched character.

The results of these studies also offer little ammunition for those who argue that online interaction is being used to 'break the binaries' in our approaches to gender (for example, Rodino 1997). Most people presented their online gender in a way that matched their 'real-life' gender. Even those who switched genders usually switched to their binary opposite (for example, men presenting as women and women presenting as men) rather than to some indeterminate form. Indeed, only 20 of the 202 total respondents in Study II (10 per cent) adopted an indeterminate or non-binary gender of any kind.

Gender-switching could not be fully accounted for by the demographic factors in the two samples we gathered. Those who switched did not differ from those who had either never switched or who had stopped switching in terms of age, sex or marital status. Heterosexuals and the non-disabled were less likely to gender-switch than people with other sexual orientations and those who reported disabilities. These findings counter speculation about gender-switching being primarily an activity of younger users (for example, Rheingold 1993) or an activity done more by males than females (Stone 1995).

Nor could we account for the phenomenon of gender-switching by looking to personality factors. Gender-switchers and non-gender-switchers did not differ on standard psychological measures of shyness, extroversion or neuroticism. MOO users as a group closely matched the norms for the more general populations. Although a wider range of demographic and personality factors obviously needs to be examined in future studies, the results of this study suggest that demographic and personality factors may be poor predictors of gender-switching.

The results of this study suggest that better predictors of gender-switching are to be found in the experiences and attitudes of those online. Although switchers and non-switchers did not differ in how long they had been using the Internet, they did differ in the particulars of their participation in MOOs. Those who switched had been using MOOs longer, spent more time on MOOs and visited more MOOs than those who did not.

The type of virtual environment one participated in was also a significant predictor of gender-switching. Those who participated in role-playing MOOs were approximately twice as likely to be gender-switching as those who participated in social MOOs. Role-playing, including the role-playing of opposite gender characters, is the primary purpose of role-playing MOOs. Participants in a role-playing MOO are explicitly engaging in a 'shared fantasy' when they are 'in character'. They are seeking something besides a 'real life' (RL) character. Social interaction that is not 'in character' is marked as 'out of character' and is usually explicitly discouraged in the various help files that guide participants and convey the MOO's rules. The 'etiquette' tutorial, for example, on Ghostwheel MOO, one of the role-playing (RP) MOOs we sampled, explains that: 'On an RP MUD, it's considered rude to ask another player their RL name, RL gender, RL location, RL age or the names of their Alts [alternative identities]. It might also be rude to volunteer your own information, because it puts an onus upon others to be mutually forthcoming.'

Thus a certain amount of gender-switching occurs simply as an out-growth of the expectations of the virtual environment and may say relatively little about the characteristics of the participants themselves.

Participants' attitudes, of course, may influence the types of MOOs they prefer as well as their willingness to experiment with gender-switching. We explored these attitudes both by seeking responses to a series of statements drawn from the literature surrounding gender-switching and by soliciting the participants' own reasons for gender-switching or not gender-switching. Three themes emerged in the analysis. First, the desire to play roles of people different from one's self, usually within the context of a role-playing game, is one of the primary reasons for gender-switching. This was the most commonly given reason in the qualitative data and a significant discriminator in the multivariate analysis of the attitude items. Second, it appears that the primary barrier to gender-switching is the belief that it is dishonest and manipulative. Statements regarding the honesty of gender-switching both in terms of one's own behaviour and in terms of expectations for others were significant discriminators in the multivariate analysis. Third, people also mentioned these same factors frequently as reasons for not gender-switching. Thus for many of the people in the group who did not switch, the largest group in both samples, gender-switching was viewed as ethically dubious and counter to the desire to be authentic online.

Although the majority of people surveyed in these two studies were not gender-switching on MOOs, it is noteworthy that a significant minority of individuals was. The social experimentation of gender-switching may have a range of effects on the lives of individuals. Future studies are required that longitudinally follow individuals who gender-switch.

Finally, we believe gender-switching for most people is best understood as an experimental behaviour rather than as an enduring expression of their sexuality or personality. Gender-switchers were more likely to endorse statements regarding the use of gender-switching as a tool for enhancing personal growth and understanding. They frequently mentioned fun and curiosity as reasons for gender-switching. And importantly, by far the most common reason people stopped gender-switching was that their curiosity had been satisfied.

The models of transgendered behaviour developed offline offer little in aiding the understanding of gender-switching behaviour online. For most of the gender-switchers surveyed, the switched gender did not represent an underlying orientation, condition or delusion. In only one instance did a gender-switching respondent indicate their MOO gender reflected their offline gender. Gender-switching on MOOs may be conceptualized as a social construction specific to the virtual environment.

There is much we still do not know about gender-switching in online environments. The data reported here looked only at one type of on-line venue, yet gender-switching occurs in chatrooms and other online social settings which may have different dynamics. We might also learn more about identity construction by studying unsuccessful attempts to gender-switch. Competent cross-gender role-playing is transparent and thus often goes unnoticed (Antunes 1995). Less competent attempts may reveal much about the assumptions of the participants and the structure of the interaction itself. Finally, although the results of this study suggest that gender-switching is often an experimental, transitory behaviour, longitudinal data on gender-switching is necessary before we can fully understand how gender-switching fits into the life history of participants in computer-mediated social environments.

Notes

1 Several lists of MOOs are available online. We used 'Gurk's MOO page' (http://www4.ncsu.edu/unity/users/a/asdamick/www/moo.html). The MOOs included in the final sample were LambdaMOO, RiverMOO, BayMOO, IdMOO, Sprawl, Meridian and Diversity University. A MOO character named 'Surveyor' was set up as a research character on each of the selected MOOs to facilitate answering questions from potential respondents.
2 The three largest social and role-playing MOOs that use the LambdaMOO core were selected from Gurk's MOO list (see Note 1) and the MUD connector (http://www.mudconnect.com). Permission was sought from the wizards of each MOO to conduct research on that MOO. Consent was obtained from five of the six MOOs. These five MOOs were LambdaMOO (social), BayMOO (social), RiverMOO (social), Ghostwheel MOO (role-play) and Angreal MOO (role-play). As in the first study, a character named 'Surveyor' was set up as a research character on each of the selected MOOs to facilitate answering questions from potential respondents.

Editors' note: To enhance accessibility for a wide academic audience and shorten the manuscript, the editors have removed the statistical test information typically included in social scientific studies of this type. Information on specific tests is available from the authors: l.roberts@psychology.curtin.edu.au or macp@u.washington.edu

References

American Psychiatric Association (1994) *Diagnostic and Statistical Manual of Mental Disorders: DSM IV*, Washington DC: American Psychiatric Association.

Antunes, S. (1995) 'Leaping into cross-gender role-play', *Interactive Fantasy*, 3: 62–7. Available online: http://www.mud.co.uk/richard/ifan195.htm (3 June 1999).

Benedikt, M. (ed.) (1994) *Cyberspace: First Steps*, Cambridge, MA: MIT Press.

Bradley, S. J. and Zucker, K. J. (1997) 'Gender identity disorder: a review of the past 10 years', *Journal of the American Academy of Child and Adolescent Psychiatry*, 36: 872–80.

Bruckman, A. S. (1992) 'Identity workshop: emergent social and psychological phenomena in text-based virtual reality', unpublished manuscript, MIT Media Laboratory, Cambridge, MA. Available online: ftp://ftp.cc.gatechedu/pub/people/asb/papers/identity-workshop.rtf (3 June 1999).

Bruckman, A. S. (1993) 'Gender swapping on the Internet', paper presented at the annual conference of the Internet Society, San Francisco, CA. Available online: ftp://ftp.cc.gatech.edu/pub/people/asb/gender-swapping.txt (3 June 1999).

Butler, J. (1990) *Gender Trouble: Feminism and the Subversion of Identity*, New York: Routledge.

Carduccio, B. J. and Zimbardo, P. G. (1995) 'Are you shy?', *Psychology Today*, 28 (6): 34–45, 64–70, 78–82.

Cheek, J. M. and Buss, A. H. (1981) 'Shyness and sociability', *Journal of Personality and Social Psychology*, 41: 330–9.

Cherny, L. and Weise, E. R. (eds) (1996) *Wired Women: Gender and New Realities in Cyberspace*, Seattle, WA: Seal Press.

Culnan, M. J. and Markus, M. L. (1987) 'Information technologies' in F. Jablin, L. L. Putnam, K. Roberts and L. Porter (eds) *Handbook of Organizational Communication*, Newbury Park, CA: Sage: 420–43.

Dibbell, J. (1998) *My Tiny Life: Crime and Passion in a Virtual World*, New York: Holt.

Eysenck, S. B. G., Eysenck, H. J. and Barrett, P. (1985) 'A revised version of the psychoticism scale', *Personality and Individual Differences*, 6: 21–9.

Germain, E. (1993) 'In the jungle of MUD', *Time Magazine*, 142 (11): 61.

Jaffe, J. M. (1995) 'Gender, pseudonyms, and CMC: masking identities and baring souls', paper presented at the 45th Annual Conference of the International Communication Association, Chicago, Illinois.

Jones, S. G. (ed.) (1995) *Cybersociety: Computer-mediated Communication and Community*, Thousand Oaks, CA: Sage.

King, D. (1993) *The Transvestite and the Transsexual: Public Categories and Private Identities*, Aldershot, UK: Avery.

McRae, S. (1996) 'Coming apart at the seams: sex, text and the virtual body' in L. Cherny and E. R. Weise (eds) *Wired Women: Gender and New Realities in Cyberspace*, Seattle, WA: Seal Press: 242–62.

O'Brien, J. (1997) 'Changing the subject', *Women and Performance*, 17. Available online: http://www.echonyc.com/~women/Issue17/art-obrien.html (3 June 1999).

Parks, M. R. (1998) 'Love and relationships on the Internet', workshop presented at the Conference on Successful Relating, University of Arizona, Tucson, AZ.

Parks, M. R. and Roberts, L. D. (1998) 'Making MOOsic: the development of personal relationships on-line and a comparison to their off-line counterparts', *Journal of Social and Personal Relationships*, 15: 517–37.

Rheingold, H. (1993) *Virtual Community: Homesteading on the Electronic Frontier*, Reading, MA: Addison-Wesley.

Roberts, L. D. (1999) 'A grounded theory of social interaction in MOOs', unpublished manuscript, School of Psychology, Curtin University of Technology.

Roberts, L. D., Smith, L. M. and Pollock, C. (1997) ' "u r a lot bolder on the net": the social use of text-based virtual environments by shy individuals', paper presented at the International Conference on Shyness and Self-Consciousness, Cardiff, Wales.

Rodino, M. (1997) 'Breaking out of binaries: reconceptualizing gender and its relationship to language in computer-mediated communication', *Journal of Computer-Mediated Communication*, 3 (3). Available online: http://ascusc.org/jcmc/vol3/issue3/rodino.html (3 June 1999).

Savicki, V., Lingenfelter, D. and Kelley, M. (1996) 'Gender language style and group composition in Internet discussion groups', *Journal of Computer-Mediated Communication*, 2 (3). Available online: http://jcmc.huji.ac.il/vol2/issue3/ (3 June 1999).

Senft, T. M. (1997) 'Introduction: performing the digital body: a ghost story', *Women and Performance*, 17. Available online: http://www.echonyc.com/~women/Issue17/introduction.html (3 June 1999).

Slouka, M. (1995) *The War of the Worlds: Cyberspace and the High-tech Assault on Reality*, New York: Basic Books.

Sproull, L. and Kiesler, S. (1991) *Connections: New Ways of Working in the Networked Organization*, Cambridge, MA: MIT Press.

Stone, R. A. (1995) *The War of Desire and Technology at the Close of the Mechanical Age*, Cambridge, MA: MIT Press.

Tamosaitis, N. (1995) 'Cross-dressing in cyberspace, you can change shape (or gender)', *Computer Life*, 2 (1): 145–7.

Turkle, S. (1995) *Life on the Screen: Identity in the Age of the Internet*, New York: Simon and Schuster.

Turkle, S. (1998) 'Drag net: from Glen to Glenda and back again: is it possible?', *Utne Reader*, 89: 50–5.

Van Gelder, L. (1996) 'The strange case of the electronic lover' in R. Kling (ed.) *Computerization and Controversy*, second edition, San Diego: Academic Press: 533–46.

Chapter 15

A camera with a view

JenniCAM, visual representation and cyborg subjectivity

Krissi M. Jimroglou

Abstract

Hailed as the originator of the digital camera 'homecam' phenomenon, Jennifer Ringley has garnered national media attention for her website, JenniCAM (Ringley 1998c), which offers viewers a constant window into the bedroom of a young woman through Internet technology. Using the JenniCAM website as my primary text, I examine how Jenni integrates flesh and machine in the formation and display of a cyborg subjectivity, a hybridized identity (re)presented through the new technology of the digital camera. Towards that end I use feminist film theory to demonstrate how the construction and display of the female body – via the medium of digital camera – transforms our readings of gendered bodies as sites of knowledge production and pleasure. I assert that JenniCAM, a cyborg subject created through the integration of the electronic image and the Internet, exposes more than just flesh. JenniCAM reveals cultural tensions surrounding epistemological conceptions of vision, gender, and identity and raises questions for future conversations regarding the role of technology in the representation and construction of gendered subjects.

Snapshot

Since its inception in April 1996, the website known as JenniCAM has blossomed into a web phenomenon, complete with fan sites dedicated to FAQs (frequently asked questions), old pictures of its creator, Jennifer Ringley, in various poses and discussion areas that monitor her daily activities. The central web page of the JenniCAM site features the most up-to-date image of Jenni's bedroom as captured by the digital camera mounted on the top of her computer. The site has other components that supplement the viewer's knowledge of Jenni and her life, for example, in 1998 Jenni expanded the presentation of her life by creating short online video clips called 'The JenniSHOW' (Ringley 1998f). These interludes feature Jenni giving tours of her apartment or answering commonly asked questions about her life via real-time streaming audio and video clips. Additionally, viewers can study cropped images of Jenni's body, read her poetry or email her at other areas of the site (Ringley 1998e). While all of these different components are not to be overlooked, they are organized around the web page that publishes the continually refreshed flow of images captured by the digital camera. JenniCAM 'guest' images upload every 20 minutes and are available for viewers free of charge. However, Jenni charges a subscription fee of US$15 per year to viewers willing to pay for access to a password-protected web page which uploads a new image every two minutes (Ringley 1998d).

Conveniently, Jenni is self-employed and works at home as a freelance website designer. Thus she can be in front of the camera for most of the day. Her daily routine, as recorded by the digital camera, is something like this: for the majority of the morning she sleeps, getting up around noon. In the afternoon, Jenni begins to work at her computer, checking the 700-plus email messages from fans or chatting with friends on the phone. Every few weeks her boyfriend comes over to visit, and they spend time together. She is often up late at night and usually goes to bed after midnight. Such is the life of Jennifer Ringley. According to a Reuters report, 'Most of the time, the photos are anything but thrilling' (Hagenbaugh 1997). In offering her viewers a glimpse at real life, JenniCAM replicates the ebb and flow of the everyday.

Although Jenni is a self-proclaimed nudist and does have sex with her boyfriend on camera, JenniCAM does not deliver sexually explicit or nude images at all times. As Jenni explains:

> This site is not pornography. Yes, it contains nudity from time to time. Real life contains nudity. Yes, it contains sexual material from time to time. Real life contains sexual material. However, this is not a site about nudity and sexual material. It is a site about real life.
>
> (Ringley 1998d)

JenniCAM has raised more than a few eyebrows since the start of the project. JenniCAM would seem to offer the perfect heterosexual male fantasy – a voyeuristic window into a woman's bedroom – and could easily be dismissed as yet another example of a sexualized woman. On the other hand, the digital window is often filled with nothing but images of Jenni's bedroom furniture and yet people continue to watch. In analysing JenniCAM, it is important not to overlook the fact that Jenni endeavours to present life as she lives it. That is, Jenni promises an unstaged display of her activity, not necessarily a staged fantasy. With the presentation of 'real life' as the project, JenniCAM offers a text that writer Simon Firth describes as 'visually fascinating, disconcertingly erotic and a provocative reflection of ourselves' (Firth 1998).

Introduction

JenniCAM brings to the fore issues at the intersection of digital camera technology, visual representation and the gendered subject. In constructing her 'real life' through the use of a new visual medium, Jennifer Ringley throws into question many identity categories often thought to be stable. Throughout this chapter, I employ Judith Butler's definition of subject construction as something that 'not only takes place in time, but is itself a temporal process which operates through the reiteration of norms'. For Butler, identity-forming categories, such as sex, are 'both produced and destabilized in the course of this reiteration' (1993: 11). In JenniCAM, we witness both the production and the contradiction of a gendered subject. It is the unique way in which JenniCAM exposes the contradictions in gender identity and desire that are of interest here. JenniCAM represents a subject that is constituted by fusing together disparate entities: the corporeal and the mechanic. In doing so, JenniCAM offers a unique presentation of subjectivity, called here 'cyborg subjectivity'. The integration of the concept of subjectivity with characteristics associated with cyborgs makes for a new definition of what it means to be a subject. Donna Haraway defines a cyborg as 'a cybernetic organism, a hybrid of machine and organism, a creature of social reality as well as creature of fiction' (1991b: 149). In Haraway's conception, cyborgs are material creatures as well as manifestations of the fantastic and the cyborg is 'resolutely committed to partiality, irony, intimacy, and perversity' (1991b: 151). These qualities are also found within JenniCAM. Through the integration of body and technology, JenniCAM is a hybrid, neither fully human nor fully machine yet constituted, in part, by both. Through Jenni's presentation of the private, she trespasses across traditional visual boundaries, always winking back at her audience. Through the playful negotiation of a subject/object position, JenniCAM emerges as a particular type of cyborg subject, one that seems to require and yet simultaneously resist certain traditional readings of female embodiment.

In the second half of this chapter, feminist film theory is used in combination with psychoanalysis to demonstrate the cyborg qualities of irony, intimacy, and perversity within JenniCAM. Feminist film theory is employed because it provides the vocabulary of the visual, of gender and of desire to discuss what is happening in this unique text. As a perverse text, JenniCAM takes on characteristics of the traditional and then turns them on their head. For example, the reading of Jenni's body by viewers is often highly sexualized and functions to perpetuate stereotypical representations of women. The images of Jenni's body lend themselves to a reading of JenniCAM through feminist film theorist Laura Mulvey's notion of the 'male gaze' (1988). However, this approach does not reveal the whole story: a psychoanalytic reading of the way in which the digital camera delivers images to audiences yields an ironic understanding of desire and self-objectification. A pre-Oedipal reading of the function of the camera through Freud's notion of fort-da (1975) and his conception of the 'deferral of meaning' allows for the pleasure of both male and female viewers and opens up room for a new conversation about subjectivity in relation to objectification. Each of these readings of JenniCAM helps to define this unique phenomenon as a cyborg subject.

Hybridity

JenniCAM challenges traditional definitions of the subject and poses a unique way to conceive of subjectivity and the agency and power that is implied therein. If subjectivity as a clean category is no longer unified or dichotomous as asserted by post-modern theorists, then this chapter takes on the project of describing an emergent subjectivity, one that is multiple and ironic. The locus of inquiry starts with the hybridized moniker: JenniCAM. Through this classification, both woman and machine become united in the creation of the cyborg subject. Haraway's cyborg counters the notion of the unified subject because it is a compilation, a combination of parts rather than a singular organism or machine. In the combination of flesh and hardware, a dynamic and unique entity arises. Within Haraway's framework, JenniCAM exists as a cyborg, disrupting boundaries and resisting monolithic definitions of the subject simply by the fact that Jenni has integrated herself with technology. Just like Haraway's cyborg, JenniCAM embraces aggregation rather than unification. In confusing dichotomous boundaries such as body/machine, private/public, and real/fiction, JenniCAM forces a rethinking of the female subject in relation to each binary opposition.

The constitution of the cyborg subject in JenniCAM through hybridity rather than through monolithic unity redefines what has once been normative. On the most fundamental level, the combination of what has been conceived of as living (organism) and non-living (machine) confuses the boundaries of what it means to be human. JenniCAM serves as a visual representation of the end of the unified body. The images of Jenni offered by the camera oscillate between a female body disconnected from her machine to the blurring of the distinction between woman and her computer. When Jenni is in her bed, getting dressed or on the phone, viewers can readily discern her body from the keyboard or computer. When Jenni sits at her computer, however, one has the sense that she has plugged her body into the machine and is connected to the mechanics of her equipment. The image of Jenni at her computer becomes an icon for that fusion, with her flesh melting into her keyboard. Fundamentally, viewers' knowledge of Jenni is shaped by the way in which the camera delivers the images. Viewers derive knowledge of Jenni's life through non-synchronous, interrupted images that change at regular intervals. The pace and narrative of Jenni's life is experienced by viewers in a timed, regimented, mechanical way rather than through serendipity or her own authored narrative. Instead, her life narrative is mechanized. This presentation of self transforms Jenni from a woman into a cyborg as her life unfolds through technology.

Perversity

Another component of being a cyborg is JenniCAM's undermining of traditional, unspoken lines of the public and private self. The erosion of the line between the private and the public composes part of the fascination with and abhorrence of JenniCAM, a perverse text. For many, Jenni is making a spectacle of herself – a 'specifically feminine danger' (Russo 1995: 53) – by transgressing notions of bourgeois femininity that uphold the woman as the guardian of morality and piety. Cultural politics have maintained a certain set of rules for the display of the female body. Jenni flouts these rules and offers herself to be looked at as both a public and a private subject. The entire world can see Jenni in her private space, her boudoir. Then again, this is nothing new, as Rebecca Schneider notes, 'The feminine is emblematic of the private sphere –

the home, the family, and consumption – while the sphere of production bears gender as a masculine domain' (Schneider 1997: 72). The image of a woman in a bedroom is, in many ways, a cultural norm. What is unusual in this instance is that it is not only the woman in front of the camera, but also the woman behind it. Jenni is both viewer and viewee: she occupies the hybrid position of both object and subject; she is composer and is composed.

One of the most common questions asked of Jenni is 'why are you doing this?' (Ringley 1998c: interview). People find it puzzling, peculiar and perverted that someone would expose herself in such a graphic, public way. Descriptions of the JenniCAM phenomenon often garner remarks of astonishment and disgust. As one Washington DC news anchor stated in reaction to a report on JenniCAM, 'Lotta strange things on that Internet' (Ringley 1998b). The aversion to JenniCAM lies in its 'profane' nature, the way in which it pushes against traditional definitions, particularly of the private and public. That JenniCAM provokes such charged responses suggests that Jenni's presentation of identity transgresses normative expressions of subjectivity. Jenni's representation of her identity stabilizes and yet disrupts the process of subject formation by repeating yet resisting cultural norms. Through this new means of representation, JenniCAM confounds 'the domains of political and linguistic "representation"' that have 'set out in advance the criterion by which subjects themselves are formed' (Butler 1990: 1) by simultaneously signifying as a woman and yet acting in a very unwomanly manner. The anxieties centred on JenniCAM suggest a breakdown in normative practices in how subjects are constituted. By acknowledging and repeating traditional representations of women, JenniCAM reiterates normative standards regarding gender. Yet JenniCAM also discloses the ideological rules that govern binary oppositions by evincing tensions and denaturalizing the formation of subjects.

References to JenniCAM in the media invariably mention the 'voyeuristic' elements of the phenomenon. As used by Freud, 'voyeurism' involves seeing what should not be seen. The object of the voyeur's gaze does not know it is being watched. Yet, Jenni anticipates and even invites the gaze of the world into her bedroom: she situates herself in front of the camera as well as behind it. Again, this dual position of viewer and viewee uncloaks the performativity involved in the production and reproduction of JenniCAM. By tempting the viewer with the fantasy of complete vision, of total knowledge, JenniCAM forces a reevaluation of the term 'voyeur.' JenniCAM uses its own images to rewrite a new relationship between the camera, the photographer, and the viewer by announcing the status of Jenni as an object yet refuting and resisting the traditional representations of objectification. By investing the object with vision and a camera, the multiple subjects of JenniCAM inhabit a space of plurality and abundance. Never pinned to positions of either subject or object, Jenni snaps her own picture, oversees her own viewing.

Psychoanalytic readings of JenniCAM

Owing to the fact that Jenni is female and that JenniCAM supplies images of her partially clothed, naked or engaged in sex at various moments, the dispute arises as to whether or not JenniCAM is simply pornography (Ringley 1998c). While the intentions and goals of this chapter do not lie in defining what is and what is not pornographic, this inquiry is put forward in order to focus on the ways in which JenniCAM is ironic, intimate and perverse – key characteristics of cyborgs. The interest of feminist film theorists in disclosing the connection between vision, vulnerability and power fosters insightful readings that open new discussions of female representation.

The tools and lexicon of psychoanalysis and the writings of feminist film theorists provide a framework for uncovering how human desire operates in the formation of the subject in JenniCAM. The often-contradictory ways in which desire has been theorized demand an explanation of JenniCAM, not as a monolithic text but as a text of diverse pleasures. First, Oedipal desires at work in JenniCAM will be examined by using Laura Mulvey's concept of the 'male gaze' (1988). Second, a discussion of what is called the pre-Oedipal desires of this text will be used to provide an explanation of the multiplicity of viewers' desires. These two uses of psychoanalysis will be juxtaposed in order to dramatize the contradictory, ironic nature of desire at work in JenniCAM.

In the first reading, the long-standing tradition of feminist film criticism that regards vision as the desire for mastery and control helps to place JenniCAM into a historical tradition of images of objectified women's bodies. In the second reading, the pre-Oedipal stage of development provides the vocabulary to show how fusing a digital camera and the World Wide Web produces the pleasures created through the simulation of the fort-da game described by Freud. In this 'game', pleasure is gained through the continual deferral of both meaning and a sense of wholeness and control. In fact, in contrast to Oedipal desire, control is given up in order to achieve pre-Oedipal pleasure. These two psychoanalytic readings of JenniCAM reveal the multiple, often contradictory, ways in which desire works, whether it be through the Oedipal fetishization of Jenni's body or the treatment of her body as the site of pre-Oedipal unity and wholeness in the fort-da game. In combination, these two different mechanisms of desire offer readings of JenniCAM that account for the pleasurable readings of both male and female viewers. Moreover, the structure of the JenniCAM site itself speaks to Jenni's awareness of the mechanisms of desires. It reveals a playful manipulation of pleasure on her part which raises questions about traditional definitions of the gendered subject.

JenniCAM as object

Given that JenniCAM is produced and made available through language, its images cannot exist outside the realm of the patriarchal binary of male and female, masculine and feminine. Consequently the knowledge produced is not neutral. Western society has a long history of objectifying women, whether it be through the fresco or the JPEG (a digitally produced picture). The 'problem' of representation brings to the fore the struggles within feminism to find a satisfactory solution. Particularly in photographic media, the situation has become one where, as feminist film theorist Mary Ann Doane notes, 'The simple gesture of directing a camera toward a woman has become equivalent to a terrorist act' (1988: 216). Is this the case in JenniCAM? For some feminists, the critique of the dominant discourses of gender through psychoanalysis continues to provide productive readings of material hegemony.

According to Laura Mulvey, women inhabit the traditional exhibitionist role and understand themselves to 'connote to-be-looked-at-ness' (1988: 62). The female body always signifies the other. In psychoanalytic theory, the marked status of the female figure is explained as representing the threat of castration because her body reveals an absence or lack of the phallus. Marked as such, women continually signify castration anxiety. According to Mulvey, the male unconscious adopts two strategies for reconciling this castration anxiety:

> The preoccupation with the original trauma (investigating the woman, demystifying her mystery), counterbalanced by the devaluation, punishment or saving of the guilty object . . . or else complete disavowal of castration by the substitution of a fetish object

or turning the represented figure itself into a fetish so that it becomes reassuring rather than dangerous.

(Mulvey 1998: 64)

The first avenue – that of the preoccupation with the female body – introduces the notion of the voyeur. In the instance of JenniCAM, there is a voyeuristic pleasure derived from the study and analysis of the body and life of a female subject, the othered body. In addition, the site of observation, Jenni's boudoir, invokes the semiotics of the most private of spaces. Thus the voyeur has crossed over into a once-secret space in an attempt to 'demystify the mystery' of woman which is the goal of Oedipal desire. In contrast to the airbrushed images of the pornographic websites easily found on the Internet, Jenni's natural body becomes the fetish, the sexualized object. Definitions of 'real' female bodies are imported and mapped on to Jenni's body, this time as a means to obtain pleasure.

Another method of escape from the fear of castration involves the fetishization of the woman in order to transform her into something pleasurable and thus repress the notion that the woman is linked to the threat. This disavowal fosters fetishistic scopophilia whereby certain objects – not necessarily connected to sexual pleasure – come to stand in for the erotic. JenniCAM plays with the notion of the fetish through the development of an auxiliary feature on the JenniCAM site. On the 'anatomy one-oh-one' portion of the website, Jenni segments her own body by cropping images of her face and torso into smaller and smaller areas. Singular web pages highlight isolated parts such as her eyes, toes, tongue and feet. In addition, Jenni writes a short paragraph on each featured body part. For example, when supplementing an image of her eyes she writes:

> I've been told (though you wouldn't know it by looking at this picture) that my eyes look like sunflowers: there's a dark blue outside ring, like the sky. There's a green middle ring, like the leaves. And in the middle is a bright yellow spot, like the petals with the iris at centre. My eyelashes are a light brown colour. And in school (elementary, that is) I could always cross my eyes better than anyone else. That's talent for you. Maybe I'll have to include a cool video of the really neat trick I can do – it usually grosses people out, but it seems worth it, doesn't it?
>
> (Ringley 1998a)

In an excessive and overt manner, Jenni breaks apart the image of her body and offers it to her viewers as a way to get to know her. The conversational discussions of her body act as a means to study and scrutinize Jenni's body, but also help viewers learn about her history, her opinions and her personality. Jenni embraces the reading of her body as a fetish as a means to introduce herself to her viewers to convey her identity.

In this example, the hegemonic portrait of the fragmented female body offered by Jenni is positioned next to an autobiographical description of the fetishized object. In contrast to the body part in isolation, these body parts are supplemented with captions written by Jenni herself. This auxiliary, explanatory text allows Jenni to author a discourse about her own body at the same time that she formulates the fetish. This autobiographical fetish reveals how Jenni reads her body as a text across which others write meaning. She does not start out by saying, 'I think my eyes look like sunflowers', rather, she uses the phrase, 'I've been told . . .'. This reference to the description of her body by others, which occurs in other descriptions of body parts as well, points to how Jenni focuses on the reading of her body by others. This integration of objectification with the creation of a subject 'I' forms a complicated text that defies the traditional readings of the female body as an object.

Multiple pleasures in JenniCAM

Although the reading of JenniCAM through the lens of voyeurism and fetishistic scopophilia is quite useful, to give the impression that desire operates through a singular mode in JenniCAM is to do an injustice to the multiple ways in which pleasure manifests itself in human experience and to make monolithic judgements about the demographics of JenniCAM spectators. In fact, these readings of JenniCAM leave out the pleasure that female viewers may receive from watching Jenni and the way in which Jenni herself plays with her own objectification. Building on the concept of desire as that which cannot be obtained, feminist film theorists writing after Mulvey (Studlar 1988) rethink the grounding of desire in the wish for control and look to the search for the return of pre-Oedipal unity as a motivation of desire. While the continual deferral of meaning is frightening, it also operates as a source of pleasure that is derived from that which is just out of reach, a situation that mirrors the viewer's engagement with JenniCAM in certain ways. In other words, the pre-Oedipal unconscious propels and motivates the repetition of certain acts in order to gain pleasure from what Freud called the fort-da, the back and forth, the loss and return of objects that signify the memory of the mother.

In *Beyond the Pleasure Principle*, Freud develops a theory of desire from his observations of his grandson's engaged play with a ball attached to a string (1975). By watching his grandson's joy from throwing a ball away from his body and then retrieving it by pulling on a string, Freud conceives of his grandson's wish for the mother's return. The figure of the mother, the source of pleasure and unity, was lost in the establishment of the infant's ego through the entrance into 'language'. The entrance into language inaugurates the infant in the world of the symbolic. At this moment, the profound loss of the prelinguistic, unified mother commences what Lacan would characterize as the continual wish to return to the earliest stage of secure meaning. Instead, language hails the endless metonymic system of deferral where one object is endlessly substituted for another. Freud believed this object (for his infant grandson, the ball) stood in for the memory of the unified mother. He theorizes that in the game, the terror of loss is endured and even repeated in order to bring about the pleasure generated by the hopeful return of the object. According to Freud, the ball-as-mother serves as a reminder of a time prior to the establishment of the symbolic order, to a moment of stasis and wholeness (Eagleton 1996). Hence, the formation of the relationship of fort-da offers an explanation of the pleasure of the repetitive in contrast to the theories of desire centred on control and mastery. If an object is endowed as a site of meaning and wholeness, the continual disappearance and reappearance of that object can be a source of intense pleasure, despite the fact that the wish for a return to wholeness is never fulfilled. Both men and women can derive pleasure from the system of fort-da as it is not dependent on the establishment of an ego.

The mapping of the fort-da game on to the functionality of JenniCAM yields a background for understanding the pleasures of such a text. Structured remarkably like the fort-da game, JenniCAM engages the viewer in the back and forth, presence and absence, of not only Jenni's body but also of the JenniCAM image itself. Jenni's body is conceived as the source of unified meaning, disappearing and reappearing at random. Her corporeality operates as a metonym of meaning. JenniCAM images are uploaded to the web and replace the old images in a continual cycle of refreshment. From one clip to the next, the image has the potential to change radically from, for example, a picture of Jenni sleeping in her bed to one where her bed is made and she is no longer present. Jenni's body is not a fixed symbol within the text: it changes and moves, disappears and reappears. In fact, the promise of witnessing Jenni's body is often not met either because she is physically not present or because the image is blurry. The viewer takes pleasure in the disappearance and return of the image; its loss and return brings great pleasure to those engaged in the fort-da pleasure of JenniCAM. The pleasure of repetition does not originate in mastery over or control of the object (Jenni's body); it stems from a search for unity, a return to a past that cannot be retrieved.

No matter how viewers hear about JenniCAM, their first glimpse of the site may or may not involve the display of Jenni's body. There is the risk that Jenni will be on vacation, out shopping, or in another room, creating the anxiety of the potential of her absence. What is critical, however, is that despite the fact that Jenni's body is not necessarily present in the production of JenniCAM, the site does not make sense without a notion of her body, her being. Thinking back to the hybridity of the name (Jenni plus CAM), the synthesis requires at the very least the promise of a corporeal Jenni. Within the psychoanalytic framework of the fort-da game, it is this promise of her return that propels the viewing of JenniCAM. The promise of her return also offers a potential answer to the question of why people watch JenniCAM, especially when there is nothing there the majority of the time. Further, her expected return can be anticipated. Although this seems insignificant, the gratification derived from anticipated pleasure should not be underestimated in JenniCAM. Aided by a timer directly below the image, the JenniCAM viewer can wait with relish to see what happens in the next sequence. Even if Jenni is not present, there is always the promise of the next reload, whether in 20 minutes or in two minutes. Without the concept of Jenni's body, whether supplemented with a visual representation of Jenni or not, JenniCAM does not make sense. Framed in this way, Jenni's body functions as the locus of meaning, as the site of plenitude and as the root of the unified meaning of JenniCAM.

The email correspondence and fan sites that are produced in order to keep track of Jenni's presence on camera buttress the concept that Jenni's body serves to provide meaning for JenniCAM. Her viewers send emails to friends or use electronic mailing lists to alert each other when something exciting or new is occurring on JenniCAM. For example, short emails like, 'Jenni is naked on Jennicam.org just now!!!!!' are dispersed to inform others of the goings-on of JenniCAM (May 1998). Through this type of behaviour, fans demonstrate the value they place on the corporeality of JenniCAM. Their excitement surrounds the possibility of witnessing Jenni's body in action and part of the pleasure becomes trying to catch Jenni in motion, to freeze her in time and space in the hope of gaining knowledge of the 'real' Jenni.

In another instance, a fan from the UK developed a 'JenniCAM activity graph' to tell viewers when Jenni is most active. At this website, a graph charts Jenni's movement patterns over the previous 24 hours, measuring the fluctuation of motion in between clips. This website's internal mechanism 'attempts to assign an activity rating to the current image, telling us just how much is going on between images. The graph shows [her activities over the course of] the last hour and the last day' (Manley 1998). This site also gives users the option of opening another smaller browser of the graph so that viewers can be conscious of Jenni's movement while doing other work.

Fan activity like this points to the deep investment viewers have in witnessing Jenni's presence. Whether naked or not, Jenni's body and, moreover, her activity, is of extreme interest to viewers. Although the first analysis signals a preoccupation with Jenni's body as a sexual object, the second seeks to track Jenni to know when she is animate. In both cases, the implication stands that without the embodied subject, JenniCAM provides little meaning to viewers. It is the presence of Jenni that viewers desire. Thus, Jenni opens up a space for conversations about desires not rooted in mastery and control but in the wish for pre-Oedipal unity.

Further, the premise on which viewers pay for access to JenniCAM also supports the use of fort-da pleasure in explaining the behaviour of viewers of JenniCAM. 'Guest' viewers receive a new image every 20 minutes without a fee while 'members' receive a new picture every two minutes by connecting to a password-protected site. The membership access does not provide anything more than a faster refresh rate of the digital images; it does not provide a secret archive of nude images of Jenni made available when one signs on and pays US$15. That is to say, what the membership provides is the opportunity to cycle through the fort-da cycle of pleasure at a faster rate. The tensions of whether or not the source of unified meaning (Jenni) will return are more quickly confirmed or quelled through membership. Thus, viewers pay a fee in order to reduce the length of time required to wait for the next return of the image. The apparatus of the digital camera in combination with the two psychoanalytic readings of JenniCAM offer identificatory positions for both male and female viewers. The viewers of JenniCAM cannot be conceived as a monolithic group, particularly given the global nature of the Internet. Offering multiple ways that pleasure functions in JenniCAM addresses this plurality. In its capacity to address various kinds of viewers, JenniCAM demands an investigation into not only the images produced but also the mechanism involved in the creation and delivery of those images.

Conclusion

JenniCAM's display of the weaving and unweaving of epistemological categories serves as 'technological drag' in the same way that Butler talks about how dressing in drag undermines the naturalization of the categories of male and female (Butler 1993). JenniCAM embraces a playfulness, an ironic stance in this subject/object position. At the same time that Jenni creates and sees, she announces her awareness of her position as something to be seen. She acknowledges her objectification through web pages like 'anatomy one-oh-one' where she posts images of specific fragmented body parts, such as her eyes, along with a narrative about her eyes. As Haraway writes, the cyborg is '[n]o longer structured by the polarity of public and private' (Haraway 1991b: 151). The cyborg has no ties to protect aspects of itself from the sphere of the social, for the cyborg exceeds the boundaries by making explicit the link between 'sexuality, vulnerability, and power' (Schneider 1997: 77).

Jenni's combination of the web and her digital camera confuses ideological rubrics, categories that implicitly bear the mark of gender. In its hybridity, JenniCAM suggests a type of 'subversive reterritorialization' of the semiotics of gender contemporaneous with the process of subject formation and evolution (Butler 1993: 19). By pushing against categories such as private/public, Jenni tacitly redefines what it means to be female within a given binary classification. In other words, Jenni may not be using the traditional tools of drag – her clothing, her makeup, etc. – to push against notions of gender, but in the production of JenniCAM she forces a questioning of the arbitrary boundaries through which identity is constituted, repeated and naturalized.

In order to imagine a new discourse, the visionary descriptions of feminist film theorists offer clues to redefining the terms of representation and subjectivity of JenniCAM. Teresa de Lauretis proscribes the invention of not only new strategies or texts but also conceiving of an entirely new 'social subject'. She suggests that the project of feminist film-makers is to ask 'how to effect another vision: to construct other objects and subjects of vision, and to formulate the conditions of representability of another social subject' (de Lauretis 1987: 135). The challenges faced by feminist film-makers to envision and imagine new relationships within the sphere of the social provide a window through which to see the potential of the medium of the Internet. Ringley may not have an overt, articulated feminist agenda, but those who follow in her footsteps may expand the uses of the digital camera as a tool for political change. The potential to stretch the definitions of vision and representation and to reconceive of the position of the object as well as the subject that is suggested by JenniCAM may prove fruitful as a tool of feminist transformation. By offering a new type of social subject, JenniCAM serves as a cairn, a memorial to the past as well as a signal of things to come. We can only wonder what new configurations of vision and gender the realm of digital cameras will bring.

JenniCAM highlights the way in which the vision of the viewer does not produce stable knowledge. Jenni is always on the move, never allowing for a final reading yet inviting the viewer to use her body as a canvas for the creation of meaning. JenniCAM muddies our understanding of the power of watching and the privilege of sight in the way in which she pushes against definitions of private and public as well as the way she exposes the shifting meanings of bodies. In closing, it is asserted that despite its seeming hegemony, JenniCAM is a text filled with play and complexity. JenniCAM offers an ironic cyborg subjectivity, one that uses the historical traditions of vision to tinker with the semiotics of representation.

References

Butler, J. (1990) *Gender Trouble*, New York: Routledge.

Butler, J. (1993) *Bodies that Matter*, New York: Routledge.

Doane, M. (1988) 'Woman's stake: filming the female body' in C. Penley (ed.) *Feminism and Film Theory*, New York: Routledge.

Eagleton, T. (1996) *Literary Criticism*, Minneapolis: University of Minnesota Press.

Firth, S. (1998) 'Live! From my bedroom', Salon 21st. Available online: http://www.salonmagazine.com/21st/feature/1998/01/cov_08feature.html (12 January 1998).

Freud, S. (1975) *Three Essays on the Theory of Sexuality*, trans. J. Strachey (ed.), New York: Basic Books.

Hagenbaugh, B. (1997) 'Woman puts herself and her apartment live on Internet', Reuters. Available online: http://www.nando.net/newsroom/ntn/info/091797/info7_22171_body.html (18 February 1998).

Haraway, D. (1991a) 'Postscript' in C. Penley and A. Ross (eds) *Technoculture*, Minneapolis: University of Minnesota Press.

Haraway, D. (1991b) *Simians, Cyborgs, and Women: The Reinvention of Nature*, New York: Routledge.

De Lauretis, T. (1987) *Technologies of Gender*, Bloomington and Indianapolis: Indiana University Press.

Manley, S. (1998) 'JenniCAM activity graph'. Available online: http://www.szyzyg.arm.ac.uk/~spm/meter.html (2 February 1998).

May, J. P. (1998) 'Nice!' Available online: futurec@uafsysb.uark.edu (10 March 1998).

Mulvey, L. (1998) 'Visual pleasure and narrative cinema' in C. Penley (ed.) *Feminism and Film Theory*, New York: Routledge.

Ringley, J. (1984a) 'Anatomy one-oh-one'. Available online: http://www.jennicam.org/~jenni/tour/ (25 April 1998).

Ringley, J. (1998b) *Eleven O'clock News*, interview, WRC-TV, Washington DC (17 March 1998).

Ringley, J. (1998c) *The Today Show*, interview, NBC, WRC-TV, Washington DC (17 March 1998).

Ringley, J. (1998d) 'JenniCam – frequently asked questions'. Available online: http://www.jennicam.org/faq/general.html (25 April 1998).

Ringley, J. (1998e) 'Jennifer: Nisi nirvana'. Available online: http://www.jennicam.org/~jenni/index.html (25 April 1998).

Ringley, J. (1998f) 'JenniSHOW'. Available online: http://www.thesync.com/jennishow/ (25 April 1998).

Russo, M. (1995) *The Female Grotesque*, New York: Routledge.

Schneider, R. (1997) *The Explicit Body in Performance*, New York: Routledge.

Studlar, G. (1988) *In the Realm of Pleasure*, Urbana: University of Illinois Press.

Chapter 16

Cyborgs or goddesses?

Becoming divine in a cyberfeminist age

Elaine Graham

Abstract

New digital and biogenetic technologies – in the shape of media such as virtual reality, artificial intelligence, genetic modification and technological prosthetics – signal a 'post-human' future in which the boundaries between humanity, technology and nature have become ever more malleable. We are more aware than ever that what we call 'nature' is open to manipulation by varieties of biotechnology such as gene therapy. Computer-assisted technologies transform perceptions of body, time and space. Dreams of merging humans and machines into new intelligent cybernetic organisms leave the realm of science fiction and enter everyday reality. As the taken-for-grantedness of what it means to be human shifts and blurs, we might consider how myth, literature and popular culture have furnished the western imagination with a gallery of fantastic and monstrous creatures on the margins of human and non-human. One contemporary example is that of the cyborg who serves as a metaphor of the various ways in which the contemporary west is currently experiencing the hybridization of human nature. One version of the cyborg popular with cultural theorists – especially feminists – has been the vision articulated in Haraway's 'A manifesto for cyborgs' (Haraway 1991a). Termed here as Haraway's 'cyborg writing', it expresses important values about gender, politics and technology; but while the cyborg subverts many of the dualisms of western culture, Haraway's comment that she would 'rather be a cyborg than a goddess' inadvertently reinforces one final, often unspoken dichotomy of modernity: that between religion and the secular. Therefore the implications for feminist theory and praxis of a recovery of the goddess are explored. To concur with Haraway, such a project is prone to an inversion of traditional gender stereotypes, enclosing women in a realm of unreconstructed 'nature' at the expense of empowering them to engage with new technologies.

Other models of 'becoming divine', however, promise more radical reconfigurations of the religious symbolic of western modernity, a symbolic that has sanctioned the equation of technology with the dis-avowal of embodied finitude in the name of a quest for transcendence. Irigaray's concept of the 'sensible transcendental' (1993b) refuses the simplistic distinctions between sacred/secular, spiritual/material and divine/human. Far from representing a female version of the patriar-chal sky-god, or even a bucolic, romanticized 'mother-goddess', there-fore, Irigaray's model of 'becoming divine' offers an exciting addition to the critical and reconstructive resources of cyberfeminism.

Introduction: mapping the post-human

In June 1998, the University of Manchester participated in a festival of special events called 'Digital Summer' to commemorate the 50th anniversary of the world's first stored program computer. The 'baby' first operated successfully on 21 June 1948 but few would have pre-dicted that its descendants would have had such a profound effect in economic and cultural terms. Computer technology has transformed the abilities of its users to store and process information; but more wide-ly, it has also changed the way we communicate, the jobs many of us do and the kinds of machines that fill our offices, shops and homes (Bolter 1984; Turkle 1984).

One other project, due for completion in the next two years, may turn out to be of similar far-reaching significance. Like the computer, the Human Genome Project is, in its own way, a kind of information technology, seeking to retrieve and classify what has been termed 'the code of codes' (Kevles and Hood 1992) – the millions of combina-tions of DNA that constitute the genetic composition of the average human person (Reiss and Straughan 1996). While both projects encode and store data, they also have the power to create new forms out of the information they record. Computer technologies can gen-erate new worlds of virtual reality and genetic intervention can manu-facture 'clones' and other genetically modified organisms. Both these forms of 'technoscience'[1] thus hold the power to observe, but also to remake, the world with far-reaching implications for present and future generations.

In one sense, none of this is entirely novel. Forms of technology – beginning with rudimentary tools of containment and projection – have been a characteristic feature of evolving human intelligence for 30 millennia (Tattersall 1998). New forms of technology have frequently been the driving force behind social changes: the history of Manchester – from where this chapter is written – is testimony to that. As the first industrial city of the modern era, it was an object of wonder as the 'manufactories' brought about changes in economic activity, social relations,[2] political culture and even religious life.

In other respects, however, this present generation may well be witnessing something unprecedented. The technoscientific innovations of the last half of the twentieth century have done more than simply introduce new patterns of work, leisure and social interaction, as in previous eras. The very category of 'nature', and human interaction with it, is brought into question by the technologies of the early twenty-first century. The boundary between the 'natural' and the 'artefactual' may never have been secure, but now it is shifting and blurring more than ever. The ubiquity of computer technology and electronic media and the advent of genetic engineering are extending and displacing the physical body into new media, such as cyberspace, and reconfiguring taken-for-granted patterns of physical space, procreation, communication and intimacy. New reproductive techniques, medical and cybernetic fusions of humans and machines and the advent of new information technologies all reveal the constructed nature of the fault-lines dividing humans from non-human animals, what we call nature and machines. It is increasingly difficult to defend an essentialist, impermeable model of human nature in the face of so many instances of the 'homogenization of the human by the technological' (Brasher 1996: 815). It may therefore be appropriate to think of these kind of developments as signifying an unprecedented phase in human history: the dawning of the age of the 'post-human'.[3]

It is easy to portray such trends as manifestations of the colonization of the 'human' by the 'mechanical': an erosion of the taken-for-grantedness of human physical and psychological integrity by invasive, deterministic technologies and the collapse of the 'spontaneity' of face-to-face communities in preference for 'artificial' interactions via electronic or virtual media. Yet these developments are as much to do with the 'enculturation' of 'nature' in ever more and novel ways as technoscience finds new methods for intervening in the stuff of life.

As the Human Genome Project, for example, consolidates it has acquired increasingly more sophisticated methods of locating, storing and encoding genetic information (Hubbard and Wald 1997). The genetic information generated by this research is extraordinarily lucrative, reflecting the degree to which commercial interests have infiltrated scientific activity and 'life itself' is commodified.

While what is called here 'the post-human condition' therefore signifies an era of new relationships between 'the human, the natural, or the constructed' (Haraway 1991b: 21), our fascination with the devices by which the very categories 'humanity', 'nature' and 'culture' are articulated is also part of a longer history. Dreams of creating forms of artificial human life by other than heterosexual reproduction extend from the ancient Greek myth of Prometheus, through the Jewish legend of the Golem of Prague, through to early modern fiction such as the classic of Gothic literature, Mary Shelley's *Frankenstein* (1992). Every age has had its own mythical figures who inhabit the boundaries between the human and the non-human, thereby calling into question the self-evidence of human distinctiveness. More recently, fictional robots, androids and smart computers offer us intriguing glimpses of machines transforming themselves from tools into sentient beings. The western imagination is therefore overflowing with fantastical, monstrous and alien beings whose ambivalent or liminal status bears witness to a perennial fascination with both the outer limits of human identity and the ultimate potential of human creativity. They are truly 'monstrous' – as in things shown and displayed – in their simultaneous demonstration and destabilization of the 'ontological hygiene' by which cultures have distinguished nature from artifice, human from non-human and normal from pathological.

In this chapter, two semi-mythical creatures – the cyborg and the goddess – serve as key figures by which some of the implications of post-human technologies for the ways in which we think about our own human identity are explored. Both the goddess and the cyborg occupy central places in contemporary feminist theory and in their different ways stimulate debate about the future of human relationships to those things we term 'nature' and 'technology' – not least the potential for reconfiguring the gendered connotations that afflict both realms. In very different ways, the cyborg and the goddess evoke all sorts of ethical and political ideals and enable new understandings of responsibility, identity and community as envisaged under the post-human condition of hybrid, non-essential human nature.

The cyborg (cybernetically-enhanced organism) is a familiar character in contemporary science fiction and has also achieved great prominence in feminist theory (Haraway 1991a; Penley and Ross 1991; Balsamo 1996). As a hybrid of the biological and the technological, the cyborg has also become a metaphor for western post-human identity but it also articulates important political, ecological and ethical issues. The goddess too, has received attention from feminists of many religious and theoretical hues who see her as a figure of renewal and empowerment. Her advocates would argue that she disrupts patriarchal polarizations between immanence and transcendence, and humanity and nature, that have traditionally sanctioned the domination and exploitation of the natural environment and, by association, the subordination of women. A goddess who is immanent, not detached and transcendent, effectively resacralizes the earth and provides powerful symbolic expression of a renewed relationship between human and non-human nature.

By way of further demonstration of their critical potential, Haraway's famous paper, 'A manifesto for cyborgs' states her preference for cyborgs over goddesses (Haraway 1991a). This pairing has often been overlooked by secular feminists commenting on Haraway's work but some of the nuances involved in this comparison need to be explored. The contention here is that the goddess has proved an evocative – if controversial – figure in some feminist theory, particularly contemporary ecofeminism and should not be underestimated as a powerful symbol of feminist empowerment, especially in new age spiritualities and woman-centred religion. Ultimately, it will be argued that the goddess as envisaged by such writers as Christ risks remaining effectively a romanticization of humanity's engagement with nature, a reversion to Edenic bliss that is no longer available in a highly technologized western context. Other evocations, however, of the goddess – or, more appropriately, the divine – are emerging. These invite us to reconceive of the very boundaries between humanity and divinity in search of a renewed ethical and political vision. With reference to the work of Irigaray (1993a, 1993b), it is suggested that such a radical reappropriation of the traditional language of transcendence and divinity is intended to rethink many of the conventions of the western symbolic of humanity, nature and culture and of challenging the seductive lure of 'technotranscendence'.

Cyborg writing

The cyborg or 'cybernetic organism' is one of the most popular models of the post-human to exercise the contemporary imagination. The term 'cyborg' was first used in a paper published in 1960 by two aeronautics experts, Manfred Clynes and Nathan Kline. Their paper speculated how technological adaptations of physical functioning might enhance human performance in hostile environments such as outer space (Clynes and Kline 1995). Subsequently, cyborg technology has been developed to restore impaired functions (such as prosthesis or implants) or to modify existing capabilities, enhancing bodies into stronger, better and faster systems. Now, technological enhancement of 'natural' human faculties are commonplace: pacemakers, forms of assisted or artificial fertilization, prosthetic limbs and synthetic organs are increasingly familiar. Besides medical and military applications of cybernetic devices to human beings, we might argue that the ubiquity of computer-mediated technology in the homes, workplaces and entertainment systems of most western societies is gradually 'borging' those of us with access to such technology. Although the cyborg's origins were, strictly speaking, speculative, it also now serves as a metaphor for the way in which humans and machines are increasingly becoming assimilated and interdependent.

Ours is an age of engineered monsters, a partial listing of which would begin with all who have undergone prosthetic surgery, had their bodies augmented by pacemakers, cochlear implants, artificial kidneys or myo-electric limbs. Such a list would also include the transsexual 'Tula' featured in a recent *Playboy* pictorial and the former Mr Universe, Steve Michalik, who used anabolic steroids – a hormonal technology – to transform himself into an androgen-addled android . . . (Dery 1992: 506).

Since Clynes and Kline's early work, the cyborg has become a prominent figure of popular science fiction. Comics, films and novels – such as the *Terminator* and *Robocop* films, the Borg species featured in several of the later *Star Trek* television series and the genre of 'cyberpunk' novels most famously represented by William Gibson's *Neuromancer* – feature many kinds of hybrid human–machines (Gray 1995). A perennial feature of the portrayal of these varieties of cyborg is that of the tension between the cyborgs' human and technological qualities, such as the struggles depicted between body and machine or emotion and rationality. For the hyper-masculine Terminator and Robocop, and many of Gibson's protagonists, prosthetic implants and enhancements, or the disembodied 'high' of cyberspace, represent technologized means of escaping the vulnerability of embodiment, an issue to which I shall return. Similarly, the 'recovering' Borg in *Star Trek: Voyager, Seven of Nine*, is ambivalent about abandoning the supposed perfection and omniscience of the cyborg collective for the bewildering contingency of human individualism.

Yet one depiction of the cyborg attempts to move beyond this dichotomy, choosing to fashion an ironic, subversive exemplar of a non-dualistic, post-gender, post-colonial, post-industrial world. This is the figure whom we encounter in Haraway's classic paper, 'A manifesto for cyborgs'. Haraway argues that the cyborg's hybrid status, as both organism and cybernetic device, calls into question the ontological purity according to which western society has defined what is normatively human. Western modernity is founded on a series of dualisms: nature/culture, female/male, primitive/civilized, body/mind, emotion/reason, sacred/secular, as well as human/technological. When the boundary between the human and the artefactual begins to dissolve, as in cyborg technology, the demarcation that separates the normatively human from the non-human also breaks down. 'Human nature', the axiom of enlightenment humanism, science and progress, is no longer a certain or secure category (Halberstam and Livingston 1995: 19). In advancing her manifesto, Haraway expresses strong preferences for certain ways of representing the world. The cyborg has no myth of origins because it has no parents and, significantly, no divine creator.[4] It is self-creating and self-sustaining, a pastiche of components rather than an organic being with a beginning and an end, thereby released from both nostalgic yearning for lost innocence and from teleological justification: A cyborg body is no innocent; it was not born in a garden; it does not seek unitary identity and so generates antagonistic dualisms without end (or until the world ends). Intense pleasure in machine skill ceases to be a sin but an aspect of embodiment. We can be responsible for machines; they do not dominate or threaten us. We are responsible for boundaries; we are they (Haraway 1991a: 173).

Thus the cyborg – or at least, Haraway's version – speaks of:

> . . . the absence of beginnings, enlightenments, and endings: the world has always been in the middle of things, in unruly and practical conversation, full of action and structured by a startling array of actants and of networking and unequal collectives.
>
> (Haraway 1992: 304)

Haraway's mood is one of exhilaration at the prospects of cyborg culture, especially in its capacity to embody a challenge to conventional categories of race, gender, nature and humanity. By virtue of their hybrid status, cyborgs call into question the impermeability of the categories by which humanity has traditionally differentiated itself from its non-human 'others'. The Scientific Revolution depended on an objectification of 'nature' as 'other' to the human project of reason, progress and domination; but contemporary technical capacities to manipulate nature, even to the very core of our genetic encoding, remind us that all of nature is a construction. Similarly, by exposing the plasticity of 'human nature', cyborgs challenge the givenness of categories of racial identity and gender difference by which humanity has so frequently been stratified. Cyborgs thus transcend the processes of dualism upon which western modernity, patriarchy and colonialism has been founded, speaking not of the hierarchy of humanity, technology and nature but one which realizes the interdependence and permeability of all these categories. In other ways, too, cyborgs do not share human hang-ups about fixed identities, exclusive communities or absolute truths: they are a paradoxical mixture of innocence and complicity which calls us to look again at the terms on which we gain our security and identity.

What is termed here as Haraway's 'cyborg writing', therefore, has three dimensions. It is writing about hybridity and indeterminacy but it is also writing from a position of immersion in, and complicity with, advanced global techno-science. This means it is firmly a first-world, late-capitalist perspective which is both a strength, in that it confronts the relative privilege of those who have access to the new technologies and a weakness, in that it does not easily afford a voice to those who do not. Thirdly, 'cyborg writing', despite its ironic overtones, contains a strong ethical element. Haraway writes partly in order to articulate renewed relationships between humanity, technology and non-human nature that do not rest on exploitation and which acknowledge the complexities of cyborg technology, indeed, the entire post-human condition. Relationships and representations for Haraway become 'articulations': speaking not of our distinctiveness and superiority over non-human nature but of our partnership and connectedness with other sentient and purposeful beings (Haraway 1992). Given that human engagement with technology is inescapable in the modern west, such ethical and political responses cannot be articulated from a pristine, detached point of objectivity but, as it were, only from the inside. There can be no 'back to nature' because the 'nature' to which we appeal is already reproduced through the medium of technoscientific represen-tation and intervention.

Haraway is adamant that the metaphorical power of her kind of cyborg rests precisely in enabling us to rethink fixed gender identities by challenging the 'naturalism' of a biologically determined dichotomy between male and female. However, there is another potential polit-ical implication of the cyborg which is a subversion of the traditional exclusion of women from participation in science and technology. Haraway seems to be implying that the ubiquity of the cyborg places all of us – and especially women – in a position of engagement and complicity with technology. The reality of an age in which, in some respects, we are all cyborgs now exposes the fragility of the ontological boundary between nature/embodiment (with which women have perennially been associated) and culture/technology (assumed to be the appropriate domain for men). She thereby subverts the gendered division of labour that has forbidden women a stake in rationality, scientific innovation and public discourse.[5] It may even inspire women to overcome the incipient 'technophobia' that often accompanies and buttresses this lack of access (Kunzru 1997).

Cyborgs or goddesses?

In the closing stages of 'A manifesto for cyborgs', Haraway makes a final statement which has been much quoted. It is worth citing in full:

> Cyborg imagery can suggest a way out of the dualisms in which we have explained our bodies and our tools to ourselves. This is a dream not of a common language, but of a powerful infidel heteroglossia. It is an imagination of a feminist speaking in tongues to strike fear into the circuits of the super-savers of the new right. It means both building and destroying machines, identities, categories, relationships, space[s,] stories. Though both are bound in the spiral dance, *I would rather be a cyborg than a goddess.*
> (Haraway 1991a: 181, author's emphasis)

It is significant to remember that the title of Haraway's piece echoes Marx and Engel's *Communist Manifesto* published in 1848. Haraway writes from a socialist-feminist standpoint and shares the secularism of a lot of post-enlightenment thought. However, her Roman Catholic upbringing constantly resurfaces in her frequent albeit ironic uses of religious imagery: look again at the references to charismatic religion – the Moral Majority – and even to Starhawk's Spiral Dance. Within a Marxist or post-enlightenment framework, the goddess – like any religious or metaphysical system – is seen as an impediment to the flourishing of human autonomy. Haraway's evocation of the goddess as 'other' to the cyborg is thus interpreted as a figure who tempts us to invest our energies in other-worldly visions, exemplifying a tendency to see power, creative will and most of all moral agency not in human efforts but in some heavenly, abstract realm.

This may well be the model of divinity on which much of the Christian tradition has assumed to rest, but I think the contemporary champions of the goddess herself would reject Haraway's 'goddess' as a misrepresentation. Contemporary goddess feminism – sometimes known as 'thealogy' – emerged in parallel with 1970s second-wave Christian feminism and is now a thriving international movement with many different emphases (Lunn 1993; Raphael 1996). Many goddess feminists trace their devotions back to prehistoric civilizations in which the veneration of resplendent female figures mirrored pacific, egalitarian societies and where women were partners, and not subordinates, to men (Gimbutas 1989). Others see the goddess as more of a metaphor for women's energy and creative power, suppressed for so long by patriarchy and misogyny (Christ 1979). While goddess feminism and its associated practices are highly eclectic, a consistent emphasis throughout is upon the goddess not as a dispassionate 'sky-god' but an immanent, intimate presence whose energy animates the entire cosmos: . . . rather than putting us in touch with a 'changeless' God who stands above the world, Goddess rituals connect us to a divinity who is known within nature and who personifies change . . . Not focused on life after death, Goddess religion calls us to hallow the cycles of birth, death and regeneration in this life' (Christ 1997: 30).

Goddess feminists would therefore challenge Haraway's antipathy to goddesses on the grounds of their putative transcendence and abstraction. Rather, the goddess of contemporary thealogians is a very different deity from the patriarchal 'sky-god' of traditional Christianity; but nevertheless thealogians are still vulnerable to Haraway's indictment that goddess aspirations run counter to the sensibility of the cyborg in other vital respects: not necessarily in terms of the otherworldliness of the goddess, but in her unreconstructed femininity. Haraway argues, for example, that the cyborg quite explicitly transgresses traditional gender boundaries and therefore challenges the identification of women with nature, embodiment and affectivity, thereby subverting their exclusion from the public domain of technology and culture (Haraway 1992, 1997). This is very different from traditions of romantic feminism which have chosen to stress women's affinity with that other oppressed 'other' of western modernity, namely nature, and constructed an oppositional politics by an appeal to women's affinity to peaceful and bodily qualities. Such themes are certainly apparent in goddess feminism, for which the goddess serves as the apotheosis of such virtues:

> The goddess, symbol of life force, natural energy and female sexuality is femininity writ large, in cosmic letters . . . [F]emale essence is reflected in the goddess, in whose power all women allegedly

participate. The survival of life on earth becomes predicated upon
. . . the radical feminization of human thought and values that is
rendered possible through a religious conversion to the goddess.

(Hewitt 1993: 149)

Yet from this we might conclude that goddess feminism is in danger
of simply performing an inversion of the traditional dualisms of patriarchy by continuing to associate women with nature and men with culture: the only difference being that the former has been emptied of its
associations with inferiority and profanity. Goddess feminism continues
to locate women in the realm of a romanticized and nostalgic 'nature'.
The Earth, women's bodies and the integrity of an imagined realm of
unadulterated nature are regarded as the springs of authentic and
redemptive experience but at the expense of reinforcing gender
dualisms that deny women access to the world of culture, knowledge
and technology.

So in its inversion of the dualisms of nature/female/immanence and
culture/male/transcendence, goddess feminism risks replicating rather
than subverting gendered ontologies. In that respect, Haraway's secular protest against the futility of invoking divine saviour figures carries
weight; but the problem with the goddess may well be not her identification with otherworldliness so much as her reinforcement of gender essentialism – not so much a 'sky-god' as an 'earth-mother'. In fact,
I think it is necessary to take another look at some of Haraway's own
assumptions in relation to the intractability of the 'sky-goddess'. In an
essay that celebrates the end of dualisms, Haraway still perpetuates one
of her own: that of the dualism between the heaven and earth. In this
way, the goddess is effectively 'othered' by the cyborg and becomes
the repository of everything negative and retrogressive. But what if,
as well as questioning the distinctions between humans/machines,
human/non-human animals and humans/nature, we also seek to
evoke the goddess to deconstruct the boundary between the spiritual
and the material, immanence and transcendence?

Why bother with this? Arguably because this dualism informs all
others. What undergirds women's being in relation to men's is a
metaphysical – or even theological – understanding of human nature
which perpetuates a final frontier between the material, embodied
world and the spiritual, immaterial realm of supposed perfection and
invulnerability. Haraway's fantastic androgynous cyborg is one solution
to overcoming many of the dualisms of western patriarchy; but there
is a compelling argument to say that the obstacles to gender equality

are so fundamental as to require a thorough-going restructuring of the very basis of the western symbolic; and that means looking again at issues of ontology.

'Techno-transcendence'

Historians of science such as Noble have argued that much of the contemporary fascination with digital and biogenetic technologies is fuelled by a patriarchal, dualistic drive to escape – literally, to 'transcend' – the contingent world of embodied finitude and continuity with non-human nature in favour of a scientific, quasi-religious 'quest' for the impermeability and total invulnerability seemingly promised by advanced technologies (Noble 1999). The fantasy of total transcendence, sanctioned in Haraway's analysis by religion and romanticism, simply exaggerates women's exclusion and plays into the hands of gender dualisms that render women ontologically unsuited to engage with machines.

This is, of course, a central concern that is more general in literature on gender and information communication technologies. Immersion in virtual technologies is believed to constitute an effacement of physical corporeality. The body is condemned as, in William Gibson's terms, mere 'meat' to be abandoned in the 'bodiless exultation' of cyberspace (Gibson 1984: 12). This reflects a deep-rooted philosophical tradition in western thought, of course: a Platonic world-view in which the physical sensory world is but a reflection of a purer, ideal realm of perfect form. For some, the advent of new information technologies represents the realization of this model. The artificial language of binary code, divorced from the everyday conventions of material communication, can aspire to the lofty perfectibility of absolute form: 'At the computer interface, the spirit migrates from the body to a world of total representation. Information and images float through the Platonic mind without a grounding in bodily experience' (Heim 1993). Physical information can be transformed into the pure forms of disembodied intelligence and data: human ontology is digitalized.

For Heim, 'the creation of computerized entities taps into the most powerful of our psychobiological urges' (Heim 1993: 66): an assumption that neatly universalizes this particular philosophical tradition of the superiority of mind over body and spirit over matter. Heim regards the flight into virtual reality as the continuation of a desire – an 'ontological continuity' (Heim 1993: 63) – to project one's physical self beyond its own limitations; to touch others, to reproduce or to create new instruments and forms of life. Allucquère Rosanne Stone elaborates, characterizing an engagement with cyberspace as 'protean', an acting out of deep-seated drives 'to cross the human/machine boundary, to penetrate and merge' (Stone 1993: 108). In describing such a desire as 'cyborg envy', Stone may well be ironically noting the gendered logic of such a model of technophilia. Yet many feminists feel ambivalent about cyberspace and virtual technologies because of its very overtones of dualism and fear of things to do with the body. Given the traditional association of women with the bodily, the affective and the realm of nature, cyberculture just looks like another attempt by patriarchy to deny these aspects of experience in favour of the virtual, the abstract and the disembodied. The exclusion of women from the digitalized world of perfect forms can be rationalized on account of the argument that their messy corporeality (and by implication, their non-rationality) compromises the circulation of pure reason.

Sensible transcendental

In order to rectify the masculinized nature of information technologies, cyberfeminists have sought an alternative symbolic for the virtual world. Plant has developed an analysis that highlights the 'secret history' of women's participation in digital technology (Plant 1995, 1996a, 1996b, 1997). She deliberately uses imagery of the Internet such as 'matrix' and 'web' to retain continuity with women's pre-industrial economic pursuits of weaving (Plant 1995; Spender 1995: 229). It is the non-hierarchical nature of cyberspace and its nature as network, which makes it a proto-feminist medium. Plant does not see the Net as erasing gender difference; rather, she celebrates the specificity of women's subjectivity, weaving a number of disparate threads into her analysis.

The retrieval of women's skills in weaving and their decisive contributions to the development of the modern computer are intertwined with psychoanalysis. Woman's absence from the computer matrix is mirrored in her representation in psychoanalysis as 'lack' or void. But these two phenomena are merely symptomatic of the effacement of the maternal (matrix–matter–mater) in the masculine search for transcendence and autonomy. Woman is the hidden necessity that underpins patriarchy's flight from contingency and connectedness (Plant 1995: 57–58); but she possesses a hidden history of her own into which the technologies of patriarchy cannot penetrate:

> Man can do nothing on his own: carefully concealed, woman nevertheless continues to function as the ground and possibility of his

quests for identity, agency and self-control. Stealth bombers and guided missiles, telecommunications systems and orbiting satellites epitomize this flight towards autonomy, and the concomitant need to defend it.

(Plant 1995: 58)

In this analysis, Plant draws upon the work of the neo-psychoanalytic philosopher Luce Irigaray. Irigaray argues that the western symbolic – the world of language, culture and society – is built on male superiority and privilege. This is derived from the work of Lacan who taught that gendered identity came about at the point of a child's entry into culture, designated by the child's acquisition of language. The infant acquires a gendered subjectivity as it undergoes the transition from the maternal, embodied pre-linguistic world – the imaginary – to locate itself in the adult world of gender difference. The rule of the phallus – the linguistic signifier related to anatomical difference – dictates the acquisition of gendered subjectivity in the transition from imaginary to symbolic so that maleness signals privilege and presence, and femaleness stands for lack, silence and invisibility:

> Women's desire . . . would not be expected to speak the same language as man's; woman's desire has . . . been submerged by the logic that has dominated the West since the time of the Greeks.
>
> (Irigaray 1993a: 25, cited in Plant 1997: 140)

Irigaray therefore argues that women can never aspire to likeness with men but only glimpse the void of their absence enclosed in phallogocentric[6] constructions. Liberal feminist politics founded on appeals to the equivalence or common humanity of women and men are belied by the total asymmetry of gender, whereby male and female within the symbolic are characterized by irreducible sexual difference. Instead, if women's representation as 'other' within the deep symbolic of patriarchy is fundamental, then it can only be radically remade into a truly woman-centred subjectivity – and politics – founded on the sexual specificity of women.

The sexual body is the foundation of women's real, lived experience because it is the ground of the very lack of symmetry in the symbolic order of patriarchy. But it also serves as the site of an alternative symbolic founded on the powers of jouissance: bodily pleasures unspeakable and irreducible to the monolithic order of the phallus. Yet because this representation of (embodied) feminine subjectivity is not available within the prevailing discourse, such an alternative is necessarily Utopian and teleological:

> Women are alienated not from some past body they have known but from a future body owed to them. These are bodies women have not yet been allowed to see, to fashion, or to listen for, even though these bodies already resist their dominant constructions, particularly where these bodies appear as holes in the dominant Symbolic.
>
> (Stockton 1994: 28)

Such a vision exists in the repressed and unvoiced arena of the maternal body; but not as a hole or void but, unexpectedly, as sacred space. Against interpretations that regard Irigaray as merely a biological essentialist, Braidotti has championed Irigaray as articulating a uniquely feminine symbolic. In referring to Irigaray's notion of the body as 'threshold of transcendence' (Braidotti 1994: 184), she seems to be hinting at the body as liminal, an inhabitant of indeterminacy and margins, in transition and fluid and it underlines Irigaray's insistence that a renewed feminist symbolic is both morphological and theological/metaphysical.

Irigaray does not see questions of ethics and politics as separate from an exploration of the nature of God. Far from representing an excursion into immateriality, and thus a denial of embodied experience, the sacred is central to Irigaray's critical and reconstructive strategy. We do not become divine by abandoning our bodies; we take our sexed bodies with us; 'spiritual becoming and corporeal becoming are inseparable' (Irigaray 1998: 203) – the immanent and the transcendent are undivided. Just as the material is inconceivable without reference to the metaphysical, so the metaphysical is irreducible to the material. Thus, Irigaray conceives as part of her reconstructive project a reworking of the western symbolic in order to find new sources of identity for women beyond phallogocentricism. Religion has been central to patriarchy's suppression of women by condemning them as profane. For Irigaray, however, this hastens the need for its reappropriation and not its rejection. Unless there is a complete reconfiguration of religion, women's effacement will continue:

> No human subjectivity, no human society has ever been established without the help of the divine. There comes a time for destruction. But, before destruction is possible, God or the gods must exist.
>
> (Irigaray 1987: 62)

Irigaray's idea of God serves as an ideal towards which women can aspire. 'God' is not a projection of our interests on to a transcendent realm but serves more as a 'horizon' which beckons us into new ways of being (Irigaray 1987: 62–3). Her notion of 'becoming divine' serves as an ideal towards which women can aspire: not a God out there against whom we measure our finitude and imperfection but 'a sensible transcendental that comes into being through us' (Irigaray 1993a: 129). Her project is therefore not to retrieve a putative female deity from prehistory but to engage in the audacious task of imagining a divinity for ourselves.

Irigaray's 'divine' beckons us beyond the ontological hygiene of fixed essences into realizing new, as yet unarticulated, possibilities for identity and community. 'God' is not conceived necessarily as a being but more as a metaphor or device which conveys the manner in which the divine represents a horizon of incompleteness and becoming – a telos – in which all human essences remain unfinished and unfixed:

> Having a God and becoming one's gender go hand in hand. God is the other that we absolutely cannot be without. In order to become, we need some shadowy perception of achievement; not a fixed objective, not a One postulated to be immutable but rather a cohesion and a horizon that assures us the passage between past and future, the bridge of a present that remembers, that is not sheer oblivion and loss, not a crumbling away of existence . . .
>
> (Irigaray 1987: 67)

Irigaray's process of 'becoming divine' is thus a Utopian eschatological rewriting of ecofeminism's mother goddess, where the maternal and the feminine is not idealized or objectified but reconfigured on women's own terms:

> If she is to become woman, if she is to accomplish her female subjectivity, woman needs a god who is a figure for the perfection of her subjectivity. . . . The impotence, the formlessness, the deformity associated with women, the way they are equated with something other than the human and split between the human and the inhuman . . . their duty to be adorned, masked, and made up, etc., rather than being allowed their own physical, bodily beauty, their own skin, their own form(s), all this is symptomatic of the fact that women lack a female god who can open up the perspective in which their flesh can be transfigured.
>
> (Irigaray 1987: 64)

In her acknowledgement of the fluid, even hybrid, nature of human identity, Irigaray is close to Haraway's celebration of the ubiquity of the cyborg. Whereas Haraway's borderland is that of humanity and technology, Irigaray's is – far more problematically for secular feminism – that of humanity and the divine, between immanence and transcendence. Haraway regards divinity as a hindrance to full personhood; Irigaray as its very guarantee. Irigaray's evocation of 'the divine' may thus be seen as an ultimate deferral of essentialism: not a projection of human finitude on to the divine – as in, classically, the work of Feuerbach – but an acknowledgement that no representation of human identity can ever be exhausted, let alone policed by any kind of fixed essence:

> . . . how can a woman maintain a margin of singleness for herself, a nondeterminism that would allow her to become and remain herself? This margin of freedom and potency (puissance) that gives us the authority yet to grow, to affirm and fulfill ourselves as individuals and members of a community, can be ours only if a God in the feminine gender can define it and keep it for us. As an other that we have yet to make actual, as a region of life, strength, imagination, creation, which exists for us both within and beyond, as our possibility of a present and a future.
>
> (Irigaray 1987: 72)

The effect of Irigaray's model of women's radical sexual difference is the construction of an alternative symbolic that eschews models of mastery, detachment and control associated with the military origins of cybernetics and the drive for disembodied perfection in the lofty realms of cyberspace. Women's traditional effacement is taken to its limit – almost parodied – into an excess and indeterminacy that prefigures the hyper-reality of virtual culture (Plant 1995: 55–63). The mirror-like transparency of women disturbs the drive towards total control and objectification that characterizes the phallogocentric fantasy of cyberspace:

> Cyberspace is the matrix not as absence, void, the whole of the womb, but perhaps even the place of women's affirmation. This would not be the affirmation of her own patriarchal past, but what she is in a future which has yet to arrive but can nevertheless already be felt . . . This fabric, and its fabrication, is the virtual materiality of the feminine; home to no-one and no thing, the passage into the virtual is nevertheless not a return to the void. . . . [T]he blind immateriality of the black hole was simply projected by man,

who had to believe that there was nothingness and lack behind the veil.

(Plant 1995: 60)

Rather than requiring our salvation to be sought in the abandonment of messy contingency in the quest for a transcendence founded upon separation, disembodiedness, universality and omnipresence, Irigaray seeks a reappropriation of theo/alogical language in order to express just the kind of decentred notion of human identity that is to be found in Haraway's cyborg. It is about liminality rather than essence and about making political sense of fragmentation and diversity. It does not seek mystical symbiosis with a perfect being but rather hopes for better things to come via a process of becoming. For Irigaray, however, controversial new concepts of divinity – as a guarantee against the reification of contingent experience – are fundamental to a renewed ethical and political vision.

Conclusion

Cyborgs and goddesses may seem strange role models for cyberfeminists as they grapple with the ambiguities of human creative will and potential. Clearly the goddess will be an altogether more contested figure than the cyborg for many cyberfeminists; although I have indicated ways in which Irigaray's vision of 'becoming divine' represents a critical departure from patriarchal religion. However, I have tried to argue that there is much to learn from fantastic encounters with semi-mythical creatures such as cyborgs and goddesses as they help us to rethink perennial questions about the nature of our engagement with, and responsibility for, nature, culture and technology. We may be entering the era of the post-human, ushered in by the new digital and genetic technologies; but the ethical and existential issues raised retain a degree of continuity with the concerns of the cultures who first dreamed of gods and goddesses, monsters and other fantastic creatures on the margins of human imagining. In the way that they are indeterminate and in the way that they avoid ontological or essential purity, those who seek to become both cyborg and divine embody the disturbing reminders of difference which are at the heart of a supposedly unitary or single identity. They suggest that any post-human ethic will not be about the creation of human essences or nostalgic communities but about the pleasures and risks of multiple allegiances, divided loyalties and nomadic sensibilities.

Notes

1 'Technoscience' encapsulates Haraway's conviction that scientific practices and institutions do not simply observe but actually serve as agents in the construction of knowledge. Much of her work examines the way in which a science and technology, as social phenomena, actually generate the cultural metaphors by which we understand what it means to be human (Haraway 1997: 279–80). 'If organisms are natural objects, it is crucial to remember that organisms are not born; they are made in world-changing techno-scientific practices by particular collective actors in particular times and places. . . . In its scientific embodiments as well as in other forms, nature is made, but not entirely by humans; it is a co-construction among humans and non-humans' (Haraway 1992: 297).

2 In his study of early Victorian Manchester, Frederick Engels draws a parallel between the geographical separation of workers and factory owners and the social segregation; thus begins a language of social 'class' unknown to the experience of no less unequal but more homogeneously conceived communities (Engels 1958).

3 I examine the advent of the post-human, and its representation in popular culture in *Representations of the Posthuman: Monsters, Aliens and Others in Popular Culture* (Graham 2001).

4 Haraway expresses antipathy to psychoanalysis for this reason, see Penley and Ross (1991).

5 Traditionally, patriarchal science has equated machines with women to symbolize male mastery over nature and technology. For further discussion of cyberfeminism, see Plant (1997).

6 Phallogocentric is intended to capture the synthesis of phallic privilege and logocentricism or the primacy of language under the Law of the Father.

References

Balsamo, A. (1996) *Technologies of the Gendered Body: Reading Cyborg Women*, Durham, NC: Duke University Press.

Bolter, J. D. (1984) *Turing's Man: Western Culture in the Computer Age*, London: Duckworth.

Braidotti, R. (1994) *Nomadic Subjects: Embodiment and Sexual Difference in Contemporary Feminist Thought*, New York: Columbia University Press.

Brasher, B. E. (1996) 'Thoughts on the status of the cyborg: on technological socialization and its link to the religious function of popular culture', *Journal of the American Academy of Religion*, 59 (4): 809–30.

Christ, C. P. (1979) 'Why women need the goddess: phenomenological, psychological, and political reflections' in C. P. Christ and J. Plaskow (eds) *Womanspirit Rising: A Feminist Reader in Religion*, San Francisco: Harper and Row: 273–87.

Christ, C. P. (1997) *Rebirth of the Goddess: Finding Meaning in Feminist Spirituality*, Reading, MA: Wesley-Addison.

Clynes, M. E. and Kline, N. (1995) 'Cyborgs and space' in C. H. Gray (ed.) *The Cyborg Handbook*, London: Routledge: 29–34.

Dery, M. (1992) 'Cyberculture', *The South Atlantic Quarterly*, 91 (4): 501–23.

Engels, F. (1958) [1842] *The Condition of the Working Class in England*, trans. W. O. Challoner and W. H. Henderson (eds) Stanford: University of California Press.

Graham, E. (2000) *Representations of the Posthuman: Monsters, Aliens and Others in Popular Culture*, Manchester: Manchester University Press.

Gibson, W. (1984) *Neuromancer*, London: Victor Gollancz.

Gimbutas, M. (1989) 'Women and culture in goddess-oriented old Europe' in C. P. Christ and J. Plaskow (eds) *Weaving the Visions: New Patterns in Feminist Spirituality*, San Francisco: Harper and Row: 63–71.

Gray, C. H. (1995) *The Cyborg Handbook*, London: Routledge.

Halberstam, J. M. and Livingston, I. (eds) (1995) *Posthuman Bodies*, Bloomington: Indiana University Press.

Haraway, D. (1991a) 'A manifesto for cyborgs: science, technology, and socialist-feminism in the late twentieth century' in D. Haraway (ed.) *Simians, Cyborgs and Women: The Reinvention of Nature*, London: Free Association Books: 149–82.

Haraway, D. (1991b) 'The actors are cyborg, nature is coyote, and the geography is elsewhere: postscript to "cyborgs at large"' in C. Penley and A. Ross (eds) *Technoculture*, Minneapolis: University of Minnesota Press: 21–6.

Haraway, D. (1992) 'The promises of monsters' in L. Grossberg, C. Nelson and P. Treichler (eds) *Cultural Studies*, New York: Routledge: 295–337.

Haraway, D. (1997) *Modest_Witness@Second_Millennium.FemaleMan©_Meets_OncoMouse™*, London: Routledge.

Heim, M. (1993) 'The erotic ontology of cyberspace' in M. Benedikt (ed.) *Cyberspace: First Steps*, Cambridge, MA: MIT Press: 59–80.

Hewitt, M. A. (1993) 'Cyborgs, drag queens and goddesses: emancipatory-regressive paths in feminist theory', *Method and Theory in the Study of Religion*, 5 (2): 135–54.

Hubbard, R. and Wald, E. (1997) *Exploding the Gene Myth*, Boston: Beacon Press.

Irigaray, L. (1987) 'Divine women' in *Sexes and Genealogies*, trans. G. Gill (ed.), New York: Columbia University Press: 57–72.

Irigaray, L. (1993a) *This Sex Which is Not One*, trans. C. Porter (ed.), New York: Cornell University Press.

Irigaray, L. (1993b) 'Women: equal or different?' in L. Irigary (ed.) *Je, Tu, Nous: Toward a Culture of Difference*, London: Routledge: 12–14.

Irigaray, L. (1998) 'Equal to whom?' in G. Ward (ed.) *The Postmodern God*, Oxford: Blackwell: 198–213.

Kevles, D. and Hood, L. (eds) (1992) *The Code of Codes: Scientific and Social Issues in the Human Genome Project*, Cambridge, MA: Harvard University Press.

Kunzru, H. (1997) 'You are cyborg'. Available online: http://www.wired.com/wired/archive/5.02/ffharaway_pr.html (3 February 1999).

Lunn, P. (1993) 'Do women need the GODDESS? Some phenomenological and sociological reflections', *Feminist Theology*, 4: 7–38.

Morton, N. (1989) 'The goddess as metaphoric image' in C. P. Christ and J. Plaskow (eds) *Weaving the Visions: New Patterns in Feminist Spirituality*, San Francisco: Harper and Row: 111–18.

Noble, D. F. (1999) *The Religion of Technology: The Divinity of Man and the Spirit of Invention*, New York: Penguin.

Penley, C. and Ross, A. (eds) (1991) 'Cyborgs at large: interview with Donna Haraway' in *Technoculture*, Minneapolis: University of Minnesota Press: 1–20.

Plant, S. (1995) 'The future looms: weaving women and cybernetics', *Body and Society*, 1 (3/4): 45–64.

Plant, S. (1996a) 'On the matrix: cyberfeminist simulations' in R. Shields (ed.) *Cultures of Internet: Virtual Spaces, Real Histories, Living Bodies*, London: Sage: 170–83.

Plant, S. (1996b) 'The virtual complexity of culture' in G. Robertson, M. Mash, L. Tickner, J. Bird, B. Curtis and T. Putnam (eds) *Future Natural: Nature/ Science/Culture*, London: Routledge: 203–17.

Plant, S. (1997) *Zeros + Ones: Digital Women + the New Technoculture*, London: Fourth Estate.

Raphael, M. (1996) 'Truth in flux: goddess feminism as a late modern religion', *Religion*, 26: 199–213.

Reiss, M. J. and Straughan, R. (1996) *Improving Nature? The Science and Ethics of Genetic Engineering*, Cambridge: Cambridge University Press.

Shelley, M. (1992) [1818] *Frankenstein or The Modern Prometheus*, W. Lesser (ed.), London: Random Century.

Spender, D. (1995) *Nattering on the Net: Women, Power and Cyberspace*, Melbourne: Spinifex.

Stockton, K. B. (1994) *God Between Their Lips: Desire between Women in Irigaray, Brontë and Eliot*, Stanford, CA: Stanford University Press.

Stone, R. A. (1993) 'Will the real body please stand up? Boundary stories about virtual cultures' in M. Benedikt (ed.) *Cyberspace: First Steps*, Cambridge, MA, MIT Press: 81–118.

Tattersall, I. (1998) *Becoming Human: Evolution and Human Uniqueness*, Oxford: Oxford University Press.

Turkle, S. (1984) *The Second Self: Computers and the Human Spirit*, London: Duckworth.

Index